Female Bladder Outlet Obstruction and Urethral Reconstruction

Nikhil Khattar • Rishi Nayyar
Arabind Panda
Editors

Female Bladder Outlet Obstruction and Urethral Reconstruction

Springer

Editors
Nikhil Khattar
Female Urology
Reconstructive Urology and
Neurovesical Dysfunction
Medanta, The Medicity
Gurugram
India

Rishi Nayyar
Department of Urology
All India Institute of Medical Sciences,
New Delhi
India

Arabind Panda
Urology and Renal Transplantation
Krishna Institute of Medical Sciences
Secunderabad, Telangana
India

ISBN 978-981-15-8523-4 ISBN 978-981-15-8521-0 (eBook)
https://doi.org/10.1007/978-981-15-8521-0

This Springer imprint is published by the registered company Springer Nature Singapore Pte Ltd.
The registered company address is: 152 Beach Road, #21-01/04 Gateway East, Singapore 189721, Singapore

To the women who have suffered from voiding difficulties and have challenged us to understand this domain of urological practice

To the clinicians and researchers on female voiding who have contributed to our understanding

Foreword

There are two mistakes one can make along the road to truth... not going all the way, and not starting.

Buddha

I was pleasantly surprised when I was requested to write a foreword for this upcoming book *Female Bladder Outlet Obstruction and Urethral Reconstruction*, co-edited by Dr. Nikhil Khattar, Dr. Rishi Nayyar and Dr. Arabind Panda. I have known Nikhil for long—a very bright young urologist, who has dedicated himself to the subspeciality of female urology. Rishi Nayyar and Arabind Panda have established themselves in the field of reconstructive urology. To be asked to write a foreword for their maiden book on female urology is truly a humbling experience. I would like to thank them for their kind gesture.

The normal physiology of voiding in women is poorly understood, as we still do not fully understand the physiology of female voiding. We recognise that many women can void with pelvic floor relaxation without detrusor contraction. There are many unanswered questions about female bladder outlet obstruction (BOO) like the role of pelvic floor in normal and abnormal voiding and the diagnostic criteria of female BOO in absence of obvious pathology like stricture or post anti-incontinence procedure. The diagnostic criteria are still evolving. Available literature too is limited and is mostly based on expert opinions. Bladder outlet obstruction in women is rare and its management complex. It is further complicated by the fact that most urologists extrapolate the treatment strategies of male outlet obstruction to treat women. Use of alpha blockers, frequent urethral dilatation in the absence of obvious stricture and bladder neck incision are common practice in the absence of good quality evidence. Urethral reconstruction in women is quite challenging as the female urethra is short with the proximal two thirds being sphincter active. Inflammatory strictures in males involve anterior urethra, and reconstruction usually does not interfere with continence; in women however, extreme care is required to preserve continence.

This book on female BOO and urethral reconstruction is most welcome as it will serve as a practical guide for the management of female voiding dysfunction. The editors of this book need to be applauded for their foresight and effort. The book boasts of India's best authors and topics covering all aspects of female voiding and urethral reconstruction comprehensively. It has been organised in two sections: the first section deals with the pathophysiology of female voiding, role of urodynamic evaluation and the common conditions causing BOO, while the second section deals with treatment and surgical procedures along with examples of clinical cases. The clinical cases are interesting and would serve as reference in daily practice.

I am sure this book would serve as a good resource to all urologists, gynaecologists and residents who manage women with voiding dysfunction. It will help improve the care of our patients.

I sincerely hope that it will stimulate further research and close scrutiny of the management strategies adopted in tackling female BOO.

I wish them all the success.

Nitin Kekre
Former Editor in Chief, Indian Journal of Urology,
Department of Urology, Naruvi Hospital
Vellore, Tamil Nadu, India

Department of Urology, Christian Medical College
Vellore, Tamil Nadu, India

Foreword

Women have long suffered from voiding difficulties secondary to outlet obstruction and urethral strictures. Until recent years these problems for many patients have been minimised and therefore under treated. Lack of recognition of these important conditions has created unnecessary distress and disruption in quality of life for those afflicted. The simple fact that these dedicated editors and authors have created this excellent textbook, *Female Bladder Outlet Obstruction and Urethral Reconstruction*, demonstrates a progressive change in collective understanding of the impact of these very treatable conditions for the improvement of urologic care for women.

The authors address the many different causes of bladder outlet obstruction in women and delineate in detail both nonsurgical and surgical treatment options for these conditions. This makes this work an excellent addition to the library of every urologist and gynaecologist who manages these patients, not only those trained in reconstructive techniques.

It is a distinct privilege to write this Foreword on a topic that I feel passionately about, alongside editors Drs. Nikhil Khattar, Rishi Nayyar, and Arabind Panda, subject matter experts that have dedicated their careers to reconstructive and female urology. This comprehensive text is a novel contribution to the contemporary urologic archives, poised to enhance female urologic education from trainees to seasoned practitioners for the benefit of our patients and communities.

Kurt A. McCammon
Department of Urology
Eastern Virginia Medical School
Norfolk, VA, USA

Devine Chair in Genitourinary Reconstructive Surgery
Eastern Virginia Medical School
Norfolk, VA, USA

Preface

The urological focus over more than a century of scientific evidence recording has been towards male urinary tract symptoms and has overlooked the voiding difficulties in women. On the contrary, the incontinence was always evident and got the required attention of clinicians, researchers and the industry alike. It appears as if the absence of a prostate and a long urethra in women made researchers and experts forget about the diseases and conditions affecting the female bladder outlet and made hard for them to consider female bladder outlet obstruction (BOO) as a diagnosis. The symptoms, however continued to puzzle clinicians. Even in males, it is increasingly being recognised that transurethral resection of the prostate often does not always give the desired results and other causes of voiding dysfunction have to be considered in these cases. In younger males too, where prostate is not yet a concern, the development of voiding symptoms forces one to look at other voiding dysfunction aetiologies once a stricture is ruled out. Similarly, in women voiding dysfunction has to be recognised and evaluated but here the anatomical causes are far too less.

Female bladder outlet obstruction is increasingly being recognised as a much more common cause of voiding abnormalities in women unlike a few years back when it was considered rare unless there were obvious causes like prolapse or an obstructing sling. The functional causes are gaining prominence and understanding is increasing. Female urethral strictures which hitherto were considered rare are also increasingly being diagnosed and the number of female urethroplasty is increasing. We are moving away from era of repeated urethral dilatation in women to provide definitive urethral reconstruction options. Female stricture, sling and pelvic organ prolapse-related obstructions along with selected cases of primary bladder neck obstructions are few surgically treatable conditions causing bladder outlet obstruction. To have one such diagnosis, one will encounter multiple times a higher number of women with BOO as the functional causes are far more common. Hence, it requires a deeper understanding of all voiding symptoms, their overlap with storage dysfunctions and their association with other common conditions like overactive bladder or recurrent urinary tract infection in order to address the voiding issues in women. The first part of the book has chapters beginning with what is different in female voiding at physiological level and why definitions of male BOO cannot be applied to women and therefore how female BOO definitions have evolved over the last three decades. After giving an overview of all major causes of female BOO, the first part ends with a working algorithm to apply in clinical practice.

The second part addresses the therapeutic options for female BOO. The identified functional issues may respond to either pharmacotherapy or biofeedback and physiotherapy or rarely may require one of the minimally invasive procedures or neuromodulation. Cases with anatomical luminal narrowing require formal reconstruction. For this, a clear understanding of the anatomy of the urethra with regard to sphincteric and female sexual anatomy is a prerequisite. There are multiple urethroplasty techniques competing with each other, but the supremacy of one over the other is not yet established. Each technique is described in detail. Finally, the second part ends with principles of management of pelvic fracture urethral injuries and advancements in anastomotic urethroplasty techniques.

This book has been compiled because we felt that there is a dearth of organised literature addressing the voiding issues in women. The high-quality evidence, the standardisation of workup, etc. have not yet been widely used for voiding problems in women, and a clinician is always faced with a lack of clarity about how to go further. We hope that this book provides the necessary stimulus to female urologists and urogynaecologists to understand and probe the subject deeper and give their patients best possible care.

Gurugram, India — Nikhil Khattar
New Delhi, India — Rishi Nayyar
Secunderabad, India — Arabind Panda

Acknowledgements

We acknowledge

Our institutions (Medanta—The Medicity Gurugram, AIIMS New Delhi, KIMS Secunderabad), for providing clinical cases which were challenging enough to inspire us to embark on this project.

Our teachers, they made us what we are.

Our departments (past and present), with astute clinicians as professional colleagues, with whom our discussions over the years, helped our understanding of this subject.

Our families, who allowed us to put our efforts in the hours which by right belonged to them and for taking on the hardships of our being engaged with this assignment.

Our patients, who through their challenging complains, inquisitiveness and feedback helped us learn about their problems.

Our authors, amongst whom there are our teachers and our colleagues, who believed in this project and came aboard and enriched the work with their clinical experience and ever-present enthusiasm for learning more.

Our publisher, Springer and their team who are the key to make reach this work to our readers.

Our colleagues who gave their critical inputs at various stages.

Each other for seeing this through!

and

You, the reader!

Nikhil Khattar, Rishi Nayyar, Arabind Panda
Editors

Overview

This book focuses on a hitherto poorly understood topic of female micturition and outlet obstruction. In an environment of increasing contemporary interest in female urethral surgery, we hope this book will help clinicians to make a proper diagnosis and impart appropriate treatment. In this background, the book has two broad parts.

Part I: Pathophysiology and Differential Diagnoses of Female Bladder Outlet Obstruction

This part begins with "**Physiology of Female Voiding: Are There Many Normals?**" It delves into the basics of voiding and different physiological patterns of female voiding and their implications. Lower tract urinary symptoms are an unreliable guide to predict an obstruction in women. More than a third of women with these symptoms may harbour an underlying bladder outlet obstruction. Moreover, other common clinical conditions such as overactive bladder, recurrent urinary tract infections or bladder pain syndrome have overlapping symptoms and may also have associated obstruction. These issues have been discussed under "**Female Bladder Outlet Obstruction: Whom to Work Up and What to Look for?**" The diagnosis once suspected is not easy to prove as there is a poor consensus on the definition of bladder outlet obstruction (BOO) in women. Unlike men, objective criteria to diagnose BOO on the basis of uroflowmetry and video-urodynamics in women are lacking. "**Controversies in Diagnosis of Bladder Outlet Obstruction in Women: A Urodynamic Perspective**" provides a detailed account of evolution of definitions from urodynamic cut-offs to increasing significance of radiological appearance of urethra.

The causes of BOO can be classified broadly as either functional or anatomical. "**Dysfunctional Voiding in Women**" and "**Primary Bladder Neck Obstruction as a Cause for Female Bladder Outlet Obstruction Syndrome**" delve into the contemporary understanding of the two most prominent functional causes of obstruction in women. Whereas dysfunctional voiding is considered to be an acquired learned behaviour of inappropriately contracting/failing to relax the external sphincter/pelvic floor during voiding, primary bladder neck obstruction is a functional obstruction due to smooth muscle dyssynergia of the bladder neck during voiding without a neurogenic or anatomical cause. **Fowler's Syndrome** is a rare functional cause of painless retention of urine occurring in young women with no obvious organic cause. Although a persistently hypertonic and non-relaxing external sphincter is thought to cause increased urethral afferent activity which in turn inhibits bladder afferent signalling leading to detrusor underactivity, still it deserves its space along with all functional obstructions in women.

Pelvic Organ Descent as a Cause of Bladder Outlet Obstruction is a surprisingly common condition affecting up to 41% of the women between 50 and 70 years. The storage symptoms also are more common in women with prolapse. Both the storage and voiding symptoms respond well to prolapse reduction. **Female Urethral Stricture** and urethroplasty in females have gained recent interest with newer urethroplasty techniques being described for various types of strictures. Female urethral stricture remains a rare disease and the clinical presentation overlaps with other functional causes of obstruction. The diagnosis is highly dependent on actual demonstration of a fibrotic ring on endoscopy. **Bladder Outlet Obstruction After Sling Surgery for Stress Urinary Incontinence** is the commonest indication for a salvage procedure after incontinence surgery. A high index of suspicion is the key to early diagnosis. Interventions can be challenging and are best handled at high volume referral centres.

The part concludes with an effort to come up with a **Working Algorithm for Female Voiding LUTS** based on the understanding developed from previous chapters. It gives a broad outlook to stepwise rational management of female LUTS in outpatient clinic, based upon current literature and clinical practices.

Part II: Treatment Modalities for Female Bladder Outlet Obstruction and Urethral Reconstruction

Pharmacotherapy for Female Bladder Outlet Obstruction is not as well studied as in men. There is no FDA-approved agent for management of voiding dysfunction in women. Nevertheless, several agents are clinically being used based on results of small-scale studies in women and experience of use in similar pathologies in men. High-quality randomised controlled trials are warranted in this nascent and orphaned area. **Urethral Dilatation and Minimally Invasive Surgical Options for Female Bladder Outlet Obstruction** discusses the contemporary role of urethral dilatation, bladder neck incision, intra-sphincteric botulinum toxin injections and sacral neuromodulation.

Applied Anatomy of Urethra for Female Urethral Reconstruction makes an attempt to answer the less discussed questions—Where exactly is the female external sphincter?; What keeps continence preserved in dorsal approaches and what keeps it intact in ventral ones?; Can the urethrotomy be extended into the bladder neck without jeopardising the continence?; After complete obliteration or transection, what keeps the two ends of the urethra vascularised?; Which anatomical structures are responsible for female sexual function?; What bed provides vascular support to the graft on dorsal and ventral sides?. Such understanding is instrumental to decide on the correct surgical procedure besides improving the outcomes of urethral reconstruction in females. This lays the foundation for next five chapters on various surgical approaches to urethral reconstruction for female urethral stricture, namely **Dorsal (Anterior) Onlay Urethroplasty, Ventral (Posterior) Onlay Augmentation Urethroplasty, Dorsal (Anterior) Inlay technique, Ventral (Posterior) Inlay technique and finally Labial and Vaginal Flaps in Female Urethroplasty for Female Urethral Stricture.**

Pelvic fracture associated urogenital injury is an important but uncommon cause of urethral stricture in females. These are complex injuries and often involve the bladder neck and the genital tract as well. **Female Pelvic Fracture Associated Urethral Injury and Stricture: Principles of Management** lays down the basics of management in such patients, and **Female Anastomotic Urethroplasty** elaborates on the technique(s) of anastomotic repair and nuances of dealing with obliterative strictures in women.

Abbreviations

ACC	Anterior cingulate cortex
ATP	Adenosine triphosphate
AUA	American Urological Association
AUR	Acute urinary retention
BBD	Bowel-bladder dysfunction
BCR	Bulbo-cavernosus reflex
BMG	Buccal mucosal graft
BN	Bladder neck
BNI	Bladder neck incision
BoNT	Botulinum neurotoxin
BOO	Bladder outlet obstruction
BOOIf	BOO index for females
BPS	Bladder pain syndrome
BPS/IC	Bladder pain syndrome/Interstitial cystitis
BWT	Bladder wall thickness
CAFTs	Cardiovascular autonomic function tests
CAH	Congenital adrenal hyperplasia
CIC	Clean intermittent catheterisation
CISC	Clean intermittent self-catheterisation
CRD	Complex repetitive discharges
CUR	Chronic urinary retention
DB	Decelerating bursts
DESD	Detrusor external sphincter dyssynergia
DHIC	Detrusor hyperreflexia with impaired contractility
DO	Detrusor overactivity
DRE	Digital rectal examination
DSD	Detrusor sphincter dyssynergia
DU	Detrusor underactivity
DV	Dysfunctional voiding
DVIU	Direct visual internal urethrotomy
DWT	Detrusor wall thickness
EAU	European Association of Urology
EEA	End to End anastomosis
EMG	Electromyography
EUS	External urethral sphincter
FS	Fowler's syndrome
FUS	Female urethral stricture

GABA	Gamma-aminobutyric acid
HTNRS	High tension non-relaxing sphincter
ICS	International Continence Society
IPSS	International Prostatic Symptom Score
KUB	Ultrasonogram of kidney ureter and bladder region
LGIT	Lower gastrointestinal tract
LUT	Lower urinary tract
LUTS	Lower urinary tract symptoms
MCUG	Micturating cystourethrography
MFR	Maximum flow rate
MRI	Magnetic resonance imaging
MUCP	Maximal urethral closure pressure
NANC	Nonadrenergic-noncholinergic
NNT	Numbers needed to treat
NO	Nitric oxide
NT	Neurotransmitters
OAB	Overactive bladder
OBoNT	Onabotulinum toxin A
PAG	Periaqueductal gray
PBNO	Primary bladder neck obstruction
Pclo	Urethral closure pressure
PCOD	Polycystic ovarian disease
PFC	Prefrontal cortex
PFMT	Pelvic floor muscle therapy
PFMT/PFME	Pelvic floor muscle training/exercises
PFR	Peak flow rate
PFUI	Pelvic fracture urethral injury
PGE2	Prostaglandin E2
PMC	Pontine micturition centre
POP	Pelvic organ prolapse
POP-Q	Pelvic organ Prolapse Quantification Scale
PPV	Positive predictive value
PRES	Poor relaxation of external sphincter
PSC	Pontine storage centre
Pura	Urethral pressure
PVR	Post-void residue
Qave	Average flow rate
RCT	Randomised controlled trial
RGU	Retrograde urethrography
SMA	Supplementary motor area
SMR	Skeletal muscle relaxants
SNM	Sacral neuromodulation
SPC	Suprapubic cystostomy
SUI	Stress urinary incontinence
TVL	Total vaginal length
UAB	Underactive bladder
UD	Urethral dilatation
UDI-6	Urinary Distress Inventory (short form)

UDS	Urodynamic study
UPP	Urethral pressure profilometry
USG	Ultrasonogram
UTI	Urinary tract infection
UUI	Urge urinary incontinence
VCUG	Voiding cystourethrography
VD	Voiding dysfunction
VIBMGU	Ventral inlay buccal mucosal graft urethroplasty
VQI	Volume-Normalised Flow Rate Index
VUDS	Video-urodynamic studies
VVF	Vesicovaginal fistula

Contents

Part I Pathophysiology and Differential Diagnoses of Female Bladder Outlet Obstruction

1 **Physiology of Female Voiding: Are There Many Normals?** 3
Pawan Vasudeva and Niraj Kumar

2 **Female Bladder Outlet Obstruction: Whom to Work Up and What to Look for?** 9
Nikhil Khattar

3 **Controversies in Diagnosis of Bladder Outlet Obstruction in Women: A Urodynamic Perspective** 23
Nikhil Khattar and Vijay Madduri

4 **Dysfunctional Voiding in Women** 35
Mayank Mohan Agarwal

5 **Primary Bladder Neck Obstruction in Women** 53
Maneesh Sinha, Ankit Singla, and Venkatesh Krishnamoorthy

6 **Fowler's Syndrome of Recurrent Painless Retention in Women** 61
L. N. Dorairajan and Sidhartha Kalra

7 **Pelvic Organ Descent as a Cause of Bladder Outlet Obstruction** 77
Arabind Panda and Nikhil Khattar

8 **Female Urethral Stricture** 87
Rishi Nayyar, Devanshu Bansal, and Bharti Uppal Nayyar

9 **Bladder Outlet Obstruction After Sling Surgery for Stress Urinary Incontinence** 99
Sanjay Sinha

10 **Working Algorithm for Female Lower Urinary Tract Symptoms** 111
Rishi Nayyar, Nikhil Khattar, and Arabind Panda

Part II Treatment Modalities for Female Bladder Outlet Obstruction and Urethral Reconstruction

11 Pharmacotherapy for Bladder Outlet Obstruction in Females 123
Mayank Mohan Agarwal

12 Urethral Dilatation and Minimally Invasive Surgical Options for Female Bladder Outlet Obstruction 131
T. Manasa

13 Applied Anatomy for Female Urethral Reconstruction 141
Nikhil Khattar and Rishi Nayyar

14 Dorsal (Anterior) Onlay Urethroplasty for Female Urethral Stricture 161
Rishi Nayyar, Prashant Kumar, and Bharti Uppal Nayyar

15 Ventral (Posterior) Onlay Augmentation Urethroplasty for Female Urethral Stricture 169
Hemant Kumar Goel, Varun Katiyar, and Varun Gunavanthe

16 Dorsal (Anterior) Inlay Technique for Buccal Mucosal Graft for Female Urethroplasty 175
Arabind Panda

17 Ventral (Posterior) Inlay Technique for Female Urethroplasty 183
Prasant Nayak and Swarnendu Mandal

18 Labial and Vaginal Flaps for Female Urethroplasty 189
Divakar Dalela and Ravi Lohani

19 Female Pelvic Fracture Associated Urethral Injury and Stricture: Principles of Management 201
Rishi Nayyar, Devanshu Bansal, and Bharti Uppal Nayyar

20 Female Anastomotic Urethroplasty 211
S. B. Viswaroop and Ganesh Gopalakrishnan

Editors and Contributors

About the Editors

Nikhil Khattar works as Associate Director of Female and Reconstructive Urology at Medanta—The Medicity, Gurgaon, India, and has dedicated himself to these areas of urology. He formerly worked as Professor of Urology at Dr. RML Hospital, New Delhi, where he took on many research projects and thesis concerning his area of interest. He has more than 25 publications to his name in peer-reviewed journals and has delivered numerous invited lectures in national and international conferences. He is also a core member of the Urological Society of India's panels for national guidelines on urinary incontinence and urethral stricture and a member of Female and Functional Urology Subsection of the Urological Society of India.

Rishi Nayyar (M.S., M.Ch., F.M.A.S., M.A.M.S., F.I.M.S.A.) is serving as Associate Professor in the Department of Urology at All India Institute of Medical Sciences, New Delhi, which is an apex institute of national eminence. Being committed to academics, teaching and research, he has been instrumental in training more than 25 residents in urology and 10 research projects. He has a keen interest in reconstructive and minimally invasive urology. He has published nearly 60 papers in various national and international peer-reviewed journals and has won several national and international awards. He is also an active reviewer for 18 indexed international and national journals of repute, besides serving as an editorial committee member for the *Indian Journal of Urology*. He is a core member of Reconstructive Urology subsection of Urological society of India

Arabind Panda is currently Senior Consultant Urologist, Krishna Institute of Medical Sciences, Hyderabad. He was formerly the Professor of Urology at the Christian Medical College hospital, Vellore, India. He completed his urological training in 2009 and has been focusing mainly on reconstructive urology and endourology. He has been an associate editor of the *Indian Journal of Urology* for the past 7 years. He is particularly interested in reconstructive surgery of the urethra, both male and female, particularly in difficult posterior urethroplasty apart from vesicovaginal and rectourethral fistulas. He was awarded the 2014 AUA/IAUA Chakrobortty fellowship by the American Urological Association and the Klinikum Luneburg German

Fellowship 2013. He has been a member of the Reconstructive and Trauma section of the Society International Urologie since 2015 and is a core group member of the Urological Society of India guideline panel on urethral strictures and a member of Female and Functional Urology Subsection of the Urological Society of India.

Contributors

Ankit Singla, MS Department of Urology, NU Hospitals, Bengaluru, India

Arabind Panda, MS, MCh Urology and Renal Transplantation, Krishna Institute of Medical Sciences, Secunderabad, Telangana, India

Bharti Uppal Nayyar, MS Department of Obstetrics and Gynecology, All India Institute of Medical Sciences, New Delhi, India

Devanshu Bansal, MS, MCh Department of Urology, All India Institute of Medical Sciences, New Delhi, India

Divakar Dalela, MS, MCh Department of Urology, King George Medical University, Lucknow, India

Ganesh Gopalakrishnan, MS, MCh, FAMS, FRCP Vedanayagam Hospital and Postgraduate Institute, Coimbatore, Tamil Nadu, India

Department of Urology, Christian Medical College, Vellore, Tamil Nadu, India

Hemant Kumar Goel, MS, MCh Department of Urology, Dr Ram Manohar Lohia Hospital and ABVIMS, New Delhi, India

L. N. Dorairajan, MS, MCh Department of Urology, JIPMER, Puducherry, India

T. Manasa, MS, MCh Ramaiah Medical College, Bengaluru, India

Maneesh Sinha, MS, MCh, DNB (Urology) Department of Urology, NU Hospitals, Bengaluru, India

Mayank Mohan Agarwal, MS, MCh Urology and Kidney Transplant Surgery, Medanta Hospital, Lucknow, Uttar Pradesh, India

Nikhil Khattar, MS, MCh Female Urology, Reconstructive Urology and Neurovesical Dysfunction, Medanta, The Medicity, Gurugram, India

Niraj Kumar, MS, MCh Department of Urology, VM Medical College and Safdarjung Hospital, New Delhi, India

Prasant Nayak, MS, MCh Department of Urology, All India Institute of Medical Sciences, Bhubaneswar, Odisha, India

Prashant Kumar, MS, MCh Department of Urology, All India Institute of Medical Sciences, New Delhi, India

Pawan Vasudeva, MS, MCh Department of Urology, VM Medical College and Safdarjung Hospital, New Delhi, India

Rishi Nayyar, MS, MCh, FMAS, MAMS Department of Urology, All India Institute of Medical Sciences, New Delhi, India

Ravi Lohani Department of Urology, King George Medical University, Lucknow, India

S. B. Viswaroop, MS, MCh Vedanayagam Hospital and Postgraduate Institute, Coimbatore, Tamil Nadu, India

Sidhartha Kalra, MS, MCh Department of Urology, JIPMER, Puducherry, India

Sanjay Sinha, MS, MCh Apollo Hospitals, Hyderabad, India

Swarnendu Mandal Department of Urology, All India Institute of Medical Sciences, Bhubaneswar, Odisha, India

Varun Katiyar, MS Department of Urology, Dr Ram Manohar Lohia Hospital and ABVIMS, New Delhi, India

Varun Gunavanthe, MS, MCh Department of Urology, Bombay Hospital, Mumbai, India

Venkatesh Krishnamoorthy, MS, MCh, FRCS Department of Urology, NU Hospitals, Bengaluru, India

Vijay Madduri, MS, MCh Department of Urology, AII India Institute of Medical Sciences, Jodhpur, India

Part I

Pathophysiology and Differential Diagnoses of Female Bladder Outlet Obstruction

1 Physiology of Female Voiding: Are There Many Normals?

Pawan Vasudeva and Niraj Kumar

Learning Objectives To understand:

- Central neural pathways involved in normal bladder function.
- Peripheral neural pathways involved in normal bladder function.
- How it all comes together: The 'Micturition Reflex'.
- Physiological voiding patterns among women.

1.1 Introduction

Urinary bladder function essentially consists of alternate storage and voiding phases. During the storage phase, the bladder acts like a reservoir to enable storage of an adequate amount of urine at low pressure with normal sensations of filling and without any incontinence. During the voiding phase, the bladder behaves like a pump to enable voluntarily initiated voiding with a good stream leading to complete bladder emptying within a normal time span without any obstruction. This dual and somewhat antagonistic function is dependent on (a) structural characteristics and integrity of the bladder and its outlet and (b) the coordination between the complex network of neurons of the central and peripheral nervous systems [1, 2].

1.2 Basic Understanding of the Neural Pathways

1.2.1 Central Pathways

The Pontine Micturition Centre (PMC), also known as Barrington Nucleus, is from where both excitatory and inhibitory efferent impulses originate. With the development of functional brain imaging, it is now understood that the brain bladder control is regulated mainly by three brain circuits. These are responsible for analysis of afferent bladder signals and subsequent facilitation/inhibition of micturition reflexes in the brainstem. (a) ***Circuit 1***: This likely operates during normal sensation of bladder filling and is responsible for the voluntary initiation of micturition. It involves the Periaqueductal Gray (PAG) in the midbrain, which receives afferent inputs from the spinal cord. The information passes through the thalamus and insula to prefrontal cortex (PFC), which makes a decision regarding appropriateness of voiding. During storage, PAG maintains tonic inhibition of the PMC, and this inhibition is controlled by PFC. When it is desirable and socially appropriate to void, inhibition of PAG by PFC is turned off, which further leads to cessation of inhibition of PMC by PAG. Main

P. Vasudeva (✉) · N. Kumar
Department of Urology, VM Medical College and Safdarjung Hospital, New Delhi, India

N. Khattar et al. (eds.), *Female Bladder Outlet Obstruction and Urethral Reconstruction*,
https://doi.org/10.1007/978-981-15-8521-0_1

PMC output is excitatory and efferents from it travel to the intermedio-lateral grey area of S2-4 spinal cord segment to the 'parasympathetic nucleus'. PMC also has an inhibitory output to 'Onuf's nucleus'. (b) ***Circuit 2***: Involves a backup mechanism in case of strong sense of urgency. Afferent signals pass from PAG directly/via thalamus to anterior cingulate cortex (ACC), which stimulates the supplementary motor area (SMA). ACC stimulation results in increased sympathetic discharge and contraction of the urethral smooth muscles, while SMA activation leads to stimulation of the Pontine storage centre (PSC). The PSC provides direct input to 'Onuf's' nucleus. Stimulation of PSC causes contraction of the striated urethral sphincter and the pelvic floor muscles. (c) ***Circuit 3*****:** Involving the parahippocampal complex, amygdala and hypothalamus is less well defined. It may be involved in sending safety or unsafety signals to the PMC [3–8].(Fig. 1.1).

Even though there are differences in micturition behaviour of men and women, no significant differences in brain activation patterns have been noted between the two [3].

1.2.2 **Peripheral Pathways** (Fig. 1.2)

1.2.2.1 Efferent Pathways

Autonomic Pathway

Parasympathetic

Parasympathetic innervation of the lower urinary tract (LUT) (conveyed by the pelvic nerves) originates from a region termed 'the sacral parasympathetic nucleus' in the intermedio-lateral gray matter of S2-4 spinal cord segments. The preganglionic axons, which emerge, synapse with the postganglionic neurons in either the pelvic plexus (a neural network located on lateral surface of rectum) or in the intramural ganglia of the bladder and the post-ganglionic fibres then innervate the bladder. While the bladder body is densely innervated by parasympathetic nerves, the innervation is sparse in the region of bladder neck and urethra [2, 7, 8].

Parasympathetic efferent pathway is the major excitatory input of bladder and the post-ganglionic fibres release both cholinergic and

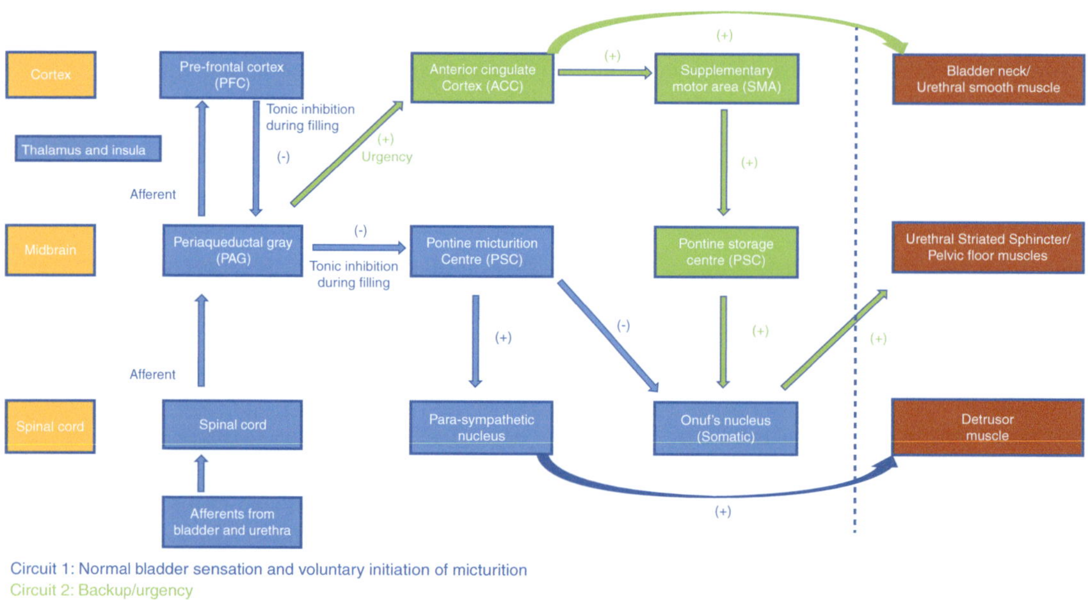

Fig. 1.1 Central pathways for control of urinary bladder functions

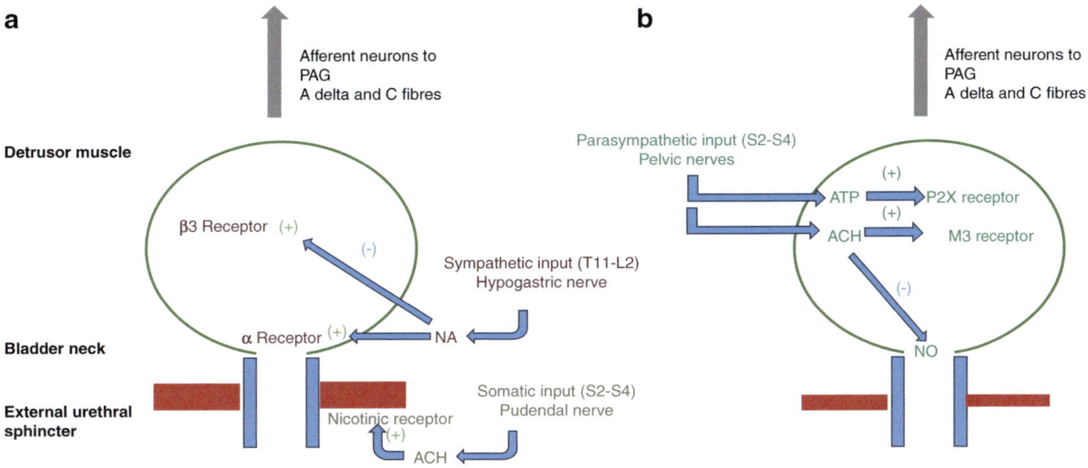

Fig. 1.2 Peripheral pathways for control of urinary bladder functions (**a**) sympathetic and somatic, (**b**) parasympathetic

non-cholinergic, non-adrenergic excitatory transmitters leading to detrusor (smooth muscle) contraction. Cholinergic transmission is predominant in human bladder and is mediated mainly by the M3 muscarinic receptor, but also by M2 receptor. The non-cholinergic excitatory transmission is mediated by adenosine triphosphate (ATP), acting on P2X purinergic receptors. Parasympathetic input to the urethral smooth muscles is inhibitory and is mediated via the release of Nitric Oxide (NO) (Fig. 1.2), which causes urethral smooth muscle relaxation [2, 7, 8].

Sympathetic

Sympathetic innervation of the LUT (conveyed by the hypogastric nerve) originates from the intermedio-lateral grey matter of the T11-L2 spinal cord segments. The pre-ganglionic axons, which emerge, enter the ganglia of the lumbar sympathetic chain. The postganglionic fibres travel in the hypogastric nerves and relay in the pelvic plexus before finally supplying the LUT.

Sympathetic efferent pathway is the major inhibitory input of bladder and the post-ganglionic fibres release noradrenaline leading to detrusor (smooth muscle) relaxation via the β3 adrenergic receptors. At the same time, noradrenaline is excitatory to the bladder base and urethral smooth muscle via α adrenergic receptors leading to contraction of the bladder neck and urethral smooth muscle [2, 7, 8].

Somatic Pathway

Somatomotor innervation of the LUT originates from the motor neurons at the level of S2-4 spinal cord segments (Fig. 1.2). Those fibres, which arise from the Onuf's nucleus, supply the striated muscles of the external urethral sphincter, while those that arise from motor nuclei medial to Onuf's nucleus supply the pelvic floor muscles. The fibres reach the periphery through the pudendal nerves and activation of the pudendal nerve leads to contraction of these muscles [2, 7, 8].

1.2.2.2 Afferent Pathways

There are two main types of afferent fibres (a) Aδ (myelinated), which sense bladder fullness (wall tension) and respond to passive distention, thereby conveying information about bladder filling and (b) C fibres (unmyelinated), which are usually silent under physiological conditions and respond primarily to noxious stimuli. Afferent fibres from the bladder are carried by pelvic and hypogastric nerves, and those from bladder neck and urethra are carried by pudendal and hypogastric nerves. Neuronal somata of these fibres are located in the dorsal root ganglia at S2-4 and T11-L2 spinal cord segments [2, 7, 8].

1.3 Micturition Reflex

During storage phase, the bladder acts as a low-pressure reservoir. Sensory afferents carried via pelvic hypogastric and pudendal nerves convey information about filling. As discussed, via the circuit 1, PFC provides tonic inhibition to the PAG and hence to PMC inhibiting conscious awareness to bladder filling ('unconscious filling'). As the filling increases, beyond a certain threshold, the person becomes aware and it becomes 'conscious filling'. The first sensation of filling, first desire to void and the strong desire to void are appreciated at about 40%, 60% and 90% of bladder capacity, respectively. During the storage phase, it is the sympathetic tonus conveyed via the hypogastric nerve, which keeps the detrusor relaxed and the bladder neck/urethral smooth muscles contracted. The external sphincter progressively contracts with bladder filling. A point in time comes when the PFC perceives timing to be safe and appropriate for voiding [1, 9].

At this time the tonic inhibition of the PAG ceases, in turn inhibition of PMC ceases resulting in (a) activation of parasympathetic neurons of sacral micturition centre resulting in detrusor contraction, (b) reduction of sympathetic tone to bladder neck and urethral smooth muscle, (c) Relaxation of urethral smooth muscle mediated by parasympathetic stimulation and NO release, (d) activation of GABAergic and glycinergic inhibitory interneurons resulting in inactivation of Onuf's nucleus and relaxation of striated sphincter. It is to be noted that voluntary relaxation of external urethral sphincter precedes the detrusor contraction. What ensues in the voiding phase is essentially that the detrusor is contracting and the outlet (comprising relaxed bladder neck smooth muscle, urethral smooth muscle and striated sphincter muscle) is relaxed to facilitate normal voiding. Once the bladder is emptied, PMC shuts off parasympathetic stimuli, detrusor relaxes and sympathetic mediated closure of outlet ensues [1, 9].

1.4 Voiding Patterns Among Women

Three physiological patterns of voiding have been reported among women (Fig. 1.3).

1.4.1 Voiding by Detrusor Contraction and Urethral Relaxation

Majority of continent women (and close to 40% of patients with stress urinary incontinence) void using this mechanism. This involves initial lowering of the urethral pressure (The drop in peak urethral closure pressure is usually ≥25 cm H_2O from pre-voided urethral closure pressure) followed by a detrusor contraction (≥15 cm H_2O during voiding represents an adequate detrusor contraction). A strong correlation exists between the detrusor contractility and the urethral resistance, which implies that the detrusor force gets adjusted to the amount of urethral resistance. **Hence women, consequent to anatomical differences in the bladder outlet, require a sig-**

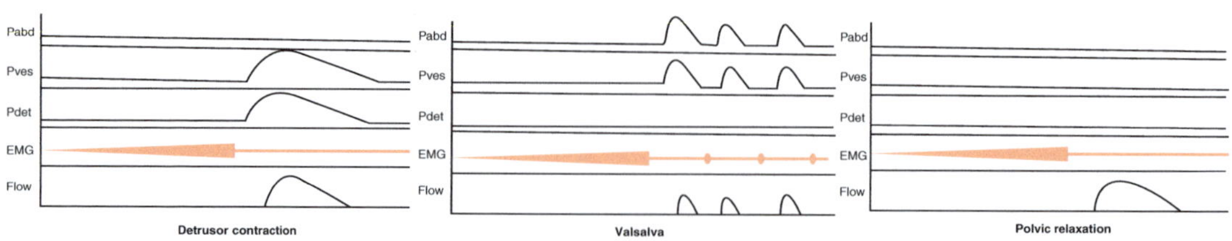

Fig. 1.3 Physiological voiding patterns among women (used with permission from "Urodynamics for Urogynecologists; A Pocket Guide for Clinical Practice" Author Vignoli G, Chapter 1, Springer 2018)

nificantly lower detrusor pressure for voiding when compared to men who have to deal with a relatively high resistance zone of prostatic urethra [10, 11].

It stands to reason then that the pressure flow nomograms developed to classify men as being either obstructed or not obstructed (and also at the same time, the severity of obstruction) cannot be extrapolated and applied to women.

1.4.2 Voiding by Valsalva and Urethral Relaxation

Nearly 40% of women with stress urinary incontinence and also some continent women void by a combination of urethral relaxation aided by Valsalva manoeuvre (An increase in intra-abdominal pressure of ≥10 cm H_2O represents use of abdominal strain). In these women, the flow is not driven by the detrusor pressure (Pdet) but by the vesical pressure (Pves), which brings up the question whether Pves instead of Pdet should be utilized while approaching female voiding dysfunction in Valsalva voiders. Maximum flow rate (Qmax), the other variable involved while defining bladder outlet obstruction, also needs to be interpreted carefully in this subset, as it is well known that straining leads to an artificially high Qmax in most cases [10, 12].

1.4.3 Voiding by Urethral Relaxation Alone in the Absence of Detrusor Contraction/Valsalva

Over 25% of women with stress urinary incontinence and also some continent women void by urethral relaxation alone without any significant contribution from either a detrusor contraction or Valsalva manoeuvre. With urethral relaxation alone being enough to empty the bladder, this may be seen as an 'energy-saving' mechanism of the body [10].

The three types of voiders cannot be normally differentiated on uroflowmetry, although an interrupted pattern may be suggestive of a Valsalva voider. For women who void with (B) or (C) mechanism as described, it does not necessarily mean that they have a detrusor that is acontractile. If urethral resistance were to increase, many of these women would generate a detrusor contraction to overcome the outlet resistance. This was demonstrated by Bhatia et al. who showed that nearly 50% of women who voided without a detrusor contraction did develop a good detrusor contraction after undergoing a stress urinary incontinence procedure and consequent increase in urethral resistance [13]. Simultaneously, it can be argued that as the amount of detrusor pressure these women would produce on encountering an obstruction has not been studied separately, hence applying uniform definition of female bladder outlet obstruction to all types of voiders may not be appropriate.

1.5 Applied Physiology/Clinical Implications

From the foregoing discussion, it seems reasonable to draw the following observations:

1. Since there is heterogenicity in the way/the mechanism with which women empty their bladder, defining obstruction universally in all women based on high detrusor pressure combined with a low flow rate is erroneous. At maximum, such a definition can only be applied to the subset of Type A voiders. For obvious reasons, it cannot be extrapolated to Type B and C voiders, in whom, a detrusor contraction is not involved in bladder emptying.
2. Men have a considerably higher urethral resistance than women and so it stands to reason that even if we have to define obstruction in women in the same way as we did in men, i.e. high detrusor pressure combined with a low flow, the nomograms from men cannot be extrapolated to women.
3. It is incorrect to presume that a woman who voids without a detrusor contraction has an acontractile bladder. On the contrary, she may be having a very effective pelvic floor relax-

ation. In the event of an increase in urethral resistance, many of the same women would demonstrate effective detrusor contractions.
4. Absence of detrusor contraction may be a risk factor for post sling voiding dysfunction as not all women would demonstrate effective detrusor contraction consequent to an increase in urethral resistance.

1.6 Conclusion

While the neural pathways and micturition reflex are essentially the same for both men and women, structural differences in the outlet allow women to empty their bladders with lesser effort/pressure and a generally higher flow when compared to men. Unlike normal men, all of whom void by detrusor contraction, three distinct forms of voiding are considered normal in women. This heterogeneity in what is a normal voiding mechanism/pattern must be incorporated into clinical decision making when evaluating women with suspected voiding dysfunction.

Key Learning Points

- Despite a difference in voiding behaviours of men and women, there are no significant differences in brain activation patterns during storage and voiding.
- As compared to men, women require lower detrusor pressure to overcome urethral resistance and, consequently, the pressure flow nomograms for diagnosing obstruction in men cannot be applied to women.
- There are three predominant physiological patterns of voiding in women with possible clinical implications.
- Voiding without detrusor contraction does not necessarily mean that detrusor is acontractile.

References

1. Sullivan MP, Yalla SV. Physiology of female micturition. Urol Clin North Am. 2002;29(3):499–514. vii
2. Bortolini MA, Bilhar AP, Castro RA. Neural control of lower urinary tract and targets for pharmacological therapy. Int Urogynecol J. 2014;25(11):1453–62.
3. Arya NG, Weissbart SJ. Central control of micturition in women: brain-bladder pathways in continence and urgency urinary incontinence. Clin Anat. 2017;30(3):373–84.
4. Blok BF, Sturms LM, Holstege G. Brain activation during micturition in women. Brain. 1998;121. (Pt 11:2033–42.
5. Fowler CJ, Griffiths D, de Groat WC. The neural control of micturition. Nat Rev Neurosci. 2008;9(6):453–66.
6. Blok BF, De Weerd H, Holstege G. Ultrastructural evidence for a paucity of projections from the lumbosacral cord to the pontine micturition center or M-region in the cat: a new concept for the organization of the micturition reflex with the periaqueductal gray as central relay. J Comp Neurol. 1995;359(2):300–9.
7. Yoshimura N, de Groat WC. Neural control of the lower urinary tract. Int J Urol. 1997;4(2):111–25.
8. de Groat WC, Yoshimura N. Anatomy and physiology of the lower urinary tract. Handb Clin Neurol. 2015;130:61–108.
9. Vignoli G. Physiology of micturition in female. In: Urodynamics for urogynecologists, vol. 2018. New York, NY: Springer, Champions; 2018. p. 1–15.
10. Rud T, Ulmsten U, Andersson KE. Initiation of voiding in healthy women and those with stress incontinence. Acta Obstet Gynecol Scand. 1978;57(5):457–62.
11. Bhatia NN. Dynamics of voiding in women. Curr Opin Obstet Gynecol. 2000;12(5):383–6.
12. Rademakers K, Apostolidis A, Constantinou C, et al. Recommendations for future development of contractility and obstruction nomograms for women. ICI-RS 2014. Neurourol Urodyn. 2016;35(2):307–11.
13. Bhatia NN, Bergman A, Karram M. Changes in urethral resistance after surgery for stress urinary incontinence. Urology. 1989;34(4):200–4.

2 Female Bladder Outlet Obstruction: Whom to Work Up and What to Look for?

Nikhil Khattar

Learning Objectives

- To understand the symptoms that should raise suspicion of BOO in a female.
- To know other conditions that should prompt an evaluation for BOO in a female.
- To know what to look for during examination of women with suspected BOO.
- To appropriately apply investigations required to make a conclusive diagnosis.
- To understand the importance of complete urethral inspection before cystoscopy.

2.1 Introduction

Bladder outlet obstruction (BOO) in women can present in myriad ways. Apart from women presenting with an obvious slow stream, recurrent retention or obstructive uropathy where looking for BOO is imperative, there are other subtle presentations where it is prudent to rule out outlet obstruction. This chapter focusses on the obvious and not-so-obvious presentations with real-life examples and illustrations.

N. Khattar (✉)
Female Urology, Reconstructive Urology and Neurovesical Dysfunction, Medanta, The Medicity, Gurugram, India

2.2 Relation Between BOO and Voiding Dysfunction

That the 'bladder is an unreliable witness' [1] is even more applicable to women than men as the presenting symptoms may be bizarre. Very few women with voiding problems present with isolated voiding symptoms. Instead, they present with a mixture of both storage and voiding symptoms or storage symptoms alone. **Whereas storage and voiding 'symptoms' may be two separate compartments, there is a definite overlap between storage and voiding 'dysfunctions'** (Fig. 2.1). Moreover, underactive bladder may present with symptoms similar to BOO. As women with BOO represent a subset of all patients diagnosed with voiding dysfunction (VD), any woman presenting with lower urinary tract symptoms (LUTS) should be assessed for presence of BOO to enable us to widen the net to include all possible presentations.

2.3 Voiding Dysfunction

International Continence Society (ICS) defines female VD as 'abnormally slow and/or incomplete micturition, based on abnormally slow urine flow rates and or abnormally high post-void residuals, ideally on repeated measurement to confirm abnormality' [2]. It is a finding for which symptoms may or may not be directly

N. Khattar et al. (eds.), *Female Bladder Outlet Obstruction and Urethral Reconstruction*,
https://doi.org/10.1007/978-981-15-8521-0_2

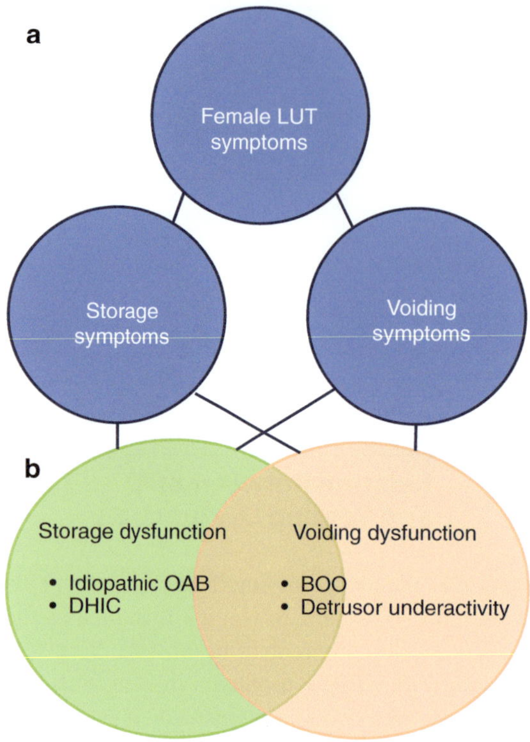

Fig. 2.1 (**a**) A Lower urinary tract symptom may be a storage or a voiding symptom with no overlap among them, but (**b**) the storage and voiding dysfunctions have a considerable overlap. Thus, women presenting with only storage symptoms may have underlying voiding dysfunction

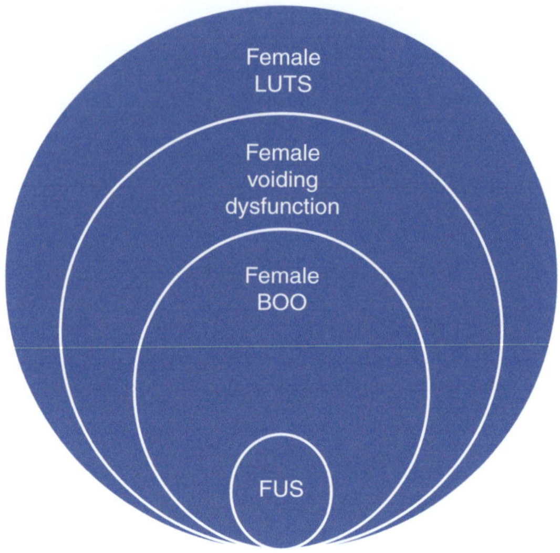

Fig. 2.2 Female VD represents a significant proportion of overall female LUTS of which less than half have urodynamic BOO. Functional causes far outnumber the anatomical causes of BOO and FUS is just a small proportion of all BOO

suggestive. In a large review of urodynamic traces of 1914 women with voiding symptoms and slow flow (excluding large-grade cystoceles, neurogenic bladder and prior history of sling surgery for incontinence) [3], urodynamic BOO was diagnosed in 810 (42%) and bladder dysfunction was diagnosed in 1048 (55%) women. Of the 810 women with urodynamic BOO, the distribution of aetiology was as follows: Anatomical Obstruction in only 6% (stricture in 30 and cystocele in 19) and Functional BOO in the rest with dysfunctional voiding (DV) and primary bladder neck obstruction (PBNO) as the most common causes of functional obstruction. The 1048 patients with bladder dysfunction had detrusor underactivity, hypersensitive bladder and detrusor hyperactivity, and inhibited contractility as chief causes. The data gives a glimpse of the high prevalence of urodynamic BOO in women with voiding symptoms without a history of sling surgery or obvious pelvic organ prolapse (which were considered as the only causes of female BOO till recently). It also emphasises that functional obstructions are many times more common than anatomical causes especially female urethral strictures (FUS) (Fig. 2.2).

2.4 Whom to Workup?

2.4.1 Symptoms of Voiding Dysfunction in Women

Straining, interrupted urinary stream, poor or weak flow of urine, suprapubic pressure with feeling of incomplete evacuation and a need to sit for prolonged periods on toilet seat in order to evacuate are some common voiding symptoms women present with. Having to stand and void is another symptom, which should alert the physician for evaluation for BOO in women [4]. The symptoms of underactive bladder and BOO are overlapping and urodynamics is required to reach a conclusion [5]. It can't be overemphasised that the symptoms should be present for at least 4–6 weeks before a woman is labelled as VD and subjected to invasive investigations as transient voiding symptoms are common during a urinary tract infection (UTI) or local vaginal pathologies like vaginitis.

There are only a few studies in women correlating symptoms with urodynamic bladder outlet obstruction, but they do give some insight on the way these women might present.

Kuo [6], in a retrospective analysis of 1605 women with lower urinary tract dysfunction who underwent urodynamic studies (UDS), divided the presenting symptoms as storage, voiding, pain or post micturition symptoms (terminal dribbling, feeling of incomplete evacuation and post void dribbling). **Less than 1% Women with urodynamic voiding disturbances presented with voiding symptoms alone**. Rather, they presented with either only storage symptoms or both storage and voiding symptoms. Among patients with functional BOO, those with pelvic floor dysfunction (i.e. DV and poor relaxation of pelvic floor) more commonly presented with frequency as their main symptom, whereas patients with bladder neck dysfunction presented with dysuria as their predominant symptom.

Malde et al. [7] retrospectively analysed data of 1014 women who had presented with lower urinary tract symptoms and had undergone extensive evaluation and detailed documentation of each of their voiding symptom along with a video-urodynamic study in all patients and MRI, urethral pressure profilometry (UPP) or cystourethroscopy, as indicated, to complete the diagnosis and to classify them to either a functional or an anatomic obstruction. Out of 192 women diagnosed with urodynamic BOO, anatomical obstruction was present in 64% of patients (anti-incontinence surgery 21%, Female urethral stricture (FUS) 20%, cystocele 12%, urethral diverticulum 9%, and a paraurethral cyst in 1%), whereas 36% had a functional obstruction (non-relaxing or dysfunctional sphincter). Storage symptoms, including day-time frequency (69%) and nocturia (67%), were the most common presenting symptoms, and surprisingly urgency urinary incontinence was recorded in 45% of women. Voiding lower urinary tract symptoms (LUTS), namely feeling of incomplete emptying and poor flow were observed in only 64% and 60%, respectively, and were more frequent in anatomical rather than functional obstruction, whereas history of retention requiring catheterisation was more common in functional obstruction. Urethral pain and recurrent urinary tract infection (UTI) were other common complaints (22% each) and were significantly more common in urethral stricture.

Many validated questionnaires have come up for assessment of female voiding dysfunction. Bristol Female Lower urinary tract symptom (BFLUTS) score was developed in 1996 [8] and later adopted by ICS. Although it was mainly developed for assessment of incontinence in women, it has sub-domains of voiding symptoms and impact of LUTS on sexual health too and has thus been adopted by ICS for use in women. International prostatic symptom score (IPSS) has also been validated for use in women [9].

Urinary distress inventory (short form) (UDI-6) [10] is a simple six-question form in which there are three questions related to incontinence and one each for frequency, pain and bladder emptying. Question no. 5 on the UDI-6 enquires for incomplete emptying ('Do you experience any problem in emptying your bladder?'). An answer in 'Yes' to a single straight question (question no. 5 of Urinary distress inventory UDI-6) better predicted presence of voiding dysfunction as confirmed with a free uroflowmetry ≤12 ml/s, and an ultrasound post void residue (PVR) of ≥100 ml than a directed questionnaire with voiding symptoms in women with history of anti-incontinence surgery [11]. In another study of 128 women evaluated with UDI-6 questionnaire and subsequent urodynamic study, 55% of the 29 women with most bothersome symptom as 'problem emptying the bladder' were found to be urodynamically obstructed. Interestingly, 25% of 99 women in whom emptying the bladder was not the most bothersome symptom, also had urodynamic BOO [12]. Therefore, whereas a single question can predict the presence of VD in a woman, it justifiably cannot predict presence of urodynamic BOO. This brings into question the superiority of various female voiding symptom questionnaires over simple questions in the clinic!

Underactive bladder also presents with similar symptoms of a feeling of decreased interrupted urinary stream, hesitancy and incomplete emptying of the bladder. In addition, enuresis and a palpable bladder are more common [5]. Moreover, there is a very thin line between definitions of underactive detrusor and BOO in women and both can often even co-exist making treatment decisions more difficult.

In conclusion, we can infer that **there are no symptoms specific for voiding dysfunction and a free uroflowmetry with an ultrasound for PVR should be obtained in all women complaining of any voiding difficulty**. Let us also examine the coexistence of BOO in other urinary symptoms where there is no overt voiding difficulty

2.4.2 Common Conditions, Which May Have Underlying BOO in Women

2.4.2.1 Overactive Bladder (OAB)

A significant proportion (between 35% and 42%, depending on the definition of urodynamic BOO used in the study) of women presenting with significant OAB symptoms (both wet and dry) *without any voiding symptoms* may be having urodynamic BOO [13, 14]. An additional 3–8% may be diagnosed with an underactive bladder during the urodynamic studies. Because a clinical diagnosis of OAB, on deeper evaluation, can uncover a plethora of conditions, it has rightly been termed as a 'symptom in search of a disease' rather than a disease itself [15]. All prominent guidelines on OAB, including AUA 2019, EAU 2019 and Indian guidelines 2019, recommend selective use of uroflowmetry or PVR only in patients with a suspected VD. But an underlying VD cannot be ruled out with symptoms alone. Should such huge percentages prompt an upfront uroflowmetry for each clinical diagnosis of OAB is yet to be studied, but this fact should certainly be considered while evaluating women with refractory OAB. During UDS in these patients, the voiding phase should be carefully studied (Fig. 2.3). Nevertheless, we feel a free uroflow must be obtained in all treatment naïve women with clinical diagnosis of idiopathic OAB.

2.4.2.2 Stress Urinary Incontinence (SUI)

Although it is known that voiding dysfunction and a possible BOO should be the first suspicion in any woman complaining of any alteration in voiding pattern after anti-incontinence surgery [16], treatment naïve women with a clinical diagnosis of 'uncomplicated' SUI have been also found to be having voiding dysfunction(Fig. 2.4). **Around 25% of 'uncomplicated' SUI may have VD** [17] **and 13–15% may have urodynamic BOO** [18].

The implication of this finding is debatable. While some authors believe that it may be important predictor for post sling voiding dysfunction and hence an additional need to counsel such patients [17], others believe that there is no statistically significant impact on the outcome [19].

2.4.2.3 Recurrent UTI

Women with history of recurrent UTI have also been found to have **voiding dysfunction as revealed by a Qmax of <15 ml/s or elevated PVR in approximately 50–60% patients**. BOO due to dysfunctional voiding or an underactive bladder are almost equally likely in these women [20]. A recent prospective case–control study found voiding dysfunction in as many as 90% of women with recurrent UTI evaluated. Dysfunctional voiding and bladder neck dysfunction were common findings. Only 11% however became free of recurrent infections after individualised treatment of their VD [21].

2.4.2.4 Bladder Pain Syndrome (BPS/ IC)

Women suspected of symptoms of painful bladder syndrome (BPS/IC) may also be harbouring BOO. This was first brought to light by Cameron and Gajewski in 2009 in a retrospective study of 274 women with PBS/IC who had undergone a

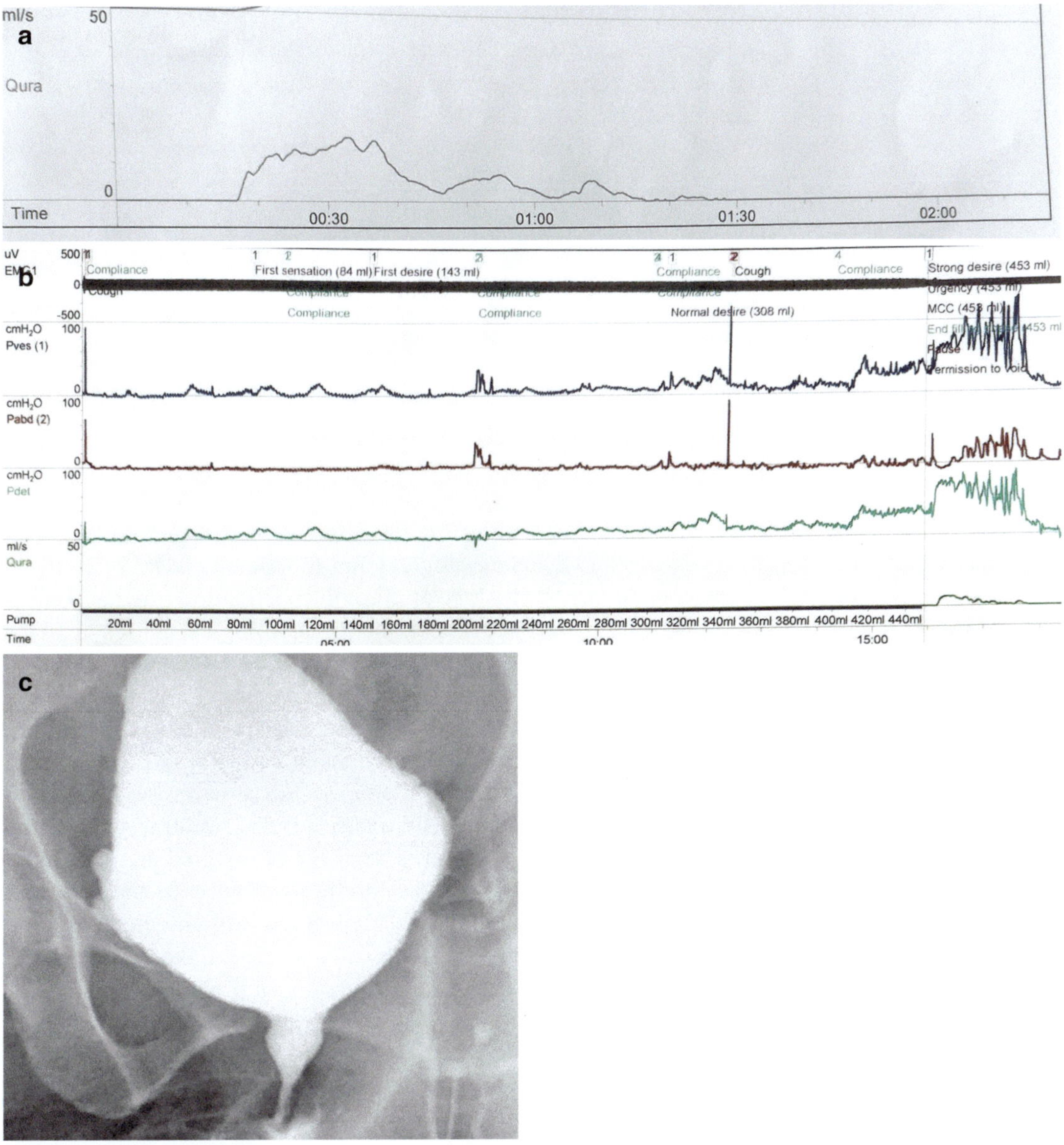

Fig. 2.3 A 58-year-old lady presented with symptoms of severe wet OAB, refractory even after two years of anticholinergic therapy. She had no voiding symptoms. (**a**) Her free uroflowmetry revealed an obstructive pattern with a *Q* max of 16 ml/s and (**b**) UDS confirmed detrusor overactivity with urodynamic evidence of BOO (Pdet@ Qmax 66 cm H2O). (**c**) Final diagnosis of dysfunctional voiding was made after voiding cysto-urethrogram showed ballooning of proximal urethra and urethra was normal on calibration

UDS study as well. Surprisingly, **urodynamic BOO was evident in 48.1% of the subjects** [22]. Routine use of UDS in patients suspected of PBS/IC, however, is not recommended because it is extremely painful and most of the urodynamic findings may be because of catheterisation-induced response of the pelvic floor during the study [23]. **As the final common pathway of urothelial dysfunction is shared between most lower urinary tract dysfunctions including BOO, PBS/IC, OAB and recurrent UTI** [24]**, it is not surprising to have overlap of symptoms between these conditions, especially in delayed and ignored presentations**.

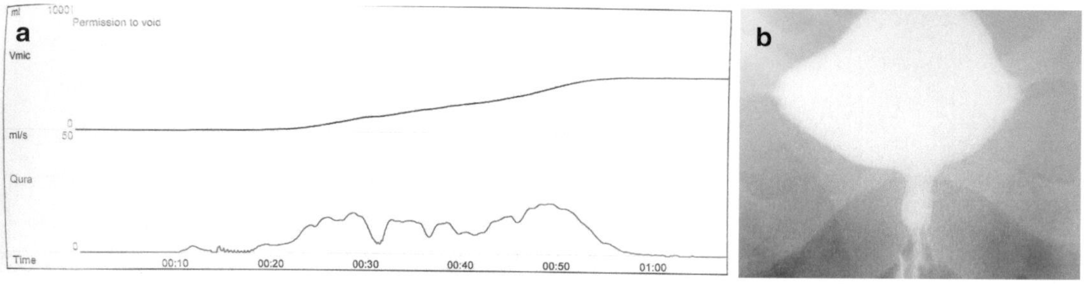

Fig. 2.4 (**a**) A 45-year female with history of stress predominant mixed incontinence of 2 years' duration without any voiding symptoms showed poor flow on uroflowmetry. Urethra was normal on calibration with 18 Fr. On her UDS, apart from demonstrable urodynamic stress incontinence, voiding phase showed a Pdet@Qmax of 38 cm H_2O with a *Q* max of 12.9 ml/s. (**b**) Her voiding cystourethrogram also demonstrated an area of urethral dilatation at the mid-urethral level confirming a functional urodynamic BOO. Her voiding dysfunction did not increase after successful mid-urethral sling surgery

Table 2.1 Aetiology of female BOO

Functional BOO
(a) Dysfunctional voiding (DV) and poor relaxation of external sphincter (PRES)
(b) Primary bladder neck dysfunction (PBNO)
(c) Fowler's syndrome
Anatomical BOO
Intrinsic anatomical
(a) Female urethral stricture
(b) Urethral divericulum
Extrinsic anatomical
(a) Periurethral benign or malignant lesions
(b) Post sling obstruction (c) Meatal stenosis (d) Labial adhesions
Positional anatomical
(a) Anterior pelvic organ prolapse (cystocele)
(a) Retroverted gravid uterus

2.5 What to Look For?

A knowledge of the common causes of BOO in women (Table 2.1) and their frequency will direct the focus areas during examination and further investigations.

2.5.1 Clinical Evaluation

Besides detailed subjective and objective assessment of lower urinary tract symptoms in women, leading questions should be asked in an effort to differentiate between anatomical, neurological and functional causes of BOO. A history of chronic constipation often accompanies functional or neurological causes of BOO. Dyspareunia may also be associated. A clinical examination of the genitalia can often reveal external causes like meatal stenosis, significant prolapse, perimeatal condyloma [25] or labial adhesions [26]. The anterior vaginal wall should be palpated for urethral tenderness, which may be a sign of infected urethral diverticulum or a urethral stricture. In addition, palpation of urethra in an infected urethral diverticulum can also reveal expressible pus at the meatus. If history of previous incontinence surgery is present, an attempt can be made to palpate the sling and to rule out any exposure. The lateral vaginal walls should be palpated for the tone of the pelvic floor muscles. They can be especially prominent in dysfunctional voiding and other pelvic floor dysfunctions. Pelvic floor dysfunctions also have chronic constipation as an associated feature and one may be able to feel fecoliths from the posterior vaginal wall.

2.5.2 Uroflowmetry and PVR

As per the ICS definition of VD as stated above [2], i.e. 'abnormally slow and/or incomplete micturition, based on abnormally slow urine flow rates and/or abnormally high post-void residuals…' **a uroflowmetry and a PVR assessment should be the first ordered investigations whenever a voiding dysfunction is suspected** on the basis of pointers mentioned above. Although presence of significant PVR (amount debatable) may represent a voiding dysfunction and warrant a detailed workup, certainly the absence of it does not rule out the presence of VD and BOO [27].

There are two widely used criteria in various studies to define an abnormal uroflow in women: (**a**) A peak flow rate (PFR) <15 ml/s and a PVR >50 ml with a minimum pre-void bladder volume of 150 ml have been used in many studies describing abnormal voiding across numerous studies in both men and women. (**b**) Liverpool nomogram has been specifically developed for women across a wide range of voided volumes (150–600 ml) where less than 10th centile curve is considered abnormal.

In a prospective study, Costantini et al. [28] compared both the above uroflowmetry cut-offs with four different cut-offs on a pressure flow study for diagnosing female BOO described till then including [29–32] in 348 consecutive women who underwent complete urodynamic evaluation for their LUTS. Both the uroflowmetry cut-off methods had a sensitivity of 50–100% and specificity of >70% for diagnosing BOO and both the methods were in good agreement. **Uroflowmetry can hence be recommended as a good screening test for diagnosing female VD**. It is recommended though to repeat the test and confirm the patterns before subjecting for more invasive tests because of factors like comfort of the patient while voiding and privacy provided. A recent study, however, concluded that a single uroflow in women may be reliable enough [33] provided she confirms that her micturition during the uroflow was representative of her usual void.

To more specifically screen women of Asian origin, PGIMER nomogram can be applied to uroflow results, which takes into account the voided volumes and can be adjusted for age too [34].

2.5.3 Uroflow with EMG

Electromyography (EMG), along with Uroflowmetry, adds a new dimension to the usefulness of uroflowmetry. It has been extensively used in paediatric patients, but reports in adults are sparse. It is non-invasive and avoids any artefacts of pelvic floor spasm because of intubated voiding that can develop during a pressure flow study. In a retrospective study, which included 26 women with voiding dysfunction, flow + EMG gave insights on the pathophysiology of pelvic floor, which could not have been known on plain uroflow study [35]. More studies will be required to explore its full potential in adult functional urology.

2.5.4 Does Ultrasound Bladder Wall Thickness Help in Diagnosing Women with BOO?

Usefulness of bladder or detrusor wall thickness (DWT) has been studied as a surrogate marker to diagnose BOO in men. In a systematic review of all non-invasive tests to predict BOO in men with LUTS [36], bladder/detrusor wall thickness of >2.9 mm was found to have a specificity of close to 100% in diagnosing urodynamic BOO (most studies used the criteria of bladder outlet obstruction index, BOOI >40 for defining urodynamic BOO in this review). However, such correlation of DWT with BOO in women is not yet established. In a retrospective study [37], records of 686 women who underwent UDS for their LUTS were retrieved. In this study, the DWT (measured with perineal ultrasound at a volume of 50 cc) was not associated with objective voiding dysfunction or even obstruction coefficients and urethral resistance factor that defined urodynamic BOO. The authors have speculated that unlike in men, the increased DWT in women represents effect of isometric contractions in storage phase against a closed outlet like in detrusor overactivity (DO) rather than as an effect of isotonic contractions against increased urethral resistance during voiding phase. There has been no further study to assess that relation for women. Apart from being retrospective in nature, the major flaw in this study has been the volume at which DWT was measured. DWT decreases rapidly till a fill volume of 250 ml and thereafter hardly changes till capacity [38]; therefore, measurement below 250 ml is expected to be unreliable. To overcome this effect, most authors in the systematic review by Malde et al. as above [36], used a higher bladder volume, e.g. 50% of capacity, or at capacity, or at a mean of values at multiple points during filling. Although measurement of DWT has also been debated as a non-invasive marker of DO and some studies inconsistently find it increased with urodynamic DO, the reproducibility is poor and confounding effect of BOO on DWT in these studies remains a major factor [39]. Yet another study noted that BWT decreased after relief of obstruction by urethrolysis in 62 women who had developed iatrogenic obstruction following incontinence surgery [40]. Therefore, in the absence of further studies, ultrasonographic documentation of increased bladder wall thickening should be considered as a marker of voiding dysfunction in women.

2.5.5 Is Urethral Calibration Contributory to Diagnosis?

There is no clear consensus for a normal or a narrow urethra in women. Various researchers have defined different cut-offs for abnormal urethral calibre in women ranging from <20 Fr to <12 Fr, and a calibre of less than 14 Fr has been the most common definition for diagnosing a female urethral stricture [41]. Moreover, because of the anxiety spasm, which can be more pronounced when pelvic floor dysfunctions are the cause of BOO, office calibration can give a false impression of having a stricture and may lead to an unwarranted urethral dilatation. **The role of urethral calibration is to rule out any luminal anatomical obstruction, which has to be finally confirmed on urethroscopy.** Calibration with 14 Fr is author's preference.

2.6 Video-Urodynamics (or Pressure-Flow Studies + VCUG): The Cornerstone of Evaluating Female VD

The final diagnosis of a BOO rests on a high-pressure low-flow pattern on a pressure-flow study. When coupled with a voiding image as a video-urodynamic study, this has been considered as the present gold standard for establishing the correct diagnosis of any VD in a female [42]. Since it is an invasive investigation, it should be undertaken when thorough evaluation with symptoms, clinical examination, bladder diary, free uroflow, and an ultrasound for PVR have already been done. If there is no facility for video UDS, a separate VCUG should be done before a pressure flow urodynamic study. The study should be performed in the supervision of the treating physician in a relaxed atmosphere with adequate privacy. ICS best practice guidelines should be followed. A note should be made whether the symptoms of urgency or bladder pain, if documented earlier, are reproduced during the study. If the woman normally voids in any other posture than sitting like a partial erect posture or a leaning forward posture, then that should be allowed during the voiding phase. The main aim of the study will be to characterise the type of voiding dysfunction (Urodynamic BOO versus detrusor underactivity) and to clearly establish the level of obstruction. A repeat cycle of filling should be done if the study has been inconclusive. Addition of a urethral pressure profilometry is required only in complex cases. In general, a detrusor pressure at maximum flow during the voiding phase (Pdet@Qmax) of more than 20 cm H_2O coupled with a Q max of <15 ml/s along with demonstration of an area of discrete narrowing in the urethra make a diagnosis of urodynamic BOO extremely likely. Although these are not absolute, and a dedicated chapter covers the evolution and controversies in definitions of urodynamic BOO.

The pattern of image of urethra during voiding presents the best opportunity to know the level of BOO. This can be obtained during a video urodynamic study or as a standalone voiding cystourethrography (VCUG). Video-urodynamics is not easily available at all centres and hence it is not uncommon to have the two studies done independently, which can also provide valuable information [43]. Although the advantage of a composite video-urodynamic study is a simultaneous visualisation of urethra and detrusor pressures in voiding phase and convenience to the patient, the effect of urethral tube during the voiding may alter the patterns of pelvic floor. On the other hand, a separate micturating study is free of indwelling catheter at the time of voiding. The presence of the treating physician in the radiology suite or recording the voiding on a cine mode as a video may be a mandatory requirement for a conclusive interpretation.

Both antero-posterior and lateral-oblique voiding images may be informative depending on the provisional diagnosis. Placement of a radiopaque marker at the meatus makes interpretation of level of obstruction easier. **A cystocele impinging on the urethra or a urethral diverticulum may be best seen in lateral images during voiding, whereas primary bladder neck obstruction, dysfunctional voiding or poor relaxation of external sphincter and urethral strictures are best visualised on anteroposterior imaging**.

Apart from changes in the bladder due to prolonged obstruction like irregularity of bladder wall and small diverticulae dotting the bladder outline or an occasional secondary vesicoureteric reflux, imaging of the urethra during voiding can give important clues on the level of obstruction.

Female urethral stricture produces a mid or distal urethral narrowing and proximal urethral bulge with a wide-open bladder neck (Fig. 2.5a). **The level on a voiding film may not always match with actual urethroscopy findings because of the often-present urethral hypermobility. Convexity of the urethral edges with a discrete area of narrowing is suggestive of outlet obstruction.**

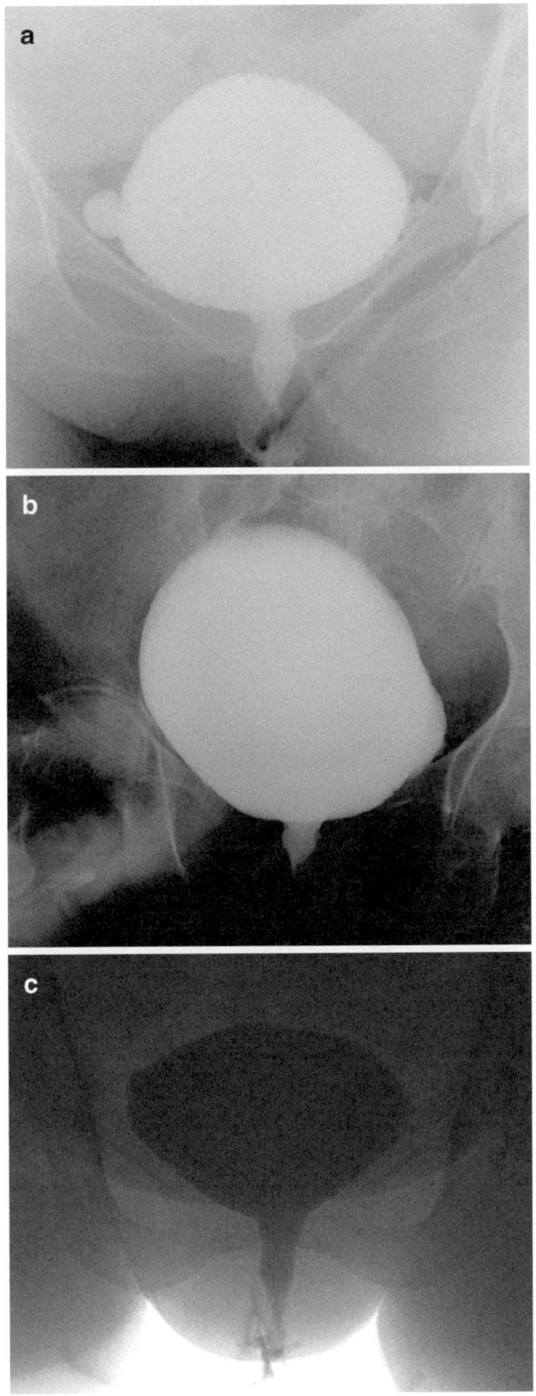

Fig. 2.5 The radiological picture of a dilated urethra only suggests an underlying BOO, but the picture is similar for anatomical and functional obstructions. (**a**) Female urethral stricture. (**b**) Dysfunctional voiding. (**c**) Poor relaxation of external sphincter (PRES). (**d**) Primary bladder neck obstruction, PBNO, can be identified by poor funnelling at the neck in voiding phase

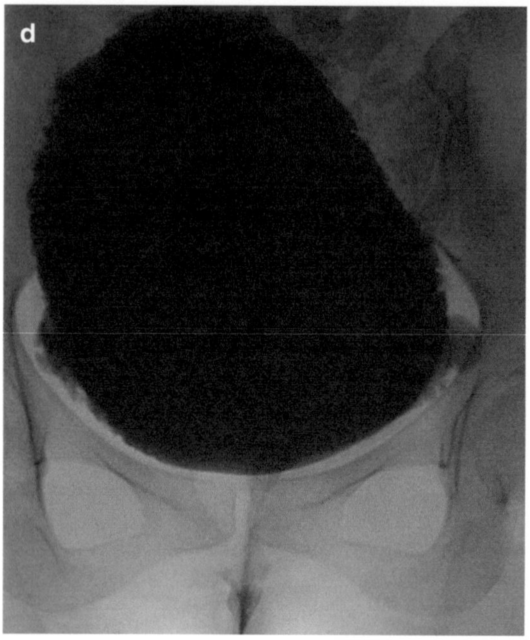

Fig. 2.5 (continued)

Dysfunctional voiding patients produce a picture very similar or even indistinguishable from that of FUS patients (Fig. 2.5b). Since the clinical presentation and pressure flow study findings also may be similar, and office calibration can be misleading, a urethroscopy under anaesthesia may be required to differentiate the two. Poor relaxation of external sphincter (PRES) is a more subtle form of functional BOO as compared to DV with less bulging of urethra on voiding image and a more distal level of narrowing in urethra [44] (Fig. 2.5c).

Poor opening at the neck on VCUG or video-urodynamics with a urodynamic obstruction is suggestive of Primary bladder neck obstruction (Fig. 2.5d). Such patients may show a frank urodynamic BOO and an anatomically normal urethra similar to DV, and hence the voiding image is the only reliable differentiating feature for diagnosing this potentially surgically treatable cause of functional BOO [45].

2.7 Investigations for Specific Situations

2.7.1 Transvaginal Sonography

Three-dimensional transvaginal sonography has been used effectively to assess sling surgery related voiding dysfunctions in women [46] and urethral diverticula. Role in voiding dysfunctions of other aetiologies is poorly defined.

2.7.2 Magnetic Resonance Imaging (MRI)

MRI of the pelvis has a definite role in specific situations like Urethral diverticulum or assessment of periurethral masses causing extrinsic compression. Role of dynamic MRI as defecography in diagnosing anterior prolapse [47] related obstruction is only investigational as it has not yet been correlated with urodynamic BOO caused by prolapse. It has however no role yet in diagnosis of female urethral stricture or functional urethral obstructions.

2.7.3 Cystoscopy

Cystoscopy has no role in the diagnosis of obstruction as such. However, once an obstruction is confirmed on video-urodynamic parameters or on an inability to catheterise, then a cystoscopy with proper visualisation of urethral lumen is instrumental to diagnose an anatomical narrowing of the lumen (stricture), to identify any urethral erosion of a sling or to confirm a urethral diverticulum. **Cystoscopy should be taken up only when adequate information has been gathered by other non/lesser invasive tests**, It may also provide another opportunity for simultaneous therapeutic procedure like urethral dilatation/urethroplasty for a stricture, bladder neck incision for a PBNO or a botulinum injection for a dysfunctional voider.

Evaluation of female urethra with a cystoscope requires meticulous care. **Being the only modality that can conclusively differentiate anatomical narrowing (stricture) and functional obstructions, it becomes absolutely mandatory to visualise the urethra completely whenever an anatomical obstruction is strongly suspected**. It should be performed under general anaesthesia. When urethroscopy is performed under local anaesthesia, the spasm of pelvic floor in anxious females or in those with a functional obstruction at pelvic floor may confound the findings. The relaxation of pelvic floor under general anaesthesia prevents labelling any of functional obstructions as a stricture and inadvertently subjecting them to lifelong dilatations. Earlier descriptions of a 'tight urethral syndrome' may well be a manifestation of female urethrocystoscopy under local anaesthesia. **A *urethral inspection* before inserting the cystoscope further is extremely informative and is recommended as a separate step to keep the context alive while performing cystoscopic examination.** A conventional beaked cystoscope is not suitable for this. Instead, **an integrated compact cystoscope, preferably 14 or 17 Fr, is better suited for this. It does not have a beak and prevents the run-off of irrigation fluid in contrast to the floor-deficient tip of conventional 3-part cystoscopy sheath**. The forward flow thus achieved allows distention of the urethra. A forward viewing (zero degree) scope is ideal.

In the absence of a dedicated female cystoscopy sheath, a Nickell's adapter is preferred. If a suitable cystoscope is not available, we have used an assembled Direct visual internal urethrotomy (DVIU) sheath with a zero-degree scope for urethral inspection, which may be adequate in cases where meatus is not narrow (Fig. 2.6).

Attempt to visualise neck of a diverticulum also requires a distended urethra but often a 30-degree lens. Having ruled out a stricture or a diverticulum, the rest of the cystoscopy can be performed with a 30-degree scope.

If an anatomical narrowing is actually identified, its extent can be further characterised with a small calibre ureteroscope or a paediatric cystoscope.

To summarise, Female bladder outlet obstruction comprises 30–40% of female voiding dysfunction. Women with any urinary symptoms (not necessarily voiding symptoms) should be screened for presence of a voiding dysfunction. Uroflowmetry is a good screening test, which may be interpreted along with an ultrasound examination of the bladder wall thickness and the post void residual volume. Functional causes for BOO are much more common than anatomic causes but can be characterised on videourodynamics (or Pressure flow study and VCUG). Office calibration is unreliable and cystoscopy with dedicated urethral inspection is the most definitive way to look for a stricture which is rare. MRI and Transvaginal sonography have specific indications and should not be ordered for all women with BOO.

Key Learning Points

- Two main causes of voiding dysfunction in women are bladder outlet obstruction and underactive bladder. Identifying voiding dysfunction therefore is the key to correctly diagnose more women with obstruction.
- As type of symptoms cannot predict an obstruction, a uroflowmetry should be obtained in all women with lower tract symptoms to rule out an underlying voiding dysfunction.
- Common conditions like overactive bladder, recurrent urinary tract infections, stress incontinence and bladder pain syndrome may have underlying undiagnosed voiding dysfunction.
- Videourodymanics is the investigation of choice to characterise a voiding dysfunction
- Functional causes are significantly more common than anatomical obstructions and strictures are rare.
- A failure to calibrate the urethra may be because of pelvic floor spasm and only a urethrocystoscopy can reliably diagnose an anatomical obstruction.

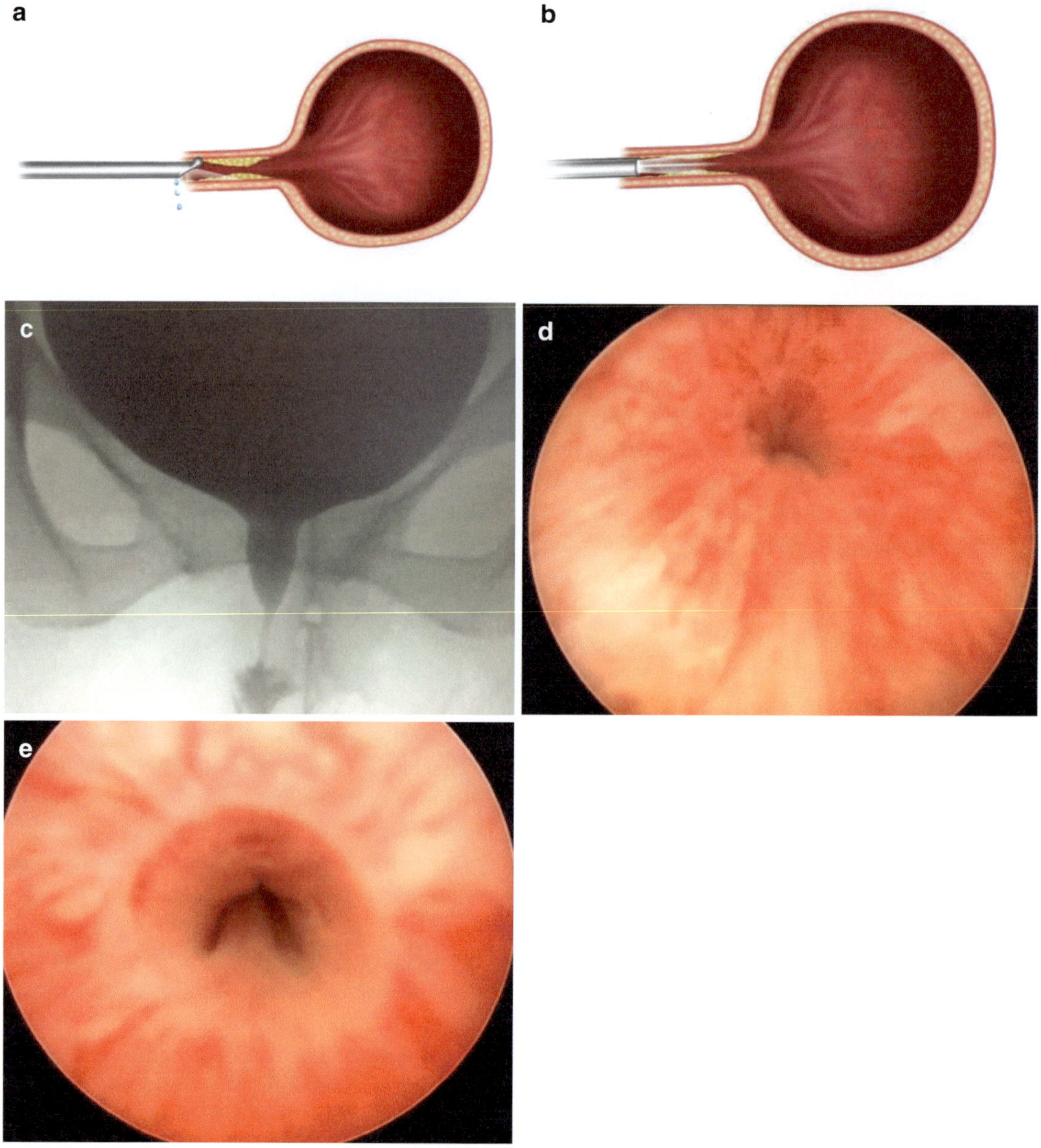

Fig. 2.6 (**a**) Conventional cystoscope sheath with its deficient floor at the tip and a 30-degree lens allows run-off of irrigant and poor distention of the female urethra and consequently inadequate inspection of the urethra. (**b**) Use of an integrated sheath or a Nickel's adapter with a 0-degree lens allows forward irrigant flow and adequate distention of urethra for proper inspection. (**c**) A woman with voiding dysfunction showed an area of narrowing in the mid-urethra on voiding cystourethrogram. (**d**) Urethroscopy with conventional sheath and 30-degree scope was unable to make a small fibrous ring prominent. (**e**) Change to a direct vision internal urethrotomy (DVIU) sheath and zero-degree lens allowed satisfactory identification

References

1. Blaivas JG. The bladder is an unreliable witness. Neurourol Urodyn. 1996;15(5):443–5.
2. Haylen BT, Maher CF, Barber MD, Camargo S, Dandolu V, Digesu A, et al. An International Urogynecological Association (IUGA)/International Continence Society (ICS) joint report on the terminology for female pelvic organ prolapse (POP). Int Urogynecol J. 2016;27(2):165–94.
3. Hsiao S-M, Lin H-H, Kuo H-C. Videourodynamic studies of women with voiding dysfunction. Sci Rep. 2017;7(1):6845.
4. Scarpero H. Urodynamics in the evaluation of female LUTS. Urol Clin North Am. 2014;41(3):429–38.
5. Gammie A, Kaper M, Dorrepaal C, Kos T, Abrams P. Signs and symptoms of detrusor underactivity: an analysis of clinical presentation and urodynamic tests from a large group of patients undergoing pressure flow studies. Eur Urol. 2016;69(2):361–9.
6. Kuo H-C. Clinical symptoms are not reliable in the diagnosis of lower urinary tract dysfunction in women. J Formos Med Assoc Taiwan Yi Zhi. 2012;111(7):386–91.
7. Malde S, Solomon E, Spilotros M, Mukhtar B, Pakzad M, Hamid R, et al. Female bladder outlet obstruction: common symptoms masking an uncommon cause. Low Urin Tract Symptoms. 2019;11(1):72–7.
8. Jackson S, Donovan J, Brookes S, Eckford S, Swithinbank L, Abrams P. The Bristol Female Lower Urinary Tract Symptoms Questionnaire: development and psychometric testing. BJU Int. 1996;77(6):805–12.
9. Hsiao S-M, Lin H-H, Kuo H-C. International Prostate Symptom Score for assessing lower urinary tract dysfunction in women. Int Urogynecol J. 2013;24(2):263–7.
10. Uebersax JS, Wyman JF, Shumaker SA, McClish DK, Fantl JA, Continence Program for Women Research Group. Short forms to assess life quality and symptom distress for urinary incontinence in women: the Incontinence Impact Questionnaire and the Urogenital Distress Inventory. Neurourol Urodyn. 1995;14(2):131–9.
11. Valdevenito JP, Flores J, Rojas RG, Manriquez V, Arribillaga L, de Benito J. Voiding symptoms obtained by open versus directed anamnesis as predictors of voiding dysfunction in women. Int Braz J Urol. 2019;45(4):798–806.
12. Lemack GE, Zimmern PE. Predictability of urodynamic findings based on the Urogenital Distress Inventory-6 questionnaire. Urology. 1999;54(3):461–6.
13. Kayigil O, Metin A, Atmaca AF. Obstructive urodynamic findings in idiopathic detrusor overactivity. Int Urol Nephrol. 2007;39(2):445–8.
14. Cho KJ, Kim HS, Koh JS, Kim JC. Evaluation of female overactive bladder using urodynamics: relationship with female voiding dysfunction. Int Braz J Urol. 2015;41(4):722–8.
15. Van Batavia JP, Combs AJ, Fast AM, Glassberg KI. Overactive bladder (OAB): a symptom in search of a disease – its relationship to specific lower urinary tract symptoms and conditions. J Pediatr Urol. 2017;13(3):277.e1–4.
16. Kobashi KC, Albo ME, Dmochowski RR, Ginsberg DA, Goldman HB, Gomelsky A, et al. Surgical treatment of female stress urinary incontinence: AUA/SUFU guideline. J Urol. 2017;198(4):875–83.
17. Topazio L, Frey J, Iacovelli V, Perugia C, Vespasiani G, Finazzi Agrò E. Prevalence of "complicated" stress urinary incontinence in female patients: can urodynamics provide more information in such patients? Int Urogynecol J. 2015;26(9):1333–9.
18. Serati M, Topazio L, Bogani G, Costantini E, Pietropaolo A, Palleschi G, et al. Urodynamics useless before surgery for female stress urinary incontinence: are you sure? Results from a multicenter single nation database. Neurourol Urodyn. 2016;35(7):809–12.
19. Nager CW. for the Urinary Incontinence Treatment Network (UITN). Re: comments on "A randomized trial of urodynamic testing before stress-incontinence surgery" (N Engl J Med. 2012;366(21):1987–1997) From the Italian Society of Urodynamics. Neurourol Urodyn. 2013;32(3):303–4.
20. Hijazi S, Leitsmann C. Clinical significance of video-urodynamic in female recurrent urinary tract infections. Int J Womens Health. 2016;8(1):31.
21. Lee P, Kuo H. High incidence of lower urinary tract dysfunction in women with recurrent urinary tract infections. Low Urin Tract Symptoms. 2020;12(1):33–40.
22. Cameron AP, Gajewski JB. Bladder outlet obstruction in painful bladder syndrome/interstitial cystitis. Neurourol Urodyn. 2009;28(8):944–8.
23. Payne C. Urodynamics for the evaluation of painful bladder syndrome/interstitial cystitis. J Urol. 2010;184(1):15–6.
24. Liu H-T, Jiang Y-H, Kuo H-C. Alteration of urothelial inflammation, apoptosis, and junction protein in patients with various bladder conditions and storage bladder symptoms suggest common pathway involved in underlying pathophysiology: urothelial dysfunction in bladder conditions. Low Urin Tract Symptoms. 2015;7(2):102–7.
25. Chae JY, Bae JH, Yoon CY, Park HS, Moon DG, Lee JG, et al. Female urethral condyloma causing bladder outlet obstruction. Int Neurourol J. 2014;18(1):42.
26. Chang C-H, Fan Y-H, Tong-Long Lin A, Chen K-K. Bladder outlet obstruction due to labial agglutination. J Chin Med Assoc. 2012;75(1):40–2.

27. Khayyami Y, Klarskov N, Lose G. Post-void residual urine under 150 ml does not exclude voiding dysfunction in women. Int Urogynecol J. 2016;27(3):467–73.
28. Costantini E, Mearini E, Pajoncini C, Biscotto S, Bini V, Porena M. Uroflowmetry in female voiding disturbances. Neurourol Urodyn. 2003;22(6):569–73.
29. Chassagne S, Bernier PA, Haab F, Roehrborn CG, Reisch JS, Zimmern PE. Proposed cutoff values to define bladder outlet obstruction in women. Urology. 1998;51(3):408–11. PMID: 9510344.
30. Romanzi LJ, Chaikin DC, Blaivas JG. The effect of genital prolapse on voiding. J Urol. 1999;161(2):581–6. PMID: 9915453.
31. Blaivas JG, Groutz A. Bladder outlet obstruction nomogram for women with lower urinary tract symptomatology. Neurourol Urodyn. 2000;19(5):553-64. PMID: 11002298.
32. Lemack GE, Zimmern PE. Pressure flow analysis may aid in identifying women with outflow obstruction. J Urol. 2000;163(6):1823–8. PMID: 10799191.
33. Lunacek L, Gärtner M, Krhut J, Mika D, Sykora R, Zvara P. Evaluation of intra-individual test–re-test variability of uroflowmetry in healthy women and women suffering from stress, urge, and mixed urinary incontinence. Int Urogynecol J. 2018;29(10):1523–7.
34. Barapatre Y, Agarwal MM, Singh SK, Sharma SK, Mavuduru R, Mete UK, et al. Uroflowmetry in healthy women: development and validation of flow-volume and corrected flow-age nomograms. Neurourol Urodyn. 2009;28(8):1003–9.
35. Jensen D, Aasen S, Talseth T. Uroflowmetry with simultaneous electromyography versus voiding video cystourethrography: a comparison of diagnostic value elucidated by a clinical sample. Scand J Urol Nephrol. 2006;40(3):232–7.
36. Malde S, Nambiar AK, Umbach R, Lam TB, Bach T, Bachmann A, et al. Systematic review of the performance of noninvasive tests in diagnosing bladder outlet obstruction in men with lower urinary tract symptoms. Eur Urol. 2017;71(3):391–402.
37. Lekskulchai O, Dietz HP. Is detrusor hypertrophy in women associated with voiding dysfunction? Aust N Z J Obstet Gynaecol. 2009;49(6):653–6.
38. Oelke M, Höfner K, Jonas U, Ubbink D, de la Rosette J, Wijkstra H. Ultrasound measurement of detrusor wall thickness in healthy adults. Neurourol Urodyn. 2006;25(4):308–17.
39. Farag FF, Heesakkers JP. Non-invasive techniques in the diagnosis of bladder storage disorders. Neurourol Urodyn. 2011;30(8):1422–8.
40. Kuhn A, Brandner S, Kuhn P, Robinson D, Raio L. Does bladder wall thickness decrease when obstruction is resolved? Int Urogynecol J. 2012;23(9):1239–44.
41. Osman NI, Mangera A, Chapple CR. A systematic review of surgical techniques used in the treatment of female urethral stricture. Eur Urol. 2013;64(6):965–73.
42. Solomon E, Yasmin H, Duffy M, Rashid T, Akinluyi E, Greenwell TJ. Developing and validating a new nomogram for diagnosing bladder outlet obstruction in women. Neurourol Urodyn. 2018;37(1): 368–78.
43. Hickling D, Aponte M, Nitti V. Evaluation and management of outlet obstruction in women without anatomical abnormalities on physical exam or cystoscopy. Curr Urol Rep. 2012;13(5):356–62.
44. Hsiao SM, Lin HH, Kuo HC. Videourodynamic Studies of Women with Voiding Dysfunction. Sci Rep. 2017;7(1):6845. PMID: 28754926; PMCID: PMC5533800.
45. Brucker BM, Fong E, Shah S, Kelly C, Rosenblum N, Nitti VW. Urodynamic differences between dysfunctional voiding and primary bladder neck obstruction in women. Urology. 2012;80(1):55–60.
46. Viereck V, Rautenberg O, Kociszewski J, Grothey S, Welter J, Eberhard J. Midurethral sling incision: indications and outcomes. Int Urogynecol J. 2013;24(4):645–53.
47. Kumar NM, Khatri G, Christie AL, Sims R, Pedrosa I, Zimmern PE. Supine magnetic resonance defecography for evaluation of anterior compartment prolapse: comparison with upright voiding cystourethrogram. Eur J Radiol. 2019;117:95–101.

Controversies in Diagnosis of Bladder Outlet Obstruction in Women: A Urodynamic Perspective

3

Nikhil Khattar and Vijay Madduri

Learning Objectives To understand that

- The definitions are evolving and there are no well-defined urodynamic cut-off values for female Bladder Outlet Obstruction (BOO).
- There is no 'Gold standard' test to confirm or rule out BOO against which to compare and measure specificity/sensitivity.
- Voiding contrast study (either a voiding cysto-urethrogram or video urodynamics) is important to reach a conclusive diagnosis.
- There is a possible role of urethral pressure profilometry in diagnosis of female BOO.
- There is an overlap in urodynamic parameters of BOO and detrusor underactivity in a woman.

3.1 Introduction

Voiding symptoms in a female can be attributed to either an obstruction to the outlet or a poor contraction of the detrusor itself. **The boundaries between female bladder outlet obstruction (BOO) and underactivity of the detrusor (DU) are blurred and still evolving.** This is in contrast to males where urodynamic criteria to distinguish between the two conditions are better established. Documentation of a poor flow on uroflowmetry is the most common starting point to look for a possible BOO in a woman with lower urinary tract symptoms. Apart from uroflowmetry, other non-invasive urodynamic markers, most importantly a high post void residual urine and a thickened bladder wall point to BOO, but none of these are definitive. Normal flow patterns and maximum flow rates (*Q*max) for women are also poorly defined and may depend on position of voiding (sitting or squatting) [1].

In a voiding cycle during filling phase, there are two distinct areas of high pressure in the urethra: one at the bladder neck (where the pressure is about two-fold higher than intravesical pressure) and one at the mid-urethra (where the pressure is about four-fold higher than intravesical pressure). During normal voiding, first, a relaxation of the striated sphincter and a drop in intra-urethral pressures occurs. This is followed by detrusor contraction, rise in intravesical pressure and expulsion of urine from bladder [2]. The amplitude of detrusor contraction is a function of the resistance provided by the urethra. **Most of the definitions of BOO are thus based on a poor flow coupled with high pressure generated by the bladder to overcome a supposed obstruction to the flow in an invasive urodynamic study (UDS). But what qualifies for a**

N. Khattar (✉)
Female Urology, Reconstructive Urology and Neurovesical Dysfunction, Medanta, The Medicity, Gurugram, India

V. Madduri
Department of Urology, All India Institute of Medical Sciences, Jodhpur, India

N. Khattar et al. (eds.), *Female Bladder Outlet Obstruction and Urethral Reconstruction*,
https://doi.org/10.1007/978-981-15-8521-0_3

poor flow or high voiding pressure is controversial in women. For few women, detrusor contractions are not necessary and just a drop in urethral pressure may be sufficient to void, or they may void with abdominal pressure with pelvic floor relaxation without generating detrusor pressure [3], making generalisation of definitions difficult, Simultaneous fluoroscopy with UDS (video UDS), a test less commonly used to diagnose male BOO, has been suggested as the main tool for diagnosis of female BOO [4, 5].

3.2 Free Uroflowmetry as a Screening Test

Since symptoms alone are unreliable in raising suspicion of BOO in a woman [6], only objective test to document a poor flow is uroflowmetry. It was evident from the beginning that poor flow alone cannot differentiate between an underactive bladder and a bladder outlet obstruction. Even the International Continence Society (ICS) definition of voiding dysfunction in a female (abnormally slow and/or incomplete micturition, based on abnormally slow urine flow rates and or abnormally high post-void residuals, ideally on repeated measurement to confirm abnormality [7]) does not objectively specify a poor flow in a woman.

Criteria for abnormal flow are arbitrary, but the consensus is a peak flow of <15 ml/s and/or a residual urine of more than 50 ml for a pre-void bladder volume of 150 ml (voided + residual) **OR** a value of peak flow rate less than tenth percentile on Liverpool Nomogram. **A voiding dysfunction can be effectively ruled out in a woman if repeated uroflow with any of the two criteria are normal** [8]. If a uroflowmetry result is repeatedly abnormal in a symptomatic woman in whom voiding dysfunction is suspected, a pressure flow study is required to differentiate between outflow obstruction and underactive detrusor.

3.3 Definitions of Female BOO

In the following sections, the evolution of the definitions for female BOO has been grouped into four subgroups—pressure flow-dependent definitions, imaging-dependent definitions, nomograms and computer-generated models. This is just for the ease of understanding of reader and does not necessarily follow a chronological order of their year of publication.

The 'high pressure-low flow' concept of BOO was first established in men with BPH and validated cut-offs were available early on. Though it was understood that same definitions cannot be translated directly to women because of anatomical differences, still there were early attempts to define female BOO by arbitrarily borrowing pressure flow cut-offs from studies in males. But very soon it was realised that a large proportion of women had BOO with significantly lower generation of detrusor pressures. Since there was no equivalent of an obstruction like BPE, where removing the obstruction in the female could help measuring the exact cut off values for BOO, the researchers worked backwards, first establishing cut offs in clinically predictable obstructions like post sling obstruction and prolapse-related obstruction (anatomical obstruction). These values were then applied for women with other LUTS, and more and more functional obstructions started being identified. The cut-offs initially determined, were refined over next several research papers. Probably the ability of a large number of women to void without generation of any detrusor pressures kept lowering the cut-off values till it was realised that in women, any radiological dilatation of urethra irrespective of the detrusor pressure generated to void would define obstruction. The radiological definition started gaining widespread acceptability and in conjunction with urodynamics (video-urodynamics) became the gold standard for diagnosing female BOO. The pressure flow cut-off criteria were still sharpened further. Concept of detrusor underactivity also evolved simultaneously and the gap in pressure cut-offs between obstruction and underactivity for women has decreased in definitions over time, and there is almost an overlap between the definitions of obstruction and detrusor underactivity. Like in males, nomograms started developing in females too. The challenge of non-invasively diagnosing BOO is being explored with computer-generated models.

3.3.1 Pressure-Flow-Dependent Definitions

Farrar et al. [9] described the urodynamic characteristics of 169 'obstructed' female patients out of their records of over 2500 patients from urogynaecology clinic. The patients with suspected neuropathic cause and bladder atonia were excluded. All patients had a poor flow of <15 ml/s and all underwent a video UDS study. They characterised these women into (a) High-pressure obstruction (Pdet@Qmax > 50 cm H_2O) and (b) Normal-pressure obstruction (Pdet@ Qmax < 50 cm H_2O). The presentations (recurrent urinary tract infections, frequency-urgency symptoms, and dysuria) in both the groups were however same. In 165 of 169 patients, the site of obstruction could be identified on the voiding films as distal urethra, whereas bladder neck did not open in four patients, and they were finally diagnosed as bladder neck obstruction. The study does not dwell into the causes of obstruction for the rest of the patients. Although it was a retrospective account, this article for the first time acknowledged and described that some of these obstructed women had a 'normal voiding pressure' in contrast to prevailing pressure flow criteria for BOO in men.

Massey and Abrams [10] were the first to suggest a pressure flow cut-off for diagnosing female BOO. This was a large retrospective account of UDS of over 5000 women where BOO was diagnosed in 2.74% of subjects (163 women) in which they used presence of any two or more of the following criteria diagnostic of BOO; (1) *Q*max <12 ml/s, (2) Pdet@Qmax > 50 cm H_2O, (3) Urethral resistance (P/F2) > 0.2 on urethral pressure profilometry (UPP) and (4) 'significant' residual urine in presence of either point numbers 3 or 4. UPP was abnormal in only one of their 163 patients. The criteria chosen were arbitrary and there was no comparison with a normal group.

Chassagne et al. [11] performed a prospective study comparing 35 'clinically obstructed' (a known apparent cause, e.g. Previous bladder neck suspension, high-grade cystocele, known stricture or extrinsic compression by a retroverted uterus) women with 135 controls (Stress urinary incontinence (SUI) patients with no risk factors for obstruction). All patients underwent a pressure flow study with electromygraphy, a separate standing voiding cystourethrography and a flexible cystoscopy. The Qmax and Pdet@Qmax were significantly different in obstructed and control groups. 'Clinical Obstruction' was taken as a surrogate for defining obstruction in the absence of clearly defined gold standard and ROC curves were drawn for ability of Qmax and Pdet@Qmax to differentiate between obstructed and unobstructed groups. A Qmax of 15 ml/s or less and a Pdet@Qmax of more than 20 cm H_2O had a sensitivity of 74% and a specificity of 91% to diagnose 'clinical obstruction'. Though the study suggested that female BOO can be present with voiding pressures as low as 20 cm H_2O, it was designed to identify only "clinical' and obvious mechanical intrinsic or extrinsic obstructions to the bladder outlet and not functional obstructions. However, the findings can possibly be extrapolated to these scenarios as well. In another study from the same group the authors, Lemack and Zimmern [12], working on a larger cohort of similarly 'clinically obstructed' females, redefined their cut-offs to a flow of 11 ml/s or less and a Pdet@Qmax of 21 cm H_2O or more. They then prospectively applied these cut-off values to 108 consecutive women undergoing video UDS evaluation for any lower tract symptoms and found urodynamic obstruction in 20%. Most of these women (77%) had no voiding complaint and instead presented with only overactive bladder symptoms and would have missed evaluation had only clinical suspicion been the driving factor for urodynamic evaluation. Refining their definition further using 'normal' women as controls instead of stress incontinent women [13], they proposed cut-offs of 12 ml/s and 25 cm H_2O for a specificity of 68% and ascribed relatively lower resistance offered by SUI women as controls in previous study as a reason for now increased Pdet@Qmax cut off when normal women acted as controls. **Thus, through repeated experiments, urodynamic values for obstruction were first defined in women with anatomic obstruction. These values were then applied to other women with only storage LUTS, revealing previously unsuspected BOO in few of them.**

Groutz, Blaivas and Chaikin [14] tried to improve upon this definition by using repeated 'free' uroflow *Q* max of 12 ml/s or less along with Pdet@Qmax of 20 cm H_2O or more from the pressure flow study. This was a retrospective study of urodynamic records of 587 consecutive women and draws criticism due to non-synchronous measurements of *Q*max and Pdet@Qmax where no attempt was made to match the pattern of free and intubated flow. The authors however claimed that the free flow was given more importance to rule out any effect of tube-induced alteration in the flow, which the authors term as 'test induced dysfunctional voiding'. Two-thirds of their patients had anatomic obstruction (anti-incontinence surgery, severe prolapse and strictures) and the rest had a functional obstruction. Only one-third of patients in this series showed obstruction on radiographic images (in the rest, the images were of poor quality), whereas in 45%, the diagnosis could be confirmed on urethrocystoscopy. Their criteria were redefined in another study by the same authors in the same year [15] based on a database of 600 patients where they also came up with a nomogram. On one hand, they stuck to free uroflow rates of 12 ml/s or less with a Pdet@Qmax of 20 cm H_2O or more, while on the other hand, they also included (a) An obvious radiographic evidence of obstruction with a sustained Pdet of 20 cm H_2O or more irrespective of free flow and (b) Inability to void during pressure flow study with a sustained Pdet of 20 cm H_2O or more (earlier studies had excluded patients who did not void during pressure flow study). The Blaivas-Groutz nomogram and its applicability are discussed in a separate section later.

In another study, apart from the traditional values of Pdet@Qmax, *Q*max, opening Pdet etc., Cormier et al. [16] also studied the area under curve of the detrusor contraction during voiding along with area under curve of detrusor contraction during voiding adjusted for voided volume and found the latter parameter to be better in segregating clearly obstructed from equivocal and equivocal from clearly unobstructed. The cut-off values they described were 5.83 cm H_2O per second per ml for obstructed and equivocal and 2.56 cm of H_2O per second per ml for separating equivocal from clearly unobstructed. This is a concept borrowed from the respiratory function studies where area under curve represents the effort or the work done by the respiratory muscles. Similarly, the area under curve of detrusor during voiding represents the effort of the entire bladder during voiding, whereas the area under curve of detrusor during voiding adjusted for volume represents the effort of bladder to void each ml of urine. So instead of relying on a cross-sectional value during the voiding curve like opening Pdet or Pdet@Qmax, the importance was given to the entire curve during the voiding phase. Though the concept was novel, the standard against which these parameters were compared was the consensus classification by two urologists by using only clinical and radiological parameters before the pressure flow study.

Overall, though the foregoing studies redefined female BOO and proved the point that female BOO parameters were indeed different than that for males, still there was a bias towards anatomically obstructed patients. Recognition that functional obstructions are a more common cause compared to anatomical obstructions came next.

Kuo [17] in a case–control study reviewed symptomatology and video UDS (with EMG) of 580 women with lower tract symptoms and matched with records of 265 mono-symptomatic

SUI and 30 freshly conducted video UDS of normal female hospital staff volunteers as controls. He defined obstruction as presence of a sustained detrusor contraction of any strength during the voiding phase along with a radiological evidence of obstruction either at the bladder neck or within the urethra along with obstructive or irritative lower tract urinary symptoms. BOO was diagnosed in 76 patients. Dysfunctional voiding was the most common cause (40/76 patients), six had high-grade prolapse and 30 had strictures at various levels, including at neck, urethral and meatal stenosis, but interestingly none had had an incontinence surgery. The sensitivities and specificities at various values of Pdet@Qmax and *Q*max to be able to diagnose BOO were then calculated. A Pdet@Qmax of 40 cm H_2O or more had a specificity of 96% to diagnose obstruction, whereas with a cut-off of Pdet@Qmax of 35 cm of H_2O, the specificity to diagnose obstruction dropped to 89%. A pressure flow cut-off of Pdet@Qmax $\geq$ 35 cm H_2O and *Q*max $\leq$15 ml/s also picked up two patients with SUI and two patients who were asymptomatic control. This cut-off had a sensitivity and specificity of 81.6% and 93.9%, respectively. At the same time, 11 obstructed patients had a *Q*max of >15 ml/s. All of them were obstructed and had a Pdet@Qmax of >40 cm H_2O. He concluded that a pressure flow cut-off of Pdet@Qmax$\geq$35 cm H_2O and *Q*max $\leq$15 ml/s was highly sensitive to pick up all BOO cases and a Pdet@Qmax$\geq$40 cm, irrespective of the flow rates, was highly specific of BOO. The study also claimed that at a pressure flow cut off of 20 or 21 cm H_2O, suggested by others, would pick up many unobstructed patients. Such a significant difference in cut-off levels from other studies was a trend also noticed by Defreitas et al [13]. when they included normal controls instead of SUI patients only. **Further deviation from that cut off could be because of moving away from a biased 'clinically obstructed' on the basis of known anti-incontinence surgery or obviously recognisable obstructions, to an unbiased application of video UDS cut off to all women with LUTS and thereby picking up more functional obstructions, which were to be later recognised as most common causes of female BOO rather than post incontinence surgeries or obvious anatomical causes.**

Again, like Blaivas and Groutz [15], Kuo's study [17] gives more importance to radiological findings in the region of urethra and bladder neck as a standard to recognise obstruction (As first described by Nitti et al. [4] and detailed in next section.) Kuo and colleagues [18] have updated their results of video-urodynamic studies in female LUTS after excluding all 'clinically obstructed' women (women with prior anti-incontinence surgery and prolapse repair) in a retrospective review of 1914 women with LUTS. Keeping the criteria for diagnosing BOO same as above, 810 women were diagnosed with female BOO. Only 49 patients (6%) had anatomic obstruction, whereas 325(40.1%) had dysfunctional voiding, 336 (41.4%) had poorly relaxing external sphincter, which is a subtype of dysfunctional voiding, and 100 (12%) had bladder neck obstruction. Using ROC curve analysis to determine cut-off on pressure flow study, they came up with a Pdet@Qmax cut-off of 30 cm H_2O for diagnosing female BOO (95% confidence interval [CI] = 0.76–0.80; sensitivity = 54.6%, specificity = 91.8%) in this subgroup of women without any obvious 'clinical obstruction'. A later study by Brucker et al. [19] compared urodynamic characteristics of anatomic and Functional obstruction in women and did not find any significant differences between the two, suggesting that **definitions for female BOO could be applied to both functional and anatomical obstructions alike. This is unlike in men where the nomograms and definitions have mainly focussed on men with prostate disease (a fixed anatomical obstruction) and cannot be generally applied to functional obstructions, which are commoner in younger males.**

3.3.2 Imaging-Dependent Definition

While all the earlier definitions had primarily tried to explore BOO from a view point of a combination of high pressure and low flow, Nitti et al.

[4] felt that it was difficult to rely only on pressure-flow criteria for diagnosing BOO in women. This emanated from the observation of patients after anti-incontinence surgery who had high clinical suspicion for BOO but were difficult to prove on pressure-flow relation. Encouraged by the improvement in symptoms after urethrolysis in such patients, they emphasised the importance of radiological image of obstruction between the bladder neck and urethral meatus rather than depending only on exact pressure-flow criteria. Similarly, they argued, many non-neurogenic voiding dysfunctions in women could be diagnosed as obstruction based on radiographic images during voiding. They reviewed Video UDS studies of 261 women with various presentations of non-neurogenic voiding dysfunction and could produce a flow during the study (they excluded patients who could not produce a flow) and **diagnosed BOO based on radiographic demonstration of obstruction between the bladder neck and distal urethra in the presence of a sustained detrusor contraction and a poor flow irrespective of the detrusor pressure generated**. Obstruction was said to be at bladder neck if the neck was closed or narrow during voiding. Urethral obstruction was diagnosed with a discrete narrowing with proximal dilatation in the urethra. BOO was diagnosed in 76 women. A Functional obstruction was identified in 49% of these patients (dysfunctional voiding in 33% and primary bladder neck obstruction (PBNO) in 16%), whereas iatrogenic obstruction due to incontinence surgery in 11%, cystocele in 21% and urethral stricture in 4%. A prospective comparative study by the same group [20] compared five contemporary definitions in 154 women with 92 evaluable video UDS and found obstruction according to Video UDS criteria in 26, the Chassagne et al. criteria in 28, the Lemack and Zimmern criteria in 18, the Defreitas et al. criteria in 13 and Blaivas and Groutz criteria in 38. The Blaivas-Grotz nomogram had overestimated obstruction, whereas the Chassagne et al. criteria had the highest concordance with the video UDS definition. They also observed that **there is a large overlap of pressure and flow values between obstructed and non-obstructed patients and that demonstrates the imprecision of absolute pressure and flow cut-offs**.

A difficulty may arise in differentiating a PBNO from an acontractile detrusor based solely on radiographic image as the neck would not show a funnelled appearance in both these conditions. A video UDS demonstrating a rise in detrusor pressure during voiding attempt would be most useful in such a scenario [4].

Thus, radiological appearance during the voiding phase of a video UDS started being recognised as the 'gold standard' for establishing the diagnosis of female BOO. But the lack of wide availability of Video UDS kept pushing the researchers to look for easy parameters to confirm/rule out BOO in women only on the basis of a pressure flow study. This led to the development of nomograms based on pressure-flow study.

In centres where Video UDS is not available, a separate voiding cystourethrogram (VCUG) may be useful to diagnose the level of obstruction at bladder neck or distal urethra [21].

3.3.3 Nomograms for Female Bladder Outlet Obstruction

The first attempt to develop a nomogram for female BOO was the Blaivas-Groutz nomogram [15]. In a retrospective review of video UDS findings in 600 women with LUTS, where, in addition to retaining their own cut-offs of *Q*max of 12 ml/s (on free uroflowmetry) and a Pdet@Qmax of ≥20 cm H_2O, they included Nitti's criteria of radiographic evidence of obstruction (but with a caveat of a sustained detrusor contraction of at least 20 cm H_2O) and also included women who could not void during the pressure flow study but produced a sustained detrusor contraction of >20 cm H_2O as their criteria of BOO. They diagnosed obstruction in 50 women who were then matched with 50 controls. Free *Q*max (from free uroflowmetry) and Pdet.max (maximum detrusor pressure generated) were used to construct the nomogram. Pdet.max was chosen because it was not significantly different from Pdet@Qmax and could be used even in patients who failed to produce a flow during the study. The nomogram could classify women into either normal or obstructed and further subclassified obstructed into mild, moderate and severe. That the Blaivas-Groutz nomogram overestimates obstruction was demonstrated in subsequent studies and was not commonly used thereafter [20, 22, 23].

Dybowski et al. [24] screened out all women who had a Qmax of ≤12 ml/s from their database of uroflow studies and called them for re-examination. Women with anatomical obstruction were excluded. Sixty-seven women were identified. All of them filled LUTS questionnaires, underwent ultrasound and urodynamic study. Obstruction was diagnosed on the basis of presence of any of the following: presence of thickened bladder wall or bladder diverticula on ultrasound, improvement in any LUTS on alpha blockers or improvement in any voiding LUTS with any form of treatment. After plotting Qmax and Pdet@Qmax for each patient on a graph, a line could be drawn, which could be described by the equation pdet(Qmax) = 1.5 × Qmax + 10 that satisfactorily separated obstructed from unobstructed group. Dybowski et al. calculated that the formula Pdet@qmax − 1.5 × Qmax>10, had 90.5% sensitivity but only a 54.3% PPV for diagnosing BOO in women. A more practical value of such nomogram would be to 'rule out' BOO. A criticism of Dybowski study would be that they excluded women with anatomical causes of obstruction. Moreover, the criteria defining obstruction were all subjective.

In a retrospective review of Video UDS data of 647 women with refractory voiding LUTS, Solomon et al. [5] designed a nomogram to diagnose female BOO. Women who failed to generate a detrusor contraction during voiding were excluded (n = 89). The first set of consecutive 185 Video UDS studies was used to develop a BOO classification system based on pressure-flow criteria and radiographic evidence (development cohort), which was then applied on the next 350 consecutive Video UDS studies to validate the findings (validation cohort). The obstructed groups identified were functional obstruction, intrinsic anatomical (stricture, urethral diverticulum, etc.), extrinsic anatomical (secondary to incontinence surgery), and positional anatomical (prolapse; confirmed with oblique voiding films). The non-obstructed groups were cystocele without obstruction, SUI where demonstration of incontinence was possible during VUDS and SUI where demonstration of incontinence was not possible during the VUDS. Obstruction was defined according to radiographic criteria described by Nitti et al. After assessing the pressure flow plots of development cohort, the values of Qmax and Pdet@Qmax were plotted against each other and cluster analysis enabled to identify a line between obstructed and unobstructed defined by the equation PdetQmax = 2 × Qmax. Applying this on the validation cohort showed sensitivity and specificity of 0.95 and 0.85, respectively. Both the cohorts were pooled together and again Qmax andPdet@Qmax were plotted to form a nomogram, which could categorise each set of Qmax and Pdet@Qmax values in <10% to >90% likelihood of BOO. Line with equation Pdet@Qmax = 2.2 × Qmax represents a line corresponding to 50% likelihood of BOO with sensitivity and specificity of 0.86 and 0.93, respectively. Using the same, a BOO index for females **(BOOIf)** was described as **Pdet@Qmax-2.2 ×** ***Q*****max**.

The study concluded that BOOIf < 0 was unlikely a Female BOO, whereas BOOIf > 5 represents a 50% likelihood of female BOO and BOOIf > 18 represents almost certain female BOO.

This nomogram (called the **Solomon-Greewell Nomogram or the S-G Nomogram**) is in the form of a colour chart and was compared with other definitions of female BOO and was found to be in closest agreement with Nitti's radiographic definition amongst all other definitions. The authors claim nomogram to be especially useful if voiding images are not available.

The same group attempted to validate the utility of their nomogram and BOOIf after successful surgical treatment of BOO in 21 women who became asymptomatic after surgery for their anatomical obstructions [25]. Both the parameters, namely probability of obstruction on SG nomogram and mean BOOIf values decreased significantly. A wider inclusion criterion, including patients who remained symptomatic after their surgery and a comparison with video UDS postoperatively as well, would have increased the significance of this study. More such better-designed studies are required where any given definition applied to define BOO is reviewed post treatment to see whether the postoperative values correlate with symptomatic relief. Since most functional obstructions cannot be cured surgically, again the values will have to be first validated in anatomical obstructions and then only they can be applied to functional obstructions.

3.3.4 Computer-Generated Models: Is It the Future?

Each uroflow curve, whether a free non-intubated flow or obtained during a pressure flow UDS, carries more information than just a Qmax, voiding time, and other traditional voiding parameters. That information was used to develop a mathematical model of micturition [26]. This model analyses all the phenomena governing micturition like detrusor structure and function (its contractile, elastic and vesicoelastic properties), urethral structure and function (elasticity of the urethra, compressive effect of sphincter or prostate on urethra and constrictive effect of a luminal narrowing), hydrodynamics of turbulent fluid within an elastic pipe and neural control [27]. Most of these phenomena have been assumed to fit one mathematical equation or the other in all past calculations when computation of multiple parameters at the same times was not feasible. The VBN software (named on the initials of researchers) computes all these observations at once. It has been evaluated and found to be in good agreement with traditional cut-offs for female BOO [28]. They describe two new parameters 'k' for detrusor contractility and 'u' for urethral compression both of which can be calculated on a pressure flow study. Patients on regular follow-up visits who are at risk of developing recurrent BOO can have subsequent k and u values calculated on a free uroflow only with reasonable certainty for defining BOO. They have come up with a nomogram for BOO in women and have described a new term 'Woman Obstruction Index' (WOI = Pdet@Qmax − 0.5 Qmax), which can be calculated just like AG number, the cut-offs for which are yet to be described after more studies on obstructed women [29]. The details of the mathematical model are complex and beyond the scope of this chapter.

3.4 Urethral Pressure Profilometry for Diagnosing Female BOO

UPP can be used to diagnose as well as localise the obstruction in female. Early studies had laid the foundation for its utilisation in diagnosing complex cases. The average closure pressures at mid-urethra level in seated females is up to 110 cm H_2O [2]. A very high maximum urethral closure pressure (MUCP: which is the highest closure pressure difference between urethral and bladder pressures) on resting UPP (in excess of 150 cm H_2O) may be seen in dysfunctional voiding syndrome [30]. During micturitional UPP (MUPP), the obstruction can be diagnosed with a drop of >5 cm H_2O at any point in the urethra while pulling the transducer and the distance from bladder neck helps in localising the site. During a normal void, there is no pressure gradient in any part of female urethra on MUPP. **MUPP can accurately differentiate between PBNO and dysfunctional voiding** [31].

Although UPP was described much before standard pressure flow studies developed [32], its utility remained limited to conditions, which precluded proper pressure flow studies like neuropathic conditions. Now with increased awareness of female BOO, the use of UPP to diagnose and localise the site of obstruction is increasingly being explored. In a recent study [33], a pulsatile pattern on UPP correlated well with typical complex repetitive discharges and decelerating bursts seen on concentric needle EMG studies in women with High-tension non-relaxing sphincter (HTNRS/ Fowler's syndrome). If this is a reproducible finding, then it may make needle EMG obsolete, which is otherwise uncomfortable to the patient and yet not specific for diagnosing HTNRS.

3.5 Detrusor Underactivity

The other differential diagnosis for female voiding dysfunction is detrusor underactivity (DU), which increases in incidence with advancing age. The understanding of DU is relatively new and there is a poor consensus on definitions for females. Nevertheless, a brief review of the contemporary definitions of DU in a female is presented as there is some degree of overlap in definitions of BOO and DU. Moreover, both can coexist as well.

ICS defines DU as 'Low detrusor pressure or short detrusor contraction time, usually in combination with a low urine flow rate resulting in prolonged bladder emptying and/or a failure to achieve complete bladder emptying within a normal time span' [34]. As with the ICS definition of female BOO, the values on a pressure flow study remain undefined for DU as well.

Abarbanel and Marcus [35] identified impaired detrusor contraction in women as a Pdet@Qmax of 30 cm H_2O with a Qmax of <10 ml/s, whereas Gammie et al. [36] defined it as a *Q*max of <15 ml/s with Pdet@Qmax of <20 cm H_2O and Hsiao et al. [18] described the same as a Pdet@Qmax of <10 cm H_2O with Qmax<15 ml/s, making it evident that there is significant overlap between BOO and DU definitions based on pressure-flow studies. **The area of gray zone where the diagnosis is typically difficult to make is when Pdet@Qmax is between 20–30 cm H_2O and occasionally even both BOO and DU may coexist. It is in this zone that a voiding film is more important and a radiographic evidence of dilated urethra helps in confirming the diagnosis of a BOO rather than underactive detrusor** [37]. Bladder voiding efficiency {BVE = Voided volume ÷ (Voided volume + postvoid residual urine) × 100%} is also helpful in deciding such scenarios where a BVE of <90% would turn the diagnosis more in favour of DU [36].

To conclude, BOO as a cause for a female voiding dysfunction may be diagnosed on a pressure flow study above a certain Pdet@Qmax (most likely 35 or 40 cm H_2O) and can mostly be excluded below a Pdet@Qmax of 20 cm H_2O. There may be a co-existence of BOO and DU between Pdet@Qmax values of 20–35 cm H_2O. It is in this grey zone that radiographic evidence of obstruction is important to exclude BOO. A radiological finding of poor opening of the bladder neck can be seen in both detrusor underactivity as well as BOO, where the simultaneous rise in detrusor pressure on video-urodynamics is the only clue to a diagnosis.

Clinical Case Discussion

A 72-year female presented with LUTS predominantly urge-related symptoms and occasional poor flow. There was no history of constipation. Her symptoms had not relieved with anticholinergics. Her bladder diary showed multiple voids (16–18 visits) with an average of around 100 ml/void during the day and night with a maximal voided volume of 120 ml. Her ultrasound of kidney ureter and bladder region showed normal upper tracts, normal bladder thickness and a post void of 44 ml. Free Uroflow showed a very poor flow with a *Q*max of 3.1 ml/s with a voided volume of 98 ml (Fig. 3.1a). Her UDS (Fig. 3.1b) showed a normal filling phase till a capacity of 430 ml, normal compliance in filling phase. During attempted void, she produced a voided volume 9 ml, *Q*max 1.2 ml/s, Opening Pdet 33 cm H_2O, Pdet@Qmax 24 cm H_2O. She predominantly used an abdominal pressure to evacuate her bladder. Also, there was an increase in EMG activity just before her full capacity, which persisted throughout the voiding phase.

With detrusor overactivity ruled out, now the diagnosis was between a BOO vs detrusor underactivity, and VCUG (Fig. 3.1c) showed a discrete dilatation in urethra at mid/lower urethral level. With a working diagnosis of BOO because of poor relaxation of external sphincter (PRES), she

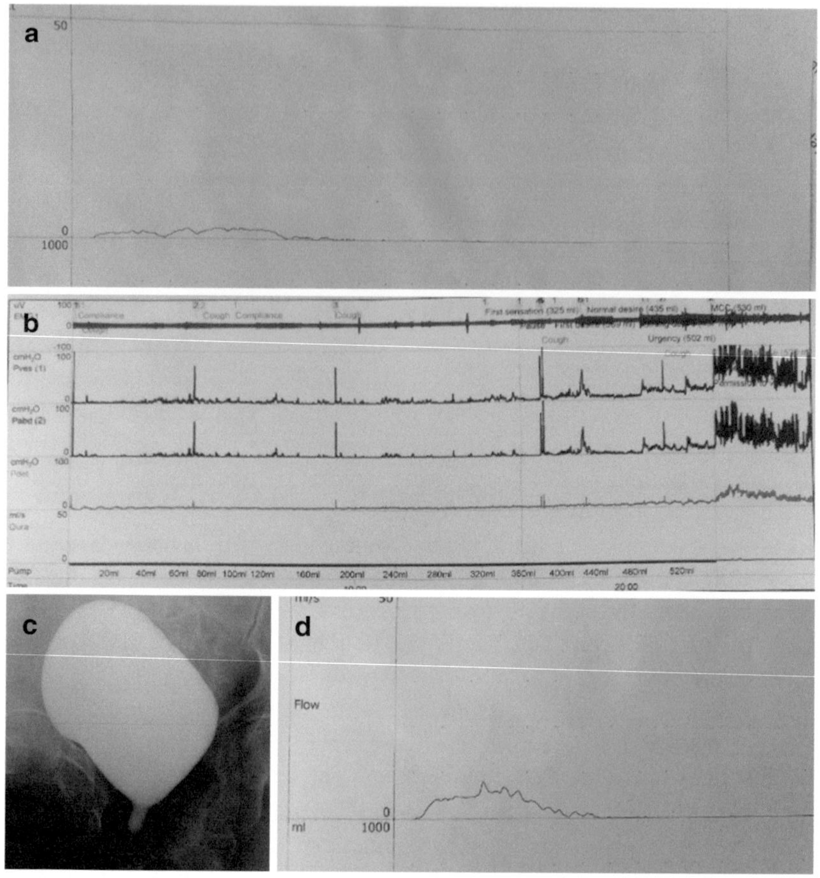

Fig. 3.1 (**a**) Uroflow. (**b**) UDS. (**c**) VCUG. (**d**) Follow-up uroflowmetry

was started on pelvic floor muscle therapy (PFMT) (with focus on relaxation) and alpha blockers. All anticholinergics were stopped. Her symptoms improved in 3 weeks and a repeat uroflow showed a *Q*max of 8.1 ml/s with a voided volume of 114 ml (Fig. 3.1d).

Key Learning Points

- The criteria for urodynamic definition of bladder outlet obstruction in women are evolving.
- The pressure flow definitions have evolved from a higher cut-off to a pressure-independent definition.
- Radiological demonstration of a dilated urethra especially with generation of any detrusor pressure may carry more importance than a set of pressure flow values.
- There is an overlap in definitions of bladder outlet obstruction and detrusor underactivity.

References

1. Gupta NP, Kumar A, Kumar R. Does position affect uroflowmetry parameters in women? Urol Int. 2008;80(1):37–40.
2. Tanagho EA, Miller ER, Meyers FH, Corbett RK. Observations on the dynamics of the bladder neck. Br J Urol. 1966;38(1):72–84.
3. Rud T, Ulmsten U, Andersson KE. Initiation of voiding in healthy women and those with stress incontinence. Acta Obstet Gynecol Scand. 1978;57(5):457–62.
4. Nitti VW, Tu LM, Gitlin J. Diagnosing bladder outlet obstruction in women. J Urol. 1999;161(5):1535–40.
5. Solomon E, Yasmin H, Duffy M, Rashid T, Akinluyi E, Greenwell TJ. Developing and validating a new nomogram for diagnosing bladder outlet obstruction in women. Neurourol Urodyn. 2018;37(1):368–78.
6. Kuo H-C. Clinical symptoms are not reliable in the diagnosis of lower urinary tract dysfunction in women. J Formos Med Assoc. 2012;111(7):386–91.
7. Haylen BT, Maher CF, Barber MD, Camargo SFM, Dandolu V, Digesu A, Goldman HB, Huser M, Milani A, Moran P, Schaer GN, Withagen MI. International Urogynecological Association (IUGA)/International Continence Society (ICS) Joint

Report on the Terminology for pelvic organ prolapse (POP). Int Urogynecol J 2016;27(2):165–94; Erratum 2016;27(4):655–84. Neurourol Urodyn. 2016;35(2):137–68.

8. Costantini E, Mearini E, Pajoncini C, Biscotto S, Bini V, Porena M. Uroflowmetry in female voiding disturbances. Neurourol Urodyn. 2003;22(6):569–73.
9. Farrar DJ, Osborne JL, Stephenson TP, Whiteside CG, Weir J, Berry J, et al. A urodynamic view of bladder outflow obstruction in the female: factors influencing the results of treatment. Br J Urol. 1975;47(7):815–22.
10. Massey JA, Abrams PH. Obstructed voiding in the female. Br J Urol. 1988;61(1):36–9.
11. Chassagne S, Bernier PA, Haab F, Roehrborn CG, Reisch JS, Zimmern PE. Proposed cutoff values to define bladder outlet obstruction in women. Urology. 1998;51(3):408–11.
12. Lemack GE, Zimmern PE. Pressure flow analysis may aid in identifying women with outflow obstruction. J Urol. 2000;163(6):1823–8.
13. Defreitas GA, Zimmern PE, Lemack GE, Shariat SF. Refining diagnosis of anatomic female bladder outlet obstruction: comparison of pressure-flow study parameters in clinically obstructed women with those of normal controls. Urology. 2004;64(4):675–9.
14. Groutz A, Blaivas JG, Chaikin DC. Bladder outlet obstruction in women: definition and characteristics. Neurourol Urodyn. 2000;19(3):213–20.
15. Blaivas JG, Groutz A. Bladder outlet obstruction nomogram for women with lower urinary tract symptomatology. Neurourol Urodyn. 2000;19(5):553–64.
16. Cormier L, Ferchaud J, Galas J-M, Guillemin F, Mangin P. Diagnosis of female bladder outlet obstruction and relevance of the parameter area under the curve of detrusor pressure during voiding: preliminary results. J Urol. 2002;167(5):2083–7.
17. Kuo H-C. Urodynamic parameters for the diagnosis of bladder outlet obstruction in women. Urol Int. 2004;72(1):46–51.
18. Hsiao S-M, Lin H-H, Kuo H-C. Videourodynamic studies of women with voiding dysfunction. Sci Rep. 2017;7(1):6845.
19. Brucker BM, Shah S, Mitchell S, Fong E, Nitti MD, Kelly CE, et al. Comparison of urodynamic findings in women with anatomical versus functional bladder outlet obstruction. Female Pelvic Med Reconstr Surg. 2013;19(1):46–50.
20. Akikwala TV, Fleischman N, Nitti VW. Comparison of diagnostic criteria for female bladder outlet obstruction. J Urol. 2006;176(5):2093–7.
21. Hickling D, Aponte M, Nitti V. Evaluation and management of outlet obstruction in women without anatomical abnormalities on physical exam or cystoscopy. Curr Urol Rep. 2012;13(5):356–62.
22. Vírseda Chamorro M, Salinas Casado J, Adot Zurbano JM, Martín García C. Puede sustituir el nomograma de Blaivas y Groutz a los estudios videourodinámicos en el diagnóstico de la obstrucción del tracto urinario inferior en la mujer? [May the Blaivas and Groutz nomogram substitute videourodynamic studies in the diagnosis of female lower urinary tract obstruction?]. Arch Esp Urol. 2006;59(6):601–6.
23. Massolt ET, Groen J, Vierhout ME. Application of the Blaivas-Groutz bladder outlet obstruction nomogram in women with urinary incontinence. Neurourol Urodyn. 2005;24(3):237–42.
24. Dybowski B, Bres-Niewada E, Radziszewski P. Pressure-flow nomogram for women with lower urinary tract symptoms. Arch Med Sci. 2014;4:752–6.
25. Lindsay J, Solomon E, Nadeem M, et al. Treatment validation of the Solomon-Greenwell nomogram for female bladder outlet obstruction. Neurourol Urodyn. 2020;39:1371–7.
26. Valentini FA, Besson GR, Nelson PP, Zimmern PE. A mathematical micturition model to restore simple flow recordings in healthy and symptomatic individuals and enhance uroflow interpretation. Neurourol Urodyn. 2000;19(2):153–76.
27. Valentini FA, Besson GR, Nelson PP, Zimmern PE. Clinically relevant modeling of urodynamics function: the VBN model: clinically relevant mathematical model of micturition. Neurourol Urodyn. 2014;33(3):361–6.
28. Valentini FA, Marti BG, Nelson PP, Zimmern PE, Robain G. Usefulness of an algebraic fitting of nomograms allowing evaluation detrusor contractility in women. Prog En Urol. 2017;27(4):261–6.
29. Valentini FA, Nelson PP, Zimmern PE. VBN-based nomograms provide critical voiding parameters which can be used for invasive or non-invasive flow interpretation of women at risk of obstruction over time: VBN-based nomograms provide critical voiding parameters. Neurourol Urodyn. 2017;36(1):37–42.
30. Mohan AM, Jaypee Brothers (Jaypeedigital). Manual of urodynamics. New Delhi: Jaypee Brothers Medical Publisher (P) Ltd; 2014. http://www.jaypeedigital.com/Book/BookDetail?isbn=9789351521877. Accessed 26 May 2020.
31. Agarwal MM, Kumar RMS. Is there a role for micturitional urethral pressure profilometry in the evaluation of voiding dysfunction in the 21st century? Curr Bladder Dysfunct Rep. 2011;6(4):193–7.
32. Sullivan MP, Comiter CV, Yalla SV. Micturitional urethral pressure profilometry. Urol Clin North Am. 1996;23(2):263–78.
33. Sihra N, Malde S, Panicker J, Kightley R, Solomon E, Hamid R, et al. Does the appearance of the urethral pressure profile trace correlate with the sphincter EMG findings in women with voiding dysfunction? Neurourol Urodyn. 2018;37(2):751–7.
34. D'Ancona C, Haylen B, Oelke M, Abranches-Monteiro L, Arnold E, Goldman H, et al. The international continence society (ICS) report on the terminology for adult male lower urinary tract and pelvic floor symptoms and dysfunction. Neurourol Urodyn. 2019;38(2):433–77.
35. Abarbanel J, Marcus E-L. Impaired detrusor contractility in community-dwelling elderly presenting with lower urinary tract symptoms. Urology. 2007;69(3):436–40.

36. Gammie A, Kaper M, Dorrepaal C, Kos T, Abrams P. Signs and symptoms of detrusor underactivity: an analysis of clinical presentation and urodynamic tests from a large group of patients undergoing pressure flow studies. Eur Urol. 2016;69(2):361–9.
37. Lin CD, Kuo HC, Yang SS. Diagnosis and Management of Bladder Outlet Obstruction in Women. Low Urin Tract Symptoms. 2016;8(1):30–7. Epub 2015 Mar 26. PMID: 26789540.

4 Dysfunctional Voiding in Women

Mayank Mohan Agarwal

Learning Objectives After reading this chapter the reader will be able to understand

- Pathophysiology of dysfunctional voiding and external urethral sphincter non-relaxation.
- Current limitations of pressure-flow studies and role of additional studies, e.g. electromyography, urethral pressure profilometry, detrusor pattern and voiding cystourethrography for diagnosis of dysfunctional voiding.
- Multi-prong systematic approach to treatment, including physical therapy, pharmacotherapy, treatment of associated problems, e.g. constipation and psychological disturbance.
- The indications and efficacy of invasive treatment.

The term **'dysfunctional voiding' (DV) is used to describe voiding dysfunction in a neurologically intact individual resulting from abnormal increased activity of pelvic floor and/or external urethral sphincter during voiding**; the latter has also been termed as poor relaxation of external sphincter (PRES) [1]. It is associated with a variety of voiding, storage and/or pelvic pain symptoms and can lead to urinary tract infection, retention of urine and, rarely, upper tract damage. The neurological counterpart of this condition is 'detrusor external sphincter dysynnergia'.

The term dysfunctional voiding was originally coined by Allen and Bright in 1978 to describe failure to coordinate detrusor and external sphincter in children. However, the condition is not limited to paediatric age group and is increasingly being described in other age groups in both sexes. DV has been described by different authors as *non-neurogenic neurogenic bladder, occult voiding dysfunction, occult neuropathic bladder, learned voiding dysfunction* and *Hinman syndrome*. Moreover, ill-understood conditions like bashful bladder of men and Fowler's syndrome of women too have abnormal pelvic floor activity and may actually be a form of DV. **Lower gastrointestinal tract (LGIT) symptoms are often associated with DV and the symptom complex is termed as *bowel-bladder dysfunction* (BBD), earlier referred to as *dysfunctional elimination syndrome* (DES).**

4.1 Epidemiology and Aetiopathogenesis

The prevalence of voiding phase dysfunction in women referred for evaluation of lower urinary tract symptoms (LUTS) widely varies from 2.0% to 25.5%. The variation is due to difference in enrolment criteria and definitions. Studies have found that a significant proportion of 'normal'

M. M. Agarwal (✉)
Urology and Kidney Transplant Surgery, Medanta Hospital, Lucknow, Uttar Pradesh, India

N. Khattar et al. (eds.), *Female Bladder Outlet Obstruction and Urethral Reconstruction*,
https://doi.org/10.1007/978-981-15-8521-0_4

women void with urethral relaxation without significant increase in detrusor pressure, often with abdominal straining [2]. Similarly, several healthy women with no clinical symptoms have been reported to have elevated post-void residue (PVR) [2–4]. At least some of these women may have been suffering from occult dysfunctional voiding. In a large study of over a thousand urodynamic studies in women with LUTS, Groutz and Blaivas found prevalence of DV to be 2% [5].

A normal lower urinary tract (LUT) function is the result of interaction among (1) inherent visco-elastic properties of the organs, (2) a highly coordinated neural activity (parasympathetic, sympathetic and somatic) as well as, particularly relevant in women, (3) an adequate pelvic floor musculoskeletal support. Pregnancy and parturition cause significant damage anatomically as well as functionally, which likely has considerable bearing on storage as well as voiding function.

Detailed discussion of neural control of LUT function is beyond the scope of this chapter. Nevertheless, a brief mention is warranted. During storage of urine, progressive distension of bladder stimulates sympathetic discharge to bladder outlet as well as somatic discharge to external urethral sphincter (bladder to urethra reflex), which, in turn, inhibit the para-sympathetic discharge to bladder (urethra to bladder reflex). Micturition reflex is simplistically described as a switch phenomenon of reflexes in which inhibitory pathways turn stimulatory and vice versa. The centre of this 'paradoxical coordination' lies in pontine micturition centre.

In cases of DV, non-relaxation of pelvic floor muscles and/or external urethral sphincter happens during voiding to a variable degree, which not only obstructs the voiding but may also cause inhibition of detrusor contraction. **DV is considered to be a learned behavioural disturbance of inability to relax external sphincter/pelvic floor muscles** triggered by events like bladder urgency, pelvic pain, sexual trauma, psychological disturbance, pelvic inflammation/infection (cystitis, pelvic inflammatory disease, etc.) and poor toilet training during early childhood. A person may have the habit of holding urine for long time either due to personal/professional reasons or recurrent urinary urgency; over a period, this habit becomes an abnormal reflex activity of persistent sphincter contraction (Fig. 4.1) [6, 7].

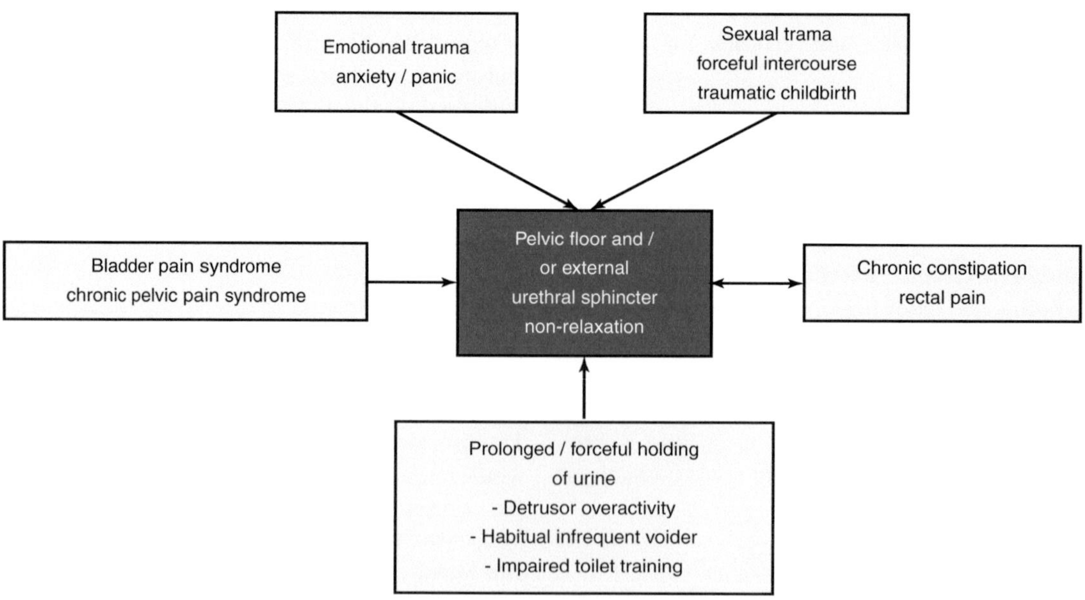

Fig. 4.1 Various trigger factors leading to pelvic floor/external urethral sphincter non-relaxation

4.2 Clinical Manifestations

In view of a large number of aetiological factors and complex pathophysiology, DV can present with a plethora of symptoms:

Voiding phase—since it is primarily a disease of the voiding phase, voiding symptoms are most often the primary presenting symptoms, viz. difficulty in initiating voiding, sensation of incomplete evacuation, intermittency, straining to void, taking awkward positions for attempts to void (not uncommonly women report trying to void in standing, crouching, etc.), and most extremely retention of urine.

Storage phase—non-relaxation of sphincter leads to changes in bladder function, directly due to obstruction per se as well as indirectly by inhibiting the detrusor contraction via urethra-to-bladder reflex often leading to elevated post-void residue (PVR). Storage symptoms are very frequent and include increased urine frequency, urgency, persistent desire to pass urine, nocturia, urge incontinence, etc.

Pain symptoms—in view of association of DV with bladder pain syndrome (BPS), chronic pelvic pain syndrome (CPPS) and 'spasm' of pelvic floor muscles, several pain symptoms are often associated, viz. lower abdominal pain, groin pain, low back pain, upper thigh pain, vaginal/introital pain, dyspareunia. Pain can be variably described as spastic, sharp, aching or burning; it can be continuous, intermittent or phasic.

Miscellaneous—Medical diseases, e.g. long-standing diabetes mellitus, peripheral neuropathy, parkinson's disease, cognitive dysfunctions, a variety of psychological disturbances, and medications, e.g. diuretics, antihistaminics, selective serotonin reuptake inhibitors (SSRI), serotonin-norepinephrine reuptake inhibitors (SNRI), etc. can be associated and/or can exacerbate the DV symptoms. Other possible associations include prior bladder, vaginal or other pelvic surgery, and pelvic radiation therapy.

Lower gastrointestinal tract (LGIT) disturbances, particularly constipation, need special mention. LUT and LGIT share a common functional neural point as well as a common pelvic floor. Therefore, it is not uncommon to have both DV and functional constipation, and both need simultaneous attention for optimum response. Moreover, in severe constipation, hard stools can cause mechanical obstruction in bladder outflow.

4.3 Approach

In view of complex aetio-pathogenesis and varied presentation, a comprehensive and detailed history and examination must precede any form of investigation(s). It is suggested to make a customized proforma to avoid missing out on any key manifestation. During the process of evaluation, emphasis must be laid to rule out occult or overt neuropathy, psychological issues, LGIT symptoms and different physical causes of pelvic pain. Specialist consults should be sought as needed, e.g. clinical psychologist, psychiatrist, gynaecologist, medical gastroenterologist and chronic pain specialist.

4.3.1 History

Detailed history of LUTS, pain symptoms, associated symptoms, e.g. psychological disturbance and constipation, is mandatory. **Effort should be made to try and elicit the trigger factor(s), if any, aggravating and relieving factors**. History of comorbidities, medications, prior surgery, radiation therapy and menstruation must be noted. A 3-day bladder diary should be requested, particularly in patients with storage symptoms—it gives important insights into functional bladder capacity, urgency, nocturnal polyuria, pain, incontinence episodes, nocturnal polyuria, etc. There are no specific features indicative of DV.

4.3.2 Examination

After the essential general physical examination, pelvic examination must always be performed, preferably in a lithotomy examination chair.

Anatomical examination—This is necessary to assess for presence and quantification of prolapse (use POP-Q system urethral hypermobility, stress incontinence, mass or discharge). However, there are no structural features, which may indicate DV.

Functional examination—Perianal and introital sensations, pelvic muscle tone, strength and duration, voluntary squeeze and relaxation of pelvic floor muscle, and bulbo-cavernosus reflex (BCR) should be assessed. BCR is elicited by checking anal sphincter contraction on squeezing clitoris, or by tug on Foley catheter in a catheterized patient. For objective assessment of pelvic floor muscles, several scales have been developed, standardized and used in clinical practice [8]. Clinicians are encouraged to implement any one scale into their clinical practice; we found modified Oxford scale easy to use and routinely use in our clinical practice (Table 4.1). Digital rectal examination (DRE) is required in patient with constipation for anal tone, faecal loading, mass and for eliciting BCR. One should take opportunity to teach awareness of contraction and relaxation of pelvic floor muscles during the examination (both DRE and vaginal). This awareness goes a long way in pelvic floor rehabilitation, an essential component of management of DV [9]. **Common findings in DV are increased pelvic muscle tone (particularly in painful conditions), absence of/weak BCR and impaired voluntary contraction and relaxation of pelvic floor**. Occasionally, a globally abnormal functional examination may be found, which indicates neuropathy requiring detailed neurological assessment. Conversely, a normal anatomical and functional pelvic floor examination doesn't rule out DV.

Table 4.1 Modified Oxford Scale [10]

	Strength	Description
1.	Nil	Lack of any discernible response in the peri-vaginal muscles
2.	Flicker	A fluttering/quivering of the muscle
3.	Weak	Contraction, which is not fluttering
4.	Moderate	Increase in pressure, compressing the examiner's fingers and incorporating a small degree of lift, as the fingers are moved in a cranial direction
5.	Good	Contraction is firm causing lifting of the PFM up and in against resistance
6.	Strong	Very strong grip of the examiner's finger and positive movement in a cranial direction against strong resistance

4.3.3 Investigations

A large majority of patients in developing countries do not undergo preventive health check-ups. Therefore, we screen for prevalent health conditions during initial visits, e.g. anaemia, chronic kidney disease and diabetes mellitus. Complete blood counts, random blood sugar, complete urine examination and cervical pap-smear examinations (as indicated) may be ordered in initial visit. Nevertheless, one should keep in mind that in a patient without symptoms of cystitis, mere presence of pyuria or bacteriuria is not a justifiable indication for antibiotic treatment.

Specific investigations for diagnosis of DV are described now. The essence of diagnosis of DV lies in demonstration of bladder outlet obstruction as a result of increased external sphincter/pelvic floor activity with no obvious neurologic cause.

4.3.3.1 Uroflowmetry

Uroflowmetry is an essential first-line investigation for patients with symptoms suggestive of DV. Components of uroflowmetry:

(a) *Quantitative*

Flow rates (maximum flow rate, Qmax; average flow rate, Qave), volumes (voided volume, VV; post-void residual urine, PVRU), and times (hesitancy, flow time, voiding time) provide initial indication of whether the flow is in normal range or not. The flow is dependent on bladder volume and there are several ways to objectively interpret flow–volume relations—flow–volume nomograms and volume–normalized flow rate index (VQI) [11]. Liverpool nomograms are widely used worldwide for this purpose; however, Indian studies have shown that this nomogram is not appropriate for Indian population. We developed and validated nomogram for Indian female population (eponymed PGIMER nomogram) and routinely use this in clinical practice [12].

VQI to flow rates is akin to what body mass index (BMI) is to body weight. We conceptualized, researched and validated the following definition:

$$VQI_{max} = Qmax / \sqrt{BV} \text{ and } VQI_{ave} = Qave / \sqrt{BV},$$

where BV = voided volume + PVR. Normal values of VQI have been defined [11] (median; interquartile range): VQI_{max} 1.39 (1.14, 1.65) and VQI_{ave} 0.79 (0.62, 0.96). One can easily understand the practical importance of VQI by the following example—intuitively, one knows that Qmax of 15 ml/s is a better-quality flow for volume of 150 ml rather than 400 ml. The objective assessment of the 'intuition' comes with applying the VQI formula; VQI_{max} would be 1.22 and 0.75, respectively. Another way would be to plot the flow versus volume on appropriate nomograms, i.e. Liverpool nomogram for Caucasian population and PGIMER nomogram for Indian population (Fig. 4.2).

(b) *Qualitative*

Qualitative assessment of uroflowmetry graph is of considerable importance. For example, a bell-shaped curve indicates normal-flow, plateau-shaped curve urethral stricture or DV (unpublished experience) and irregular intermittent curve straining (Fig. 4.3).

4.3.3.2 Uroflometry with Electromyography (EMG)

Addition of perineal EMG (representative of pelvic floor activity as a whole) to 'free-uroflometry' improves its diagnostic value to a great extent and may avoid invasive urodynamics in a significant proportion of patients (Fig. 4.4). During normal voiding, there is relative 'silence' of pelvic floor activity, which returns after voiding. In contrast, **the EMG activity would increase (intermittently or continuously) during voiding in cases of DV, or fail to relax in PRES leading to slow/staccato voiding**. However, one must be attentive and cautious in interpreting the EMG; for example, both pelvic pain and abdominal straining would increase the EMG activity even if there is no DV (Fig. 4.5).

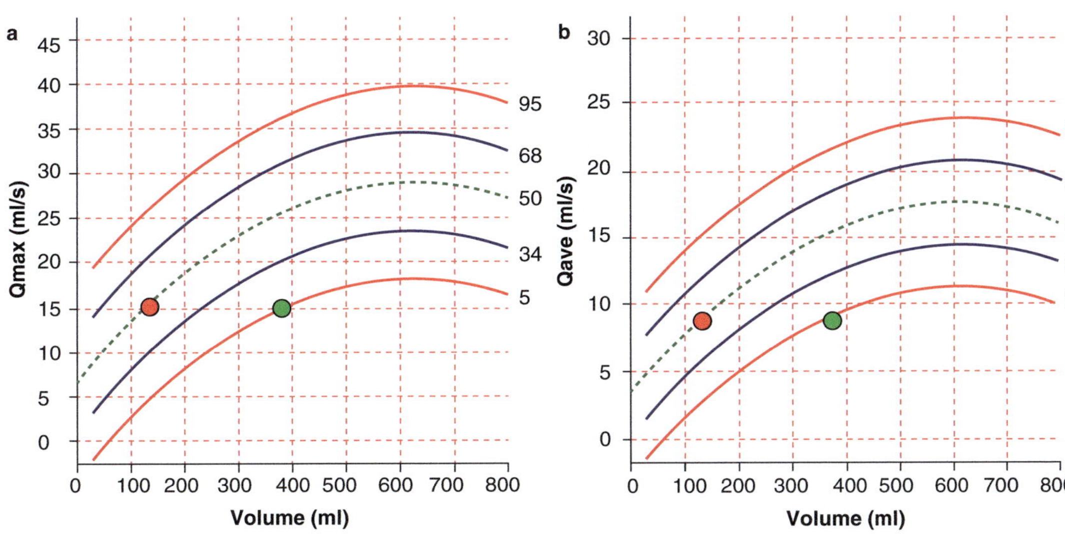

Fig. 4.2 Objective assessment of quality of flow-volume relation on PGIMER nomogram (**a**) Qmax-VV, (**b**) Qave-VV. The numbers towards right of each curve represent percentile values. Flow–volume relations (Qmax/Qave/VV) of patient 1 (green dot) and patient 2 (red dot) are 15/8/150 and 15/8/400, respectively. The relations in patient 1 are normal at 50th percentile compared to significantly subnormal below fifth percentile in patient 2

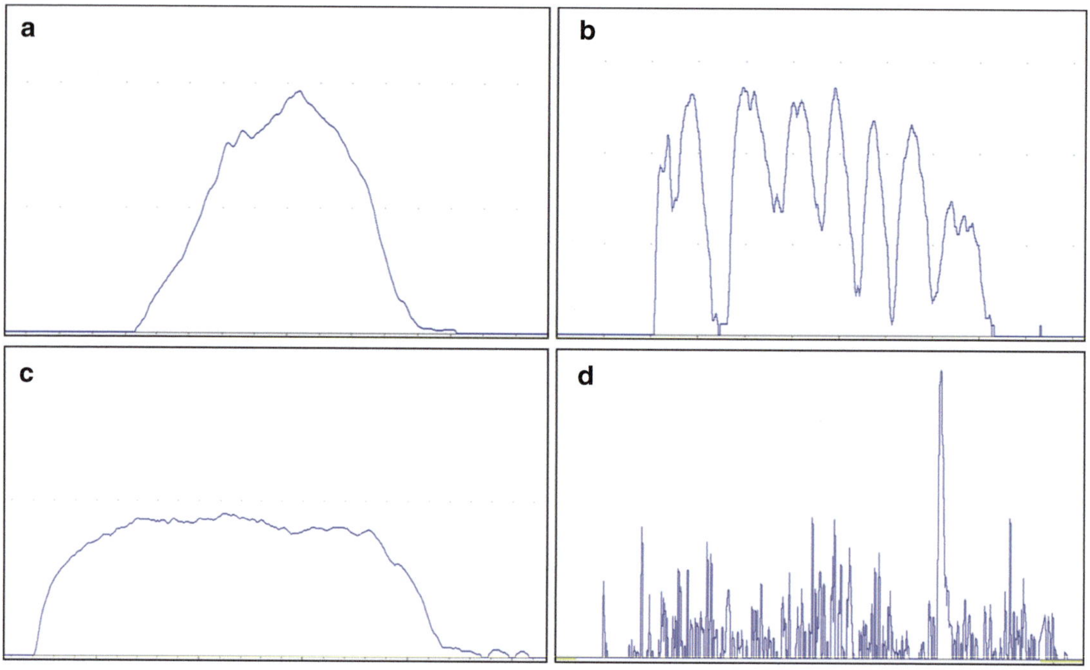

Fig. 4.3 Flow rate (ml/s)-time curve depicting (**a**) normal bell-shaped, and (**b**–**d**) abnormal voiding patterns—staccato, plateau and straining, respectively

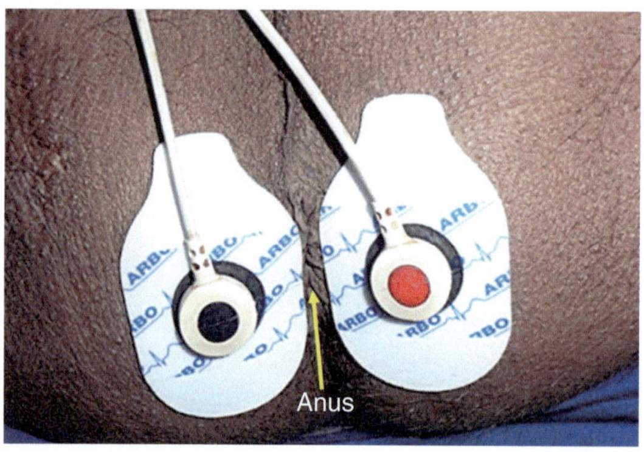

Fig. 4.4 Placement of perineal electrodes for surface electromyography. The closer the electrodes to anal verge, the better

Much work has been done on uroflow-EMG for diagnosis, biofeedback as well as monitoring of treatment-success in paediatric DV, both in boys and girls [13, 14]; however, there is dearth of literature specifically on adult population. Nevertheless, in view of similar pathophysiology, it is safe to assume that perineal EMG would add value to uroflometry.

It is evident from the discussion that interpretation of uroflowmetry can be greatly enhanced beyond flow rates, by adding VQI, VE and graph; these would also add value to interpreting follow-up uroflow of the same patient as well as for interpreting research data.

4.3.3.3 Ultrasonography of Kidney-Ureter-Bladder

There is no high quality of evidence available related to upper tract ultrasonography in DV and is generally not performed at initial visit. However, a significant minority of DV patients are at high risk of upper tract damage. Therefore, evaluation of upper tracts and bladder is of great importance. Even if not performed at initial visit, it must be considered in high-risk situations, e.g. urinary tract infection, haematuria, elevated post-void residue, incontinence coupled with voiding dysfunction and, of course elevated creatinine. Status of bladder wall thickness (BWT) has been studied and found to be clinically relevant in men with bladder outlet obstruction, detrusor under-

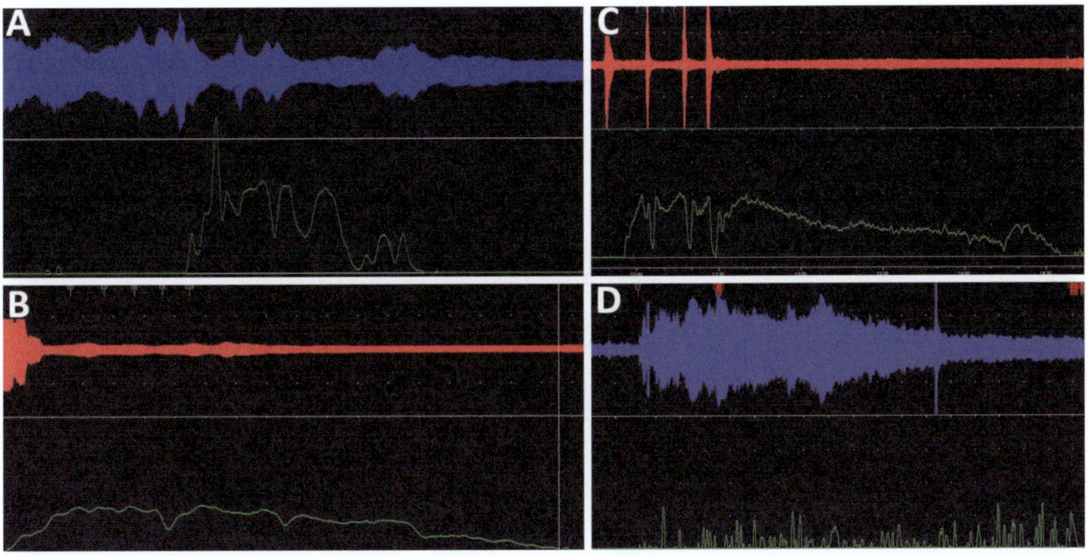

Fig. 4.5 (**a**) A typical dysfunctional voider—EMG activity and uroflow are reciprocal; (**b**) A patient with bladder neck obstruction—relative silence of EMG with slow flow; (**c**) A false positive—a patient with bladder neck obstruction with increased EMG activity due to discomfort in initial phase of voiding; (**d**) A false positive—a patient with voiding dysfunction voiding with abdominal straining

activity and overactive bladder, and children with neurogenic and non-neurogenic bladder conditions [7, 15–18]. Even in absence of consensus and standardization of BWT, one can infer the following

1. Women with thin-wall large-capacity bladder may correlate with detrusor underactivity.
2. Women with thick-walled bladder, with or without upper tract changes may correlate with poor bladder compliance and bladder outlet obstruction.
3. Women with detrusor overactivity may have thick-walled bladder even in absence of BOO.

Estimation or measurement of PVRU is of utmost importance in initial assessment of DV; an elevated PVRU may be associated with bladder dysfunction, renal dysfunction, recurrent urinary tract infection and urinary incontinence. The most accurate method would be to directly measure by catheterization; however, for obvious reasons, it is too invasive and mostly undesirable. Ultrasound estimation of bladder volume is a trade-off between accuracy and invasiveness and widely acceptable tool for this purpose. Several formulae have been studied with different levels of accuracy; formula D1 × D2 × D3 × 0.7 is widely used, easy to calculate and reasonably accurate [19]. Hand-held bladder scanners, with or without pre-measurement imaging, are widely available worldwide for the sole purpose of estimating bladder volume; however, the accuracy may be inferior to conventional ultrasound [11].

PVRU is expressed either as an absolute value or, better still, as **voiding efficiency (VE)**, which represents voided volume as percentage of total bladder volume. It can be calculated as under

$$\%\mathrm{VE} = \mathrm{VV} \times 100 / \left(\mathrm{BV} = \mathrm{VV} + \mathrm{PVR}\right).$$

For example, if a patient has PVRU of 100 ml, it would be intuitive to consider it more significant if patient voided 150 ml vis a vis 500 ml; the VE would be 60% and 83%, respectively, providing readily available objective parameter to the 'intuition'. Generally, for an asymptomatic adult woman (except elderly) PVRU of <50 ml and VE > 90% is considered normal [20, 21].

4.3.4 Multichannel Urodynamics (UDS)

Clinical picture combined with aforementioned investigations are usually sufficient to initiate presumptive conservative treatment. However, invasive testing is often required to pinpoint the diagnosis of DV, either after failure of initial therapy or, at times, even at an earlier stage. The invasive testing comprises (1) *basic UDS*—cystometry and pressure-flow study (PFS), (2) *advanced UDS*—urethral pressure profilometry (UPP), EMG of pelvic floor (perineal electrodes) or of external urethral sphincter complex (needle electrodes), (3) *uro-radiological studies*—micturating cystourethrography (MCUG), video-urodynamics (integrated UDS and fluoroscopy), perineal/rectal ultrasonography and functional magnetic resonance imaging.

As discussed before, the role of UDS would be to answer the following key questions:

1. Is there obstruction in the outflow? If there is obstruction, is it at the level of external sphincter/pelvic floor or at bladder neck? What is the degree of obstruction?
2. How are the filling sensations, capacity and compliance? Is there any detrusor overactivity?

In a large majority of men with bladder neck obstruction and prostatomegaly, diagnosis of bladder outlet obstruction (BOO) can be made by looking for 'high-pressure-low-flow voiding' in the pressure-flow relations. Various tools have been studied and validated, e.g. Abrams-Griffith nomogram and bladder outlet obstruction index, Schaefer nomogram and detrusor-adjusted mean passive urethral resistance relations factor (DAMPF). In view of fundamental differences between physiology of voiding and pathophysiology of voiding dysfunction between men and women, these concepts are not directly applicable in the latter and despite development of several formulae and nomograms, there is no universally applicable pressure-flow derivative [22]. **The situation becomes even more complex in DV in view of reflexive inhibition of detrusor activity during voiding in these patients** [23]; **many patients tend to void with abdominal straining. Therefore, diagnosis of BOO based on 'high-pressure-low-flow' becomes particularly challenging**. Additional measures are required to be able to diagnose and pinpoint the obstruction at external urethral sphincter/pelvic floor

1. **Electromyography (EMG)**—As described, an increased activity of pelvic floor EMG during voiding (in absence of abdominal straining and cystometry catheter-related pain) is suggestive of dysfunctional voiding. Absence of relaxation of EMG activity during voiding (without increase) may be indicative of PRES. It can be recorded either by perineal surface electrodes, which measure overall activity of pelvic floor, or by needle electrode placed specifically into EUS or into pubococcygeus, thus pinpointing the affected muscles. The placement of needle electrodes is a painful and cumbersome process, therefore not in common usage.
2. **Urethral pressure profilometry**—Urethral pressures (Pura) are recorded by triple lumen UPP catheter and closure pressures (Pclo) are derived by subtracting Pves from Pura (much like Pdet is derived from subtracting Pabd from Pves). Normal median resting Pclo in women ranges from 65 to 90 cm H_2O, progressively decreasing with age. In women, during voiding Pves and Pura (throughout the functional urethra) are almost equal; therefore, Pclo normally remains nearly zero during voiding all along the length of functional urethra. If resistance is encountered during voiding, Pura drops beyond the point of resistance. A decrease in Pura >5 cm H_2O below Pves indicates obstruction and the point at which the drop happens indicates the location of the obstruction (Fig. 4.6). Such finding is however not specific for DV and will even be seen in anatomical obstructions.
3. **Plateau detrusor pattern**—The pattern of detrusor contraction during normal voiding is bell-shaped. We discovered a unique pattern of detrusor contraction found in patients with

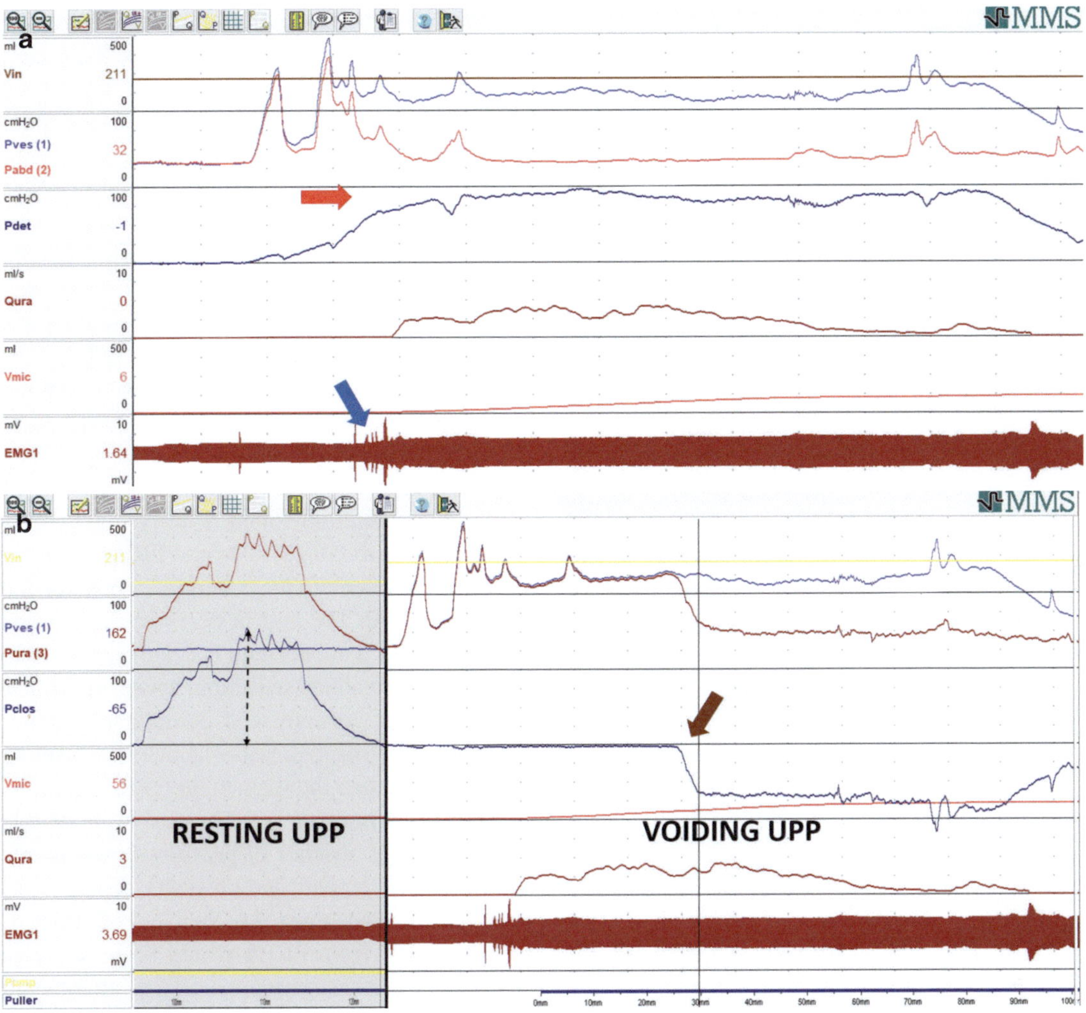

Fig. 4.6 Multichannel urodynamics of a 35-year-old woman with dysfunctional voiding (*Pves* vesical pressure, *Pabd* abdominal pressure, *Pdet (= Pves – Pabd)* detrusor pressure, *Pura* urethral pressure, *Pclo (= Pura – Pves)* urethral closure pressure, *Qura* flow rate, *EMG* perineal surface electromyography) (**a**) Pressure-flow study shows high-pressure-low flow voiding indicating obstruction, 'plateau pattern' of detrusor contraction (red arrow) and increased EMG activity of pelvic floor (blue arrow) both indicating pelvic floor non-relaxation; (**b**) Dynamic urethral pressure profilometry of the same patient—resting urethral pressure very high at 155 cm H_2O (grey background) and Pclo dropping at 25 mm from bladder neck to −75 cm H_2O (brown arrow) indicating obstruction at distal external urethral sphincter

DV, the plateau pattern [24] (Fig. 4.6). In our experience, this pattern is quite consistent and has been helpful in diagnosing DV in our clinical practice.

4. **Micturating cystourethrography**—Whether done integrated with urodynamic study or separately in uro-radiology suite, MCUG is the cornerstone of diagnosis of DV. However, fluoroscopic recording of functional urethra during voiding phase in a woman in sitting or squatting position can be a challenging task. Oblique positioning and vertical tilting of C-arm relative to the patient's pelvis is required to be able to visualize the functional urethra (Fig. 4.7). Using radiolucent urodynamic chair and fluoroscopic C-arm would be

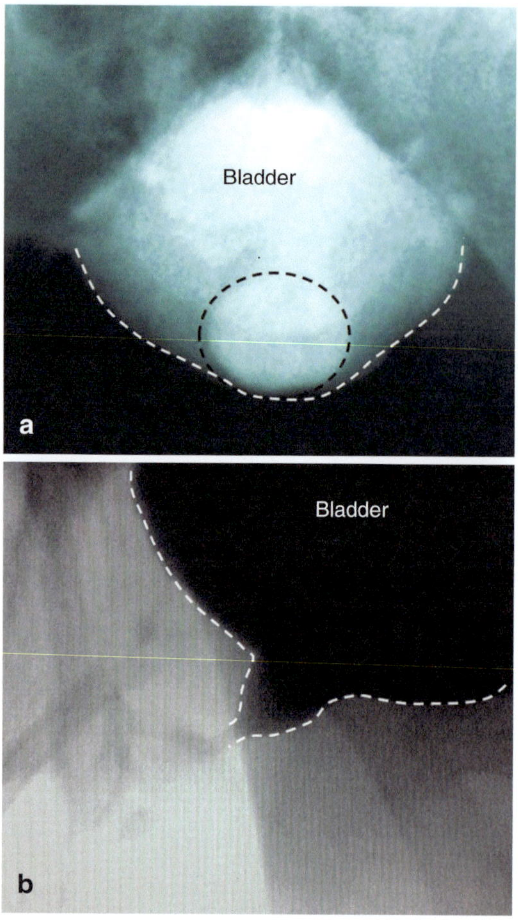

Fig. 4.7 Micturating cystourethrography of the same 35-year-old woman (depicted in Fig. 4.5) showing importance of proper position of patient in relation to the fluoroscopy. (**a**) An anteroposterior image taken with c-arm perpendicular to patient's pelvis. Note that the open bladder neck is superimposed on bladder and can easily be missed; (**b**) An oblique image taken with C-arm at 45-degree oblique position to patient's pelvis unmasking the whole length of urethra clearly revealing non-relaxation of external sphincter/pelvic floor (Reproduced with permission from Chapter 5, MAnual of Urodynamics, Mayank Mohan Agarwal, 2014. Copyright Jaypee Brothers Medical Publishers (P) Ltd.)

ideal; however, such a setup is obviously cost prohibitive. One can improvise as per availability of equipment. We routinely do such MCUG in Operation Theatre having patient squatting on the operation table using fluoroscopic C-arm for imaging. A wooden chair may come handy for the same purpose.

Little is known about the diagnostic criteria and clinical implications of differentiating pelvic floor dysfunction from external urethral sphincter. Kuo et al. have published the largest experience on this topic [1, 25, 26]. They coined the term PRES, acronym for poor relaxation of external sphincter, to differentiate from DV due to non-relaxation of pelvic floor muscles. They defined PRES as presence of low pressure-low flow in association with no increase/decrease in EMG activity of pelvic floor (that's why 'poor relaxation' term) and DV as moderate—high pressure low flow in association with increase in EMG activity; spinning top deformity on MCUG was a mandatory criterion for both the conditions. They analysed results of urodynamic studies of 1914 women and found a fairly high prevalence of both DV (17.0%) and PRES (17.6%). Detrusor overactivity occurred in 60% of the women with DV and in 5.7% of the women with PRES. Patients with DV had significantly increased bladder sensation, lower cystometric bladder capacity and compliance, higher voiding detrusor pressure and lower voiding efficiency than the women with PRES and the control individuals [1]. The limitation of this definition is absence of pressure-flow cut-offs and heavy dependence on EMG, which itself has limited accuracy. Another way of differentiating DV from PRES would be to measure voiding urethral pressure at EUS along with perineal EMG—an increased pressure with reduced EMG activity may indicate PRES and decreased pressure with increased EMG activity DV (personal communication with Dr. Aparna Hegde).

4.4 Treatment

The treatment of DV is a multi-step, multimodality and multi-disciplinary process. **Patient education is an essential part of any medical treatment, even more important in chronic conditions like DV affecting disease-specific and global quality of life**. The patient should be made to understand the normal functional anatomy and physiology of pelvic floor and pelvic organs, the chronic nature of disease process, difficulties in diagnosis, available modalities of treatment and response to therapy. During the initial encounters itself, patient must be made 'aware' of the pelvic floor, preferably through clinical pelvic examination, and importance of pelvic floor training/exercises (PFMT/PFME) must be emphasized.

4.4.1 Physical Therapy

Detailed techniques of PFMT/PFME are beyond the scope of this chapter. Nevertheless, few principles must be understood. The schedule of PFMT should be tailor-made to each individual's pelvic floor status, i.e. strength, endurance, relaxation levels. A supervised program is the key to efficacy; physical pelvic floor assessment should be done periodically and enquiry on regularity and schedule of exercises should be made. Patient should be made to understand that the exercises should be continued indefinitely to maintain strength, relaxation and responsiveness much like any other muscle in the body.

Typically, the patient is asked to perform pelvic floor squeeze for 3–10 s followed by relaxation for 10–20 s (at least twice the duration of squeeze). She is asked to perform 10–20 repetitions in one session and repeat the sessions 3–5 times a day. Particular emphasis is laid on the 'relaxation' phase and asked not trying to 'hurrying up' through the process. Recently, in a study comprising on 16 women with DV, Hegde found pelvic bulge manoeuvre to cause pelvic floor relaxation. The patients were asked to lightly blow through pursed lips (as if blowing through a drinking straw); concomitant EMG relaxation was noticed [27]. This can be of great assistance particularly if patient is unable to understand relaxation otherwise.

4.4.2 Pharmacotherapy

This is an adjunct to physical therapy during initial phase of therapy. The literature on medical therapy for DV is scattered over different age groups and both sexes, and there is dearth of high-quality evidence. Nevertheless, since pathophysiology of DV is considered to be similar across the groups; within the limits of available data, the following medications have been found effective

(a) **Alpha blockers**—Tamsulosin, a relatively alpha 1a selective alpha 1 blocker, is the most extensively studied alpha blocker in adult voiding dysfunction patients, both men and women. While most studies used urodynamic criteria to define voiding dysfunction, only few of these qualified the functional voiding dysfunction as DV. In commonly prescribed dosage of 0.2–0.4 mg once daily, a clinical response rate of 30–80% has been observed [28]. Conventionally, alpha blockers have been thought to work on bladder neck and proximal urethral smooth muscles; however, studies in children with DV have shown clear benefit of alpha blocker doxazosin at doses of 0.5–3 mg comparable to biofeedback, putting this notion into question [29]. Moreover, Reitz et al. found Tamsulosin to reduce urethral closure pressure all along the length in healthy women volunteers [30].
(b) **Skeletal muscle relaxants**—Since DV is patho-physiologically spasm of skeletal muscles, it is natural to consider skeletal muscle relaxants for its treatment. **Diazepam** was one of the first agents but went into disfavour in view of sedation and addiction. Nevertheless, it has been used lately as vaginal pessary for pelvic floor spasticity-related dyspareunia. **Baclofen** is a gamma amino butyric acid (GABA) B type receptor agonist and is widely used in various neurogenic spastic conditions. Since GABA-ergic interneurons in sacral cord are responsible for relaxation of EUS during micturition, baclofen (5–10 mg three times a day) has been used for management of neurogenic (DESD) and non-neurogenic (DV) pelvic floor spasm. In a randomized controlled placebo-controlled trial enrolling 60 women with urodynamically proven DV, Xu et al. showed a significant reduction in voiding frequency with corresponding reduction in EMG activity with baclofen at doses of 10 mg three times a day [31]. Dose-limiting

side effects are somnolence, muscle weakness and nausea. **Tizanidine** is centrally acting alpha-2 adrenergic receptor agonist, which has been used for myofascial pain syndromes since 1990s. In a randomized study, El-Hefnawy et al. found tizanidine to be more efficacious than doxazosin in children with DV [32]. There is no other such clinical study available in English medical literature. We have used tizanidine in combination with alpha blocker at doses 2–4 mg three times a day for adults with urodynamically confirmed DV refractory to alpha blocker alone and found it mild-to-moderately effective in approximately 40% (unpublished data). Similar to baclofen, somnolence is a dose-limiting side effect.

(c) **Miscellaneous**—It cannot be over-emphasized that medical management of DV is a multi-disciplinary one in which the urologist plays a key role of coordinating across specialties. Referral to medical gastroenterologist, psychiatrist, gynaecologist and chronic pain-specialist may be required from time to time, at times to rule out an alternative/sinister diagnosis.

Anticholinergics are used for urgency with or without frequency of urine if the post-void residue is less than 100–150 ml. Drug-induced constipation may worsen already-existing constipation in many of these patients and to be taken care of appropriately. In this regard **mirabegron**, a beta-3 agonist, offers advantage of efficacy similar to anti-cholinergics with safer side-effect profile. For chronic pelvic pain, **gabapentenoids**, particularly gabapentin and **tricyclic antidepressants**, amitriptyline/nortriptyline may be required. Constipation often improves with pelvic floor relaxation exercises/bulge manoeuvre; however, **laxatives and/or bulking agents** may be used as appropriate. Many of these patients are/become anxious due to poor quality of life and may need to be put on SSRIs, SNRIs, benzodiazepine, other psychoactive medications.

4.4.3 Interventional Treatment

(a) **Onabotulinum toxin A (OBoNT)**—It is a neurotoxin produced by *Clostridium botulinum*; it acts on pre-synaptic cholinergic nerve terminals decreasing acetylcholine release, by cleaving synaptosome-associated protein (SNAP-25). Intra-sphincter injection of 50–200 units OBoNT has been used for treatment of DV both in children and adults with promising results in terms of reduction in post-void residues and urethral pressures, and improvement in flow rates [33]. Kuo et al. reported largest single-centre experience of OBoNT sphincter infiltration in a cohort of 200 patients with bladder emptying failure. They reported 88.5% success rate (including 47.5% excellent result and 41% improved result) [34]. They also reported reversal of detrusor underactivity to normalcy in 48% of injected patients [23]. Most commonly, 100 units are diluted in 4-ml sterile water and injected into the EUS transperineally or transurethrally. Typically, the effect lasts for 6 months or so following which a repeat injection is required. Most studies have reported efficacy of one repeat injection [35]. Recently, in a small randomized study, Kuo et al. found efficacy of OBoNT injection similar to that of placebo (0.9% normal saline) putting its efficacy into question [36].

(b) **Sacral neuromodulation (SNM)**—Since dysregulation of sacral reflexes is central to pathophysiology of DV, it is fair to expect neuromodulation of sacral nerve pathways to be effective. SNM is a two-step process. In the first step, temporary/permanent leads are implanted in S3 foramen under fluoroscopic guidance, checked functionally, connected to external pulse generator and patient discharged for 1–3 weeks. If the patient reports ≥50% improvement, external pulse generator is surgically replaced with permanent pacemaker. In DV, SNM is best studied in children with dysfunctional elimination syndrome (DES) [37] and women with idiopathic retention [38], and has proven efficacy of 60–94% in well-selected individuals in terms of need for self-catheterization, improved flow rates, decreased post-void residues, frequency and incontinence. Battery of a successfully implanted pacemaker works for several years; however, there is 18–56% surgical revision rate for pain, lead migration, loss of efficacy and infection.

(c) **Surgery**—Surgical procedures to increase bladder compliance (augmentation cystoplasty) and/or decrease outlet resistance (sphincterotomy) are not uncommonly employed in patients of neurogenic bladder with detrusor-sphincter dyssynergia. However, data for DV patients are sparse. **External urethral sphincterotomy—**it has long been used successfully in treating patients with neurogenic Detrusor external sphincter dyssynergia (DESD). The technique evolved over time switching from lateral incisions (3 and 9 o'clock) to midline (12 o'clock) maintaining efficacy and reducing side effects such as haemorrhage and erectile dysfunction [39, 40]. Sphincteric stent (Urolume™) has also shown promising result in men with DESD, sparing irreversible sphincterotomy [41]. We could find only one report of external sphincterotomy in patients with DV—Moreno-Palacios et al. reported excellent improvement in subjective as well as objective parameters in 30 men with DV [42]. **Augmentation cystoplasty**—it is the cornerstone treatment for patients with small-capacity bladder with poor compliance with/without hydro-ureteronephrosis. It has been employed in neurogenic as well as non-neurogenic bladder conditions (Hinman syndrome, genitourinary tuberculosis, etc.). Most commonly a distal ileal segment is utilized; peritoneum, lower ureters and other bowel segments have also been used in select circumstances. For facilitating CIC, sometimes a Mitrofanoff procedure utilizing appendix or Yang-Monti principle is added.

4.4.4 Constipation [43]

LUT and LGIT share similar locale, structural concept (sphincters, reservoir and pelvic floor) as well as innervation (S2–4) and therefore work in harmony. Often DV is associated with LGIT, most commonly constipation. **It has been observed that treatment of constipation tends to improve outcome of LUT dysfunction as well** [44, 45] Therefore, urologist should familiarize oneself with basic knowledge and initial treatment of constipation.

Functional constipation is further categorized as slow transit type, evacuation disorder and constipation-predominant irritable bowel syndrome. Clinician should enquire about duration of constipation, frequency and consistency of stools, sensation of incomplete defecation, straining, associated abdominal bloating, pain and altered bowel habit. Diet pattern (especially fibre and fluid), psychological status, co-morbid medications should be enquired. Examination has been covered previously. In absence of severe constipation and of alarm features (iron deficiency anaemia, faecal occult blood, melena, haematochezia, recent change in stool calibre, new-onset constipation in patients >50 years with no prior colon cancer screening, weight loss), evaluation beyond history, examination and baseline laboratory investigations is generally not required before initiation of treatment. Initial treatment includes increased intake of fibre by diet and bulk supplements (psyllium/ispaghula) with or without osmotic agents (polyethyl glycol or lactulose). Prokinetic agents and enemas may also be prescribed as needed. Refractory constipation, severe constipation and alarm features are indications for specialist referral and further evaluation. Similar to dysfunctional voiding and urinary incontinence, sacral neuromodulation has proven efficacy in treatment of functional constipation and faecal incontinence as well.

In conclusion, DV is a chronic condition and an elusive diagnosis. A thorough clinico-urodynamic evaluation by a dedicated team is required to pin-point it. A correct diagnosis is the first step towards multi-prong, multi-disciplinary, supervised and persistent treatment. Limitation of low level of evidence of modalities of treatment and side effects must be understood by the clinical team and discussed with patient from time to time.

Case Discussion (Fig. 4.8)
A 35-year-old woman presented with difficulty in voiding with recurrent acute retention of urine (AUR) for last 3 years. The problem started after an episode of urinary tract infection with severe pelvic pain. There were no earlier lower urinary tract symptoms. She did not have any lower gastrointestinal symptoms, before or after the pain episode. At the time of presentation, she was in retention of urine and was on clean intermittent self-catheterization (CISC). She was a mother of two boys, both delivered vaginally (age of younger child 7 years), did not have any medical co-morbidity and her menstrual cycles were normal. On examination, there was no discernible prolapse and pelvic floor muscle strength was 4/5. Perineal sensations were normal; however, BCR was negative.

There hadn't been any response to alpha blockers (tried tamsulosin and alfuzosin for a cumulative period of 4 months). Uroflowmetry before last episode of AUR revealed slow flow with dribbling. Multi-channel urodynamics revealed low pressure-low flow voiding with plateau detrusor pattern. UPP and MCUG localized the obstruction at external urethral sphincter level. A diagnosis of dysfunctional voiding was made and she was initiated on trial of Tamsulosin 0.4 mg once daily, Baclofen 5 mg tid with pelvic relaxation exercises. However, there was no

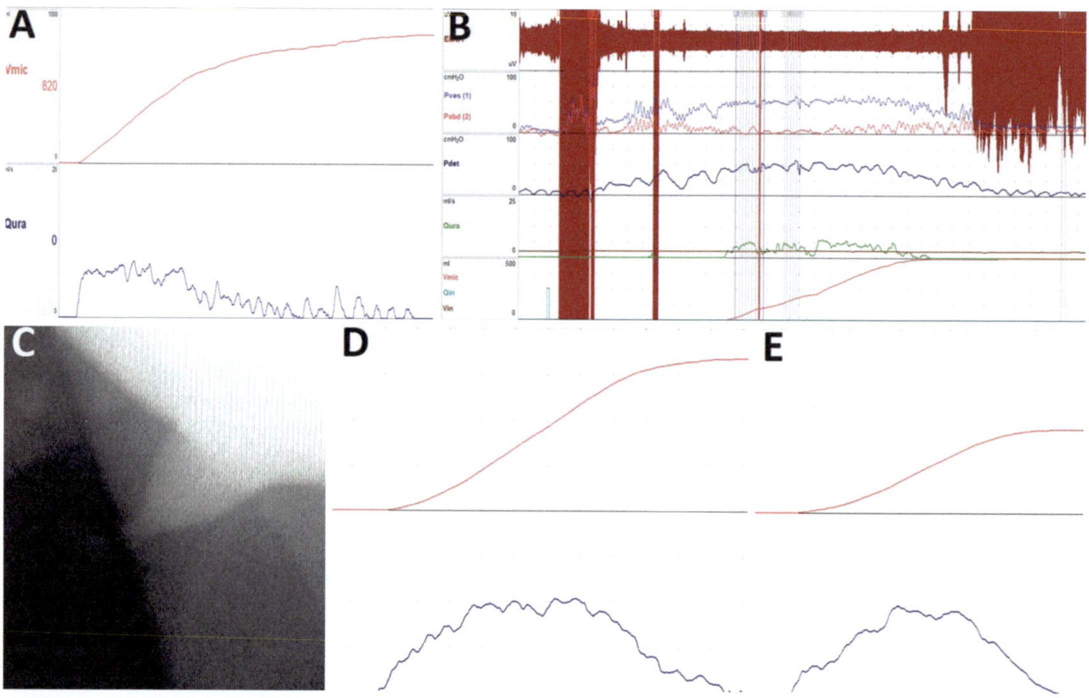

Fig. 4.8 (**a**) Uroflometry before last episode of retention of urine (Qmax/Qave/VV/PVR/cQmax/cQave 8.6/4/0/834/78/0.28/0.13); (**b**) Multichannel urodynamics revealing low-pressure low-flow voiding with plateau detrusor pattern and mild straining at the beginning and end of micturition. Non-relaxation of EMG during voiding can be made out; (**c**) Micturating cystourethrography showing spinning top urethra with wide open bladder neck and non-relaxed external urethral sphincter; (**d**) Uroflometry after placement of temporary pacemaker of sacral neuromodulation, subjectively better (12.6/7.8/420/5/0.61/0.37); (E) Uroflometry 3 months after placement of permanent pacemaker, improvement maintained (11.6/7.0/230/5/0.75/0.45)

response even after a trial for 3–4 weeks and she remained dependent on CISC. After extensive counselling she opted for trial of sacral neuromodulation; she was able to void after temporary lead placement and became free from CISC. She has continued to do well after permanent pacemaker placement. However, she needed additional surgery for lead replacement 3 months after the above in view of non-responsive pain at lead site.

Key Learning Points

- Dysfunctional voiding is a non-neurogenic voiding dysfunction caused by either increased activity or failure to relax of the pelvic floor and/or external urethral sphincter muscles during voiding. This can be demonstrated on EMG trace during a pressure flow study along with high detrusor pressures and a narrowing in mid/distal urethra on voiding film.
- It is the most common cause of functional bladder outlet obstruction in women. Clinically, it can present with voiding symptoms alone, storage symptoms alone or a combination of both. It can also present with predominant pain symptoms leading to delay in diagnosis.
- Constipation is a common accompaniment and treatment of constipation helps relieving urinary symptoms as well.
- Behavioural therapies are the cornerstone of management focussing on relearning of pelvic floor relaxation while voiding. Pharmacotherapy with alpha adrenergic blockers or skeletal muscle relaxants plays an adjunctive role.
- Intra-sphincteric injections of botulinum toxin may be effective but require repeated treatment.
- Sacral neuromodulation may be curative in well-selected patients but the need for revisions and cost may be prohibitory.

References

1. Peng C-H, Chen S-F, Kuo H-C. Videourodynamic analysis of the urethral sphincter overactivity and the poor relaxing pelvic floor muscles in women with voiding dysfunction. Neurourol Urodyn. 2017;36(8):2169–75.
2. Pauwels E, De Laet K, De Wachter S, Wyndaele J-J. Healthy, middle-aged, history-free, continent women—do they strain to void? J Urol. 2006;175(4):1403–7.
3. Gehrich A, Stany MP, Fischer JR, Buller J, Zahn CM. Establishing a mean postvoid residual volume in asymptomatic perimenopausal and postmenopausal women. Obstet Gynecol. 2007;110(4):827–32.
4. Griffiths DJ, Harrison G, Moore K, McCracken P. Variability of post-void residual urine volume in the elderly. Urol Res. 1996;24(1):23–6.
5. Groutz A, Blaivas JG, Pies C, Sassone AM. Learned voiding dysfunction (non-neurogenic, neurogenic bladder) among adults. Neurourol Urodyn. 2001;20(3):259–68.
6. Klingele CJ, Lightner DJ, Fletcher JG, Gebhart JB, Bharucha AE. Dysfunctional urinary voiding in women with functional defecatory disorders. Neurogastroenterol Motil. 2010;22(10):1094–e284.
7. Everaert K, Van Laecke E, De Muynck M, Peeters H, Hoebeke P. Urodynamic assessment of voiding dysfunction and dysfunctional voiding in girls and women. Int Urogynecol J Pelvic Floor Dysfunct. 2000;11(4):254–64.
8. Newman DKLJ. Clinical evaluation of the pelvic floor muscles. In: Baessler K, Schussler B, Burgio KL, Moore KH, Norton PASS, editors. Pelvic floor re-education: principles and practice. 2nd ed. London: Springer; 2008. p. 91–108.
9. Newman D, Laycock J. Clinical evaluation of the pelvic floor muscles. In: Pelvic floor re-education: principles and practice. London: Springer; 2008. p. 91–104.
10. Russell B, Brubaker L. Muscle function and ageing. In: Kaven B, Schussler B, Burgio KL, Moore KH, Norton PA, Stanton SL, editors. Pelvic floor re-education. second. London: Springer; 2008. p. 49–61.
11. Agarwal MM, Patil S, Roy K, Bandawar M, Choudhury S, Ravimohan M. Rationalization of interpretation of uroflowmetry for a non-Caucasian (Indian) population: conceptual development and validation of volume-normalized flow rate index. Neurourol Urodyn. 2014;33(1):135–41.
12. Barapatre Y, Agarwal MM, Singh SK, et al. Uroflowmetry in healthy women: development and validation of flow-volume and corrected flow-age nomograms. Neurourol Urodyn. 2009;28(8):1003–9.
13. Babu R, Gopinath V. Role of uroflowmetry with electromyography in the evaluation of children with lower urinary tract dysfunction. Indian J Urol. 2015;31(4):354–7.
14. Van Batavia JP, Combs AJ, Fast AM, Glassberg KI. Use of non-invasive uroflowmetry with simultaneous electromyography to monitor patient response to treatment for lower urinary tract conditions. J Pediatr Urol. 2014;10(3):532–7.
15. Kuo H, Chen Y, Chen C, Chancellor M. Transabdominal ultrasound measurement of detrusor wall thickness in patients with overactive bladder. Tzu Chi Med J. 2009;21:129–35.

16. Manieri C, Carter SS, Romano G, Trucchi A, Valenti M, Tubaro A. The diagnosis of bladder outlet obstruction in men by ultrasound measurement of bladder wall thickness. J Urol. 1998;159(3):761–5.
17. Tangal S, Gökçe Mİ, Özayar A, et al. Evaluation of a new ultrasound measurement tool for the diagnosis of dysfunctional voiding in pediatric population: full/empty bladder wall thickness ratio. Urology. 2014;83(6):1369–72.
18. Bright E, Oelke M, Tubaro A, Abrams P. Ultrasound estimated bladder weight and measurement of bladder wall thickness—useful noninvasive methods for assessing the lower urinary tract? J Urol. 2010;184(5):1847–54.
19. Yip S-K, Sahota D, Chang AM. Determining the reliability of ultrasound measurements and the validity of the formulae for ultrasound estimation of postvoid residual bladder volume in postpartum women. Neurourol Urodyn. 2003;22(3):255–60.
20. Pfisterer MH-D, Griffiths DJ, Rosenberg L, Schaefer W, Resnick NM. Parameters of bladder function in pre-, peri-, and postmenopausal continent women without detrusor overactivity. Neurourol Urodyn. 2007;26(3):356–61.
21. Haylen BT. Residual urine volumes in a normal female population: application of transvaginal ultrasound. Br J Urol. 1989;64(4):347–9.
22. Gammie A, Kirschner-Hermanns R, Rademakers K. Evaluation of obstructed voiding in the female: how close are we to a definition? Curr Opin Urol. 2015;25:292–5.
23. Kuo HC. Recovery of detrusor function after urethral botulinum a toxin injection in patients with idiopathic low detrusor contractility and voiding dysfunction. Urology. 2007;69(1):57–61.
24. Agarwal M, Jain S, Mavuduru R, Singh S, Mandal A. Plateau pattern of detrusor contraction: a surrogate indicator of presence of external sphincter dysfunction during micturitional phase of urodynamic study. Indian J Urol. 2016;32(2):137.
25. Chen Y-C, Kuo H-C. Clinical and video urodynamic characteristics of adult women with dysfunctional voiding. J Formos Med Assoc. 2014;113(3):161–5.
26. Shao IH, Kuo HC. Role of poor urethral sphincter relaxation in men with voiding dysfunction refractory to α-blocker therapy: clinical characteristics and predictive factors. Low Urin Tract Symptoms. 2019;11(1):8–13.
27. Liaw Y-M, Kuo H-C. Biofeedback pelvic floor muscle training for voiding dysfunction and overactive bladder. Incontinence Pelvic Floor Dysfunct. 2007;1(1):13–5.
28. Meyer LE, Brown JN. Tamsulosin for voiding dysfunction in women. Int Urol Nephrol. 2012;44(6):1649–56.
29. Yucel S, Akkaya E, Guntekin E, et al. Can alpha-blocker therapy be an alternative to biofeedback for dysfunctional voiding and urinary retention? A prospective study. J Urol. 2005;174:1612–5.
30. Reitz A, Haferkamp A, Kyburz T, Knapp PA, Wefer B, Schurch B. The effect of tamsulosin on the resting tone and the contractile behaviour of the female urethra: a functional urodynamic study in healthy women. Eur Urol. 2004;46(2):235–40.
31. Xu D, Qu C, Meng H, et al. Dysfunctional voiding confirmed by transdermal perineal electromyography, and its effective treatment with baclofen in women with lower urinary tract symptoms: a randomized double-blind placebo-controlled crossover trial. BJU Int. 2007;100(3):588–92.
32. El-Hefnawy AS, Helmy T, El-Assmy MM, Sarhan O, Hafez AT, Dawaba M. Doxazosin versus tizanidine for treatment of dysfunctional voiding in children: a prospective randomized open-labeled trial. Urology. 2012;79(2):428–33.
33. Apostolidis A, Dasgupta P, Denys P, et al. Recommendations on the use of botulinum toxin in the treatment of lower urinary tract disorders and pelvic floor dysfunctions: a European consensus report. Eur Urol. 2009;55(1):100–20.
34. Liao YM, Kuo HC. Causes of failed urethral botulinum toxin a treatment for emptying failure. Urology. 2007;70(4):763–6.
35. Kuo HC. Botulinun A toxin urethral sphincter injection for neurogenic or nonneurogenic voiding dysfunction. Tzu Chi Med J. 2016;28(3):89–93.
36. Jiang YH, Wang CC, Kuo HC. Onabotulinumtoxin a urethral sphincter injection as treatment for non-neurogenic voiding dysfunction – a randomized, double-blind, placebo-controlled study. Sci Rep. 2016;6(1):38905.
37. Dwyer ME, Vandersteen DR, Hollatz P, Reinberg YE. Sacral neuromodulation for the dysfunctional elimination syndrome: a 10-year single-center experience with 105 consecutive children. Urology. 2014;84(4):911–8.
38. van Kerrebroeck PEV, Marcelissen TAT. Sacral neuromodulation for lower urinary tract dysfunction. World J Urol. 2012;30(4):445–50.
39. Pan D, Troy A, Rogerson J, Bolton D, Brown D, Lawrentschuk N. Long-term outcomes of external sphincterotomy in a spinal injured population. J Urol. 2009;181(2):705–9.
40. Whitmore WF III, Fam BA, Yalla SV. Experience with anteromedian (12 O'clock) external urethral sphincterotomy in 100 male subjects with neuropathic bladders. Br J Urol. 1978;50(2):99–101.
41. Chancellor MB, Bennett C, Simoneau AR, et al. Sphincteric stent versus external sphincterotomy in spinal cord injured men: prospective randomized multicenter trial. J Urol. 1999;161(6):1893–8.
42. Moreno-Palacios J, Maldonado-Alcaraz E, Montoya-Martinez G, Serrano-Brambila E. Outcomes and complications of sphincterotomy with bladder neck incision in neurologically healthy male patients with voiding dysfunction. Arch Esp Urol. 2012;65(2):244–50.

43. Lindberg G, Hamid SS, Malfertheiner P, et al. Erratum: world gastroenterology organisation global guidelines constipation-a global perspective. J Clin Gastroenterol. 2012;46(1):90.
44. Charach G, Greenstein A, Rabinovich P, Groskopf I, Weintraub M. Alleviating constipation in the elderly improves lower urinary tract symptoms. Gerontology. 2001;47(2):72–6.
45. Loening-Baucke V. Urinary incontinence and urinary tract infection and their resolution with treatment of chronic constipation of childhood. Pediatrics. 1997;100(2):228–32.

Primary Bladder Neck Obstruction in Women

5

Maneesh Sinha, Ankit Singla, and Venkatesh Krishnamoorthy

Learning Objectives

- To understand the pathophysiology of primary bladder neck obstruction as a cause of bladder outlet obstruction in females.
- To learn the contemporary diagnostic criteria of primary bladder neck obstruction in females.
- To understand the indications and efficacy of various treatment modalities for primary bladder neck obstruction.

5.1 Introduction

Primary bladder neck obstruction (PBNO) is described as a functional failure of the bladder neck to open adequately during voiding [1]. While there are no universally accepted urodynamic criteria, most authors use a Q_{max} of 11–15 ml/s and a $P_{det}Q_{max}$ of 20–25 cm H2O to define bladder outlet obstruction (BOO). Failure of the bladder neck to open in a video-urodynamic study or a voiding cystourethrogram points to the bladder neck as the site of obstruction.

M. Sinha · A. Singla · V. Krishnamoorthy (✉)
Department of Urology, NU Hospitals, Bengaluru, India
e-mail: dr.maneesh@nuhospitals.com; dr.venkatesh@nuhospitals.com

5.2 The Normal Bladder Neck in Women

The existence of a functional bladder neck in females is not universally accepted. Foetal studies have shown that there is scant circular smooth muscle in the bladder neck in females [2]. While males have well-defined outer circular and inner longitudinal layers in their smooth muscle, females do not have a well-defined longitudinal layer [3]. Oswald reported that female bladder necks were wider with less dense smooth muscles during foetal development [4]. The bladder neck has been described as a functional rather than a distinct anatomical entity, which acts in concert with the proximal urethra in achieving continence. Surprisingly, a search of the literature did not reveal detailed anatomical studies on the adult female bladder neck.

5.3 Aetiopathogenesis

As early as 1921, Caulk had reported bladder neck obstruction in an adult female [5]. Jacobson summarized the available evidence and added 4 of his own cases to the early literature [6]. In 1963, Corrin Mayer and Moore described histopathological changes in 49 women with obstruction at the bladder neck and emphasized the presence of inflammatory infiltrates in the lamina propria. They did not note any fibrosis in these

N. Khattar et al. (eds.), *Female Bladder Outlet Obstruction and Urethral Reconstruction*,
https://doi.org/10.1007/978-981-15-8521-0_5

women. Unfortunately, the paper does not talk about smooth muscle changes at the bladder neck [7]. In 1984, Diokno described a series of three urodynamically diagnosed cases of primary bladder neck obstruction. Histologic evaluation revealed smooth muscle hypertrophy of the bladder neck in one patient treated by Y-V pasty [8].

The cause for PBNO remains largely unknown till date. Several mechanisms have been put forth for this clinical entity. Mostly, only a functional obstruction is identified. Very rarely, it has been a fibrosed bladder neck. Farrar et al. have attributed underlying detrusor instability for the outflow obstruction at all levels of the urethra, including the bladder neck [9]. Smooth muscle hypertrophy was postulated to cause obstruction in the urethra also. They treated all patients with urethral dilatation by various methods. Though they had relief of symptoms, the detrusor instability itself did not change post therapy.

George and Slade proposed that these patients fall into the group of 'anxious bladders'. In these patients, the detrusor contractions were poor but not sustained [10]. Their patients also had a high incidence of dyspepsia and anxiety disorder. Rat models of bladder outlet obstruction have reported a tonic increase in the locus coeruleus. This change is related to anxiety and sleep disorders. While they have not been specifically implicated in PBNO, they are associated with bladder dysfunction in general and may explain the increased frequency seen in patients with PBNO. These psychiatric disorders may not only point towards a pelvic pathology but may also require independent treatment [11].

Axelrod and Blaivas proposed that increased smooth muscle tone was imparting a loss of elasticity to the bladder neck and was the cause of PBNO [12].

Mayo and Deacon suggested aberrant adrenergic receptor density or smooth muscle hypertrophy of the proximal urethra to be the causes for PBNO, but it is likely that the concomitant bladder wall hypertrophy and trabeculation could have been the cause of the hypertrophic bladder neck [8, 13]. Histologic evidence of bladder neck hypertrophy was reported by Diokno in one patient after YV plasty [8].

A fibrotic bladder neck, while seen in a few cases, is not considered a primary cause but rather secondary to past infection, intervention or surgeries.

The reported occurrence in children suggests that it is either a congenital condition or acquired in early childhood. The association with anxiety may explain why a large number of patients are seen only in the post-menopausal age group.

5.4 Prevalence

Irwin estimates that 8.2% of adult women are affected by lower urinary tract symptoms [14]. A fifth of the patients seeking medical help for lower tract symptoms may have obstruction. In a specialist referral centre for video urodynamics, Malde found 19% of women with lower urinary tract symptoms (LUTS) to have BOO [15]. In a population of women with BOO, the bladder neck was the site of obstruction in 10.2%, while the remaining were due to dysfunctional voiding [1].

A lack of awareness of this condition amongst physicians leads to PBNO being easily missed in the female child. The incidence of PBNO in children of both sexes with voiding dysfunction may be as high as 6–15%. As in adults, it is more common in boys with girls constituting only 19% of children with confirmed PBNO [15, 16].

5.5 The Definition of PBNO in Women

In 1999, Nitti described BOO on video-urodynamics as radiographic evidence of obstruction anywhere between the bladder neck and urethra in the presence of raised detrusor pressures of any magnitude [17].

In 2000, Blaivas and Groutz developed their nomogram to identify BOO. The Q_{max} on a free flow and the $P_{det}Q_{max}$ were the variables used to classify women into four zones ranging from normal-to-severe obstruction [18]. In 2004, Defreitas reported that a Q_{max} of 11 ml/s and

$P_{det}Q_{max}$ of 21 cm H_2O further improved the accuracy of diagnosis [19].

While all the urodynamic controversies over definition of BOO are beyond the scope of this chapter, there is consensus that failure of the bladder neck to open during voiding must be evident on video-urodynamics for a diagnosis of PBNO. This definition does suffer from the fallacy that similar findings will be noted in an underactive detrusor where the bladder pressure generated is insufficient to adequately open the bladder neck. In males, the differentiation between the two conditions is easily achieved on evaluating detrusor pressures on pressure flow study. However, in females, this distinction sometimes becomes difficult due to overlapping detrusor pressure-based definitions of BOO and underactive bladder.

In order to avoid urodynamics in children, BOO has been defined using uroflowmetry and non-invasive electromyography (EMG). A combination of symptomatology, a lag phase (time between cessation of EMG activity and start of urinary flow) on EMG of more than 6 s and poor peak flows on repeated flow studies are used to diagnose bladder outlet obstruction. In children, a failure of alpha blocker therapy to relieve symptoms, hydronephrosis or recurrent UTI would be indications for pressure flow studies [20]. Similar studies have not been carried out in adult women and this could be an interesting area for further research.

5.6 Clinical Presentation and Diagnosis

5.6.1 History

While PBNO has no specific symptoms, it must be emphasized that a high index of suspicion of BOO must be entertained in all women presenting with LUTS or urinary tract infection (UTI). The diagnosis of BOO is not entirely objective in most cases. As many as 29% of women with BOO may present with isolated storage symptoms. Others present with mixed storage and voiding LUTS. Isolated voiding symptoms are the exception (0.5%) rather than the norm. In fact, about 37% of patients may present with burning micturition [21].

5.6.2 Examination

Local examination is done to rule out anatomical causes of BOO. An obvious prolapse or an obvious mass lesion in the periurethral area needs evaluation. Meatal stenosis is virtually unheard of in premenopausal women in the absence of an iatrogenic cause such as radiation or surgery. A palpable bladder suggests chronic retention. Examination of the spine and a focused neurological examination is necessary to rule out neurogenic bladder dysfunction. A loaded rectum on digital rectal examination points towards bladder bowel dysfunction or a neurogenic bladder. A significantly loaded rectum may be the sole cause for bladder outlet obstruction.

5.6.3 Cystoscopy

Cystoscopy reveals a normal urethra. Bladder neck itself is normal in PBNO or cases resulting from prolapse. A fibrotic or anatomically narrow bladder neck is seen only in rare cases like those which result from earlier surgical intervention or mass lesions. Trabeculations and diverticuli in the bladder may indicate evidence of chronic obstruction.

5.6.4 Ultrasound

Galica reported on the use of transvaginal ultrasound to diagnose failure of the bladder neck to open during micturition, and this correlated well with invasive video-urodynamic findings. With the bladder neck closed, the urethra and periurethral tissues appear as a cylindrical hypoechoic structure. In women with PBNO, there is no change in appearance during voiding. After bladder neck incision, there is a sonographically demonstrable change in the appearance, which the authors describe as a stem of a flower [22]. An additional finding in this study was a mean distance of 1.3 cm between the bladder neck and the vagina. This information would be valuable to the surgeon in planning a bladder neck incision.

5.6.5 Video-Urodynamics

While individual definitions vary, the final diagnosis depends on a high bladder pressure (>20–25 cm H_2O), a poor Q_{max} (<10–15 cm H_2O) along with a failure of the bladder neck to open during voiding. An absence of an increase in EMG activity suggests a diagnosis of PBNO rather than dysfunctional voiding. However, this is not a rule as increased EMG activity has been reported in 14% of women with PBNO [1]. As the activity is being measured by surface electrodes, pelvic floor muscle activity and abdominal straining can lead to an increase in EMG activity. A careful analysis has to be done by the urodynamics team to differentiate the two conditions. Urethral pressure profilometry is not indicated for a diagnosis of PBNO (Figs. 5.1 and 5.2).

5.7 Treatment

5.7.1 Medical Management

The scientific evidence supporting the use of alpha blockers in women is tentative and their use remains off label. However, they are being increasingly prescribed and a nationwide survey from Taiwan reported 1.6 times increase in the prescriptions administered to women between 2007 and 2012 [23]. The rationale for use of alpha blockers in women is based on sympathetic innervation of the bladder neck and urethra from T10–12. Resting pressures in the bladder outlet have been shown to reduce with prazosin in the mid-urethra and with tamsulosin along the entire length of the urethra [24]. Most studies on the use of alpha blockers in women tend to be small, non-randomized, single-centre studies. Response rates in improvement of symptoms have been reported in 64–67% of women on alpha blockers [25, 26]. Improvement in urodynamic parameters has also been reported by Kessler who reported a fall in $P_{det}Q_{max}$ from 45 to 35 cm H_2O and an improvement in flow rates from 9 to 20 ml/s [24]. However, use of alpha blockers in women is limited as the smooth muscle component in the bladder neck in women is scant. Therefore, clean intermittent catheterization continues to be a widely prescribed non-surgical treatment for PBNO in women. For those cases where the bladder capacity and compliance are normal with little risk for deterioration of upper tracts, timed and frequent voiding is a reasonable option. A follow-up 3–6 monthly evaluation to assess for any deterioration may be advised.

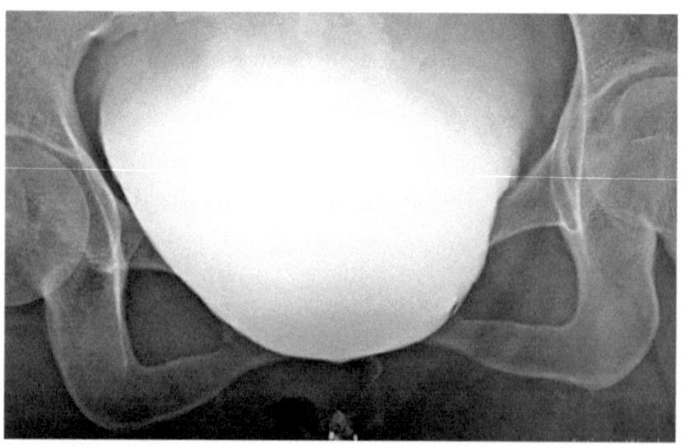

Fig. 5.1 Micturating cystourethrogram showing a closed bladder neck with a thin stream of contrast in the urethra. The radio opaque markers are at the external meatus

5.7.2 Surgical Management of PBNO

Women not responding to alpha blockers or other conservative measures should be offered surgery. Extrapolating from practices in men, women with upper tract changes, large residual volumes and recurrent urinary infections would also qualify as candidates for surgical intervention.

Bladder neck incision (BNI) offers a permanent cure to some women with PBNO. The decision for BNI should be taken with utmost caution as the literature available is still sparse. Unlike men, retrograde ejaculation is not a problem and young women can be offered a BNI. On the other hand, there is a small

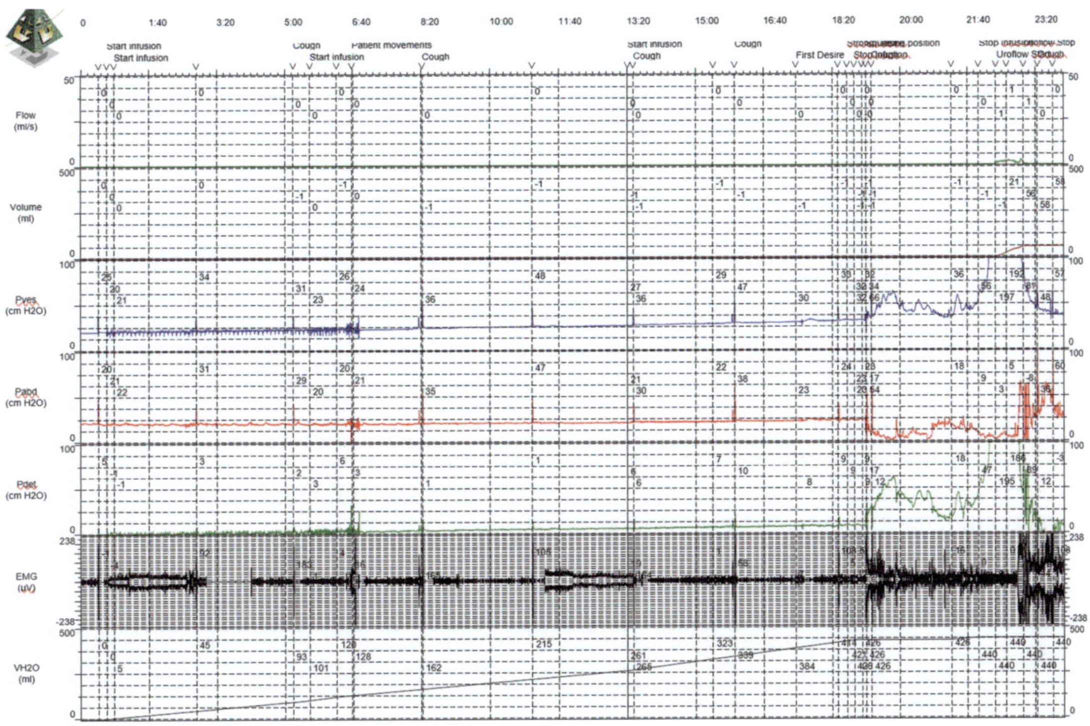

Fig. 5.2 A 28-year-old lady presented with burning micturition, frequency and poor stream of 6 months duration. The MCU in Fig. 5.1 revealed classical findings of PBNO. She underwent a single incision BNI at 6 o'clock. At 2 weeks, her peak flow rate improved from 6.3 ml/s to only 8.3 ml/s, but she had no measurable post void residue as compared to 300 ml preoperatively. At 6-month follow-up, she had persistent improvement in subjective and objective parameters

risk of stress incontinence, which must be borne in mind.

Most authors make incisions at 5 and 7 O′ clock. Some have also advocated resection of the intervening tissue. Others have reported positive outcomes even with a single incision [27–29].

In 2012, Jin et al. modified their incision technique to make four incisions at 3, 6, 9 and 12 O'clock. At 60 months all 25 of the 30 women who remained on follow-up had an improvement in symptoms and one patient who had reported stress leak had improved with pelvic floor exercises [30].

In 2014, Zhang reported improvement in multiple urodynamic parameters, including flow rate and $P_{det}Q_{max}$ with two incisions. With a follow-up of 84 patients, this study is, at present, the largest series reported in the world. In their first 63 patients, the incisions were made at 5 and 7 O′ clock. They noted three VVFs and changed the location of the incision to 2 and 10 O′ clock. No further VVFs were noted. Stress urinary leak was noted in 4.7%. The authors recommend limiting the incision to the proximal third of the urethra in order to prevent stress urinary incontinence. Bladder neck obstruction recurred in 7.14% of patients. Six patients developed recurrences requiring a repeat procedure. Five patients underwent a second BNI and one underwent a third procedure. Interestingly all 6 patients had a very high mean $P_{det}Q_{max}$ of 97.2 cm H_2O before the first procedure who then went on to have a second or even a third bladder neck incision. Urethral strictures were reported in 3.6% after BNI in this series [31]. Whether very high baseline values of $P_{det}Q_{max}$ can be used as a selection criterion for more invasive procedures like bladder neck resections at the outset may be a matter of further research.

The short length of the urethra, proximity of the vaginal mucosa and the absence of anatomical landmarks to define the extent of the incision are challenges to incision of the bladder neck in women.

We would recommend two incisions at 2 and 10 O′ clock. The length of the incision should be limited to the proximal third of the urethra. The depth should traverse the full thickness of the bladder neck muscle and reach the underlying fat.

Following BNI, these women should be kept on follow up with a 3-monthly uroflow assessment. **Long-term follow-up is recommended as recurrence may occur after years.** Worsening flow and recurrence of symptoms may be pointers to a possible recurrence and warrant re-evaluation.

Blaivas has reported a series of seven patients where incisions were made at 5 and 7 O′ clock and the intervening tissue, which he describes as similar in cystoscopic appearance to prostatic tissue, was resected. Most authors, however, feel that BNI is sufficient treatment. Resection may be reserved for recurrent bladder neck stenosis after an earlier BNI [29].

Evidence for use of Botulinum toxin in PBNO remains scanty. In 2009 Pradhan had injected Botulinum toxin into the urethra in seven women with bladder outlet obstruction and reported an improvement in flow [32]. However, he did not specify how many of his patients had PBNO. Moreover, Liao reported bladder neck obstruction to be one of the causes of failure to void after urethral injection [33]. **At present, Botulinum toxin is approved for use in overactive bladder and its use in PBNO should be limited to research settings.** Similarly, the role of neuromodulation in PBNO can only be considered investigational. A recent review on its role in female pelvic disorders did not mention PBNO as an indication [34].

In conclusion, the bladder neck in women is a functional rather than a distinct anatomical entity. A high clinical index of suspicion is essential to avoid missing patients as many women report with non-specific symptoms. Video-urodynamics remains the mainstay of diagnosis. Alpha blockers can only be used off label. In carefully selected patients, bladder neck incision can offer cure. CIC remains an option in women unwilling or unable to undergo bladder neck incision.

Clinical Case Discussion

A 28-year-old lady presented with burning micturition, frequency and poor stream 6 months duration. The MCU and UDS in Figs. 5.1 and 5.2 revealed classical findings of PBNO. She underwent a single incision BNI at 6 o'clock. At 2 weeks, her peak flow rate improved from 6.3 ml/s to only 8.3 ml/s, but she had no measurable post void residue as compared to 300 ml preoperatively. At 6-month follow-up, she had persistent improvement in subjective and objective parameters.

Key Learning Points

- After dysfunctional voiding, PBNO is the second most common cause of functional BOO in women.
- There is no consensus on aetiopathogenesis but unlike a learnt behaviour in dysfunctional voiding, PBNO is believed to result from an autonomic disturbance.
- Inability to demonstrate funnelling at bladder neck along with high detrusor pressures on a video-urodynamic study are the key to diagnosis.
- Pharmacotherapy with alpha blockers gives satisfactory symptomatic relief.
- Bladder neck incision may be curative for selected refractory cases. Risk of incontinence is minimal with proper case selection.

References

1. Brucker BM, Fong E, Shah S, Kelly C, Rosenblum N, Nitti VW. Urodynamic differences between dysfunctional voiding and primary bladder neck obstruction in women. Urology. 2012;80(1):55–60.
2. Gilpin SA, Gosling JA. Smooth muscle in the wall of the developing human urinary bladder and urethra. J Anat. 1983;137.(Pt 3:503–12.
3. Yucel S, Baskin LS. An anatomical description of the male and female urethral sphincter complex. J Urol. 2004;171(5):1890–7.
4. Oswald J, Heidegger I, Steiner E, et al. Gender-related fetal development of the internal urethral sphincter. Urology. 2013;82(6):1410–5.

5. Caulk JR. Contracture of the vesical neck in the female. J Urol. 1921;6:341–3.
6. Jacobson CE Jr. Unrecognized vesical neck obstruction in women. N Engl J Med. 1946;235(18):645–8.
7. Corrin B, Mayor D, Moor T. The pathology of bladder neck obstruction in the female patient. J Urol. 1963;90:434–9.
8. Diokno AC, Hollander JB, Bennett CJ. Bladder neck obstruction in women: a real entity. J Urol. 1984;132(2):294–8.
9. Farrar DJ, Osborne JL, Stephenson TP, Whiteside CG, Weir J, Berry J, Milroy EJ, Warwick RT. A urodynamic view of bladder outflow obstruction in the female: factors influencing the results of treatment. Br J Urol. 1975;47(7):815–22.
10. George NJ, Slade N. Hesitancy and poor stream in younger men without outflow tract obstruction—the anxious bladder. Br J Urol. 1979;51(6):506–9.
11. Saito M, Longhurst PA, Tammela TL, Wein AJ, Levin RM. Effects of partial outlet obstruction of the rat urinary bladder on micturition characteristics, DNA synthesis and the contractile response to field stimulation and pharmacological agents. J Urol. 1993;150(3):1045–51.
12. Axelrod SL, Blaivas JG. Bladder neck obstruction in women. J Urol. 1987;137(3):497–9.
13. Mayo ME. Primary bladder neck obstruction in men: variation in detrusor response. J Urol. 1982;128(5):957–9.
14. Irwin DE, Kopp ZS, Agatep B, Milsom I, Abrams P. Worldwide prevalence estimates of lower urinary tract symptoms, overactive bladder, urinary incontinence and bladder outlet obstruction. BJU Int. 2011;108(7):1132–8.
15. Malde S, Solomon E, Spilotros M, et al. Female bladder outlet obstruction: common symptoms masking an uncommon cause. Low Urin Tract Symptoms. 2019;11(1):72–7.
16. Grafstein NH, Combs AJ, Glassberg KI. Primary bladder neck dysfunction: an overlooked entity in children. Curr Urol Rep. 2005;6(2):133–9.
17. Nitti VW. Pressure flow urodynamic studies: the gold standard for diagnosing bladder outlet obstruction. Rev Urol. 2005;7(Suppl 6):S14–21.
18. Blaivas JG, Groutz A. Bladder outlet obstruction nomogram for women with lower urinary tract symptomatology. Neurourol Urodyn. 2000;19(5):553–64.
19. Defreitas GA, Zimmern PE, Lemack GE, Shariat SF. Refining diagnosis of anatomic female bladder outlet obstruction: comparison of pressure-flow study parameters in clinically obstructed women with those of normal controls. Urology. 2004;64(4):675–9; discussion 679–81.
20. Combs AJ, Grafstein N, Horowitz M, Glassberg KI. Primary bladder neck dysfunction in children and adolescents I: pelvic floor electromyography lag time—a new noninvasive method to screen for and monitor therapeutic response. J Urol. 2005;173(1):207–10; discussion 210–1.
21. Chuang FC, Huang KH, Kuo HC. Lower urinary tract symptoms and video-urodynamic characteristics of women with clinically unsuspected bladder outlet obstruction. Low Urin Tract Symptoms. 2013;5(1):23–7.
22. Galica V, Toska E, Saldutto P, Galatioto GP, Vicentini C. Use of transvaginal ultrasound in females with primary bladder neck obstruction. A preliminary study. Arch Ital Urol Androl. 2015;87(2):158–60.
23. Lin YH, Huang WY, Chang CC, Chen YF, Wu LY, Chang HC, Huang KH. Trends in the use of antimuscarinics and alpha-adrenergic blockers in women with lower urinary tract symptoms in Taiwan: a nationwide, population-based study, 2007–2012. PLoS One. 2019;14(10):e0220615.
24. Kessler TM, Studer UE, Burkhard FC. The effect of terazosin on functional bladder outlet obstruction in women: a pilot study. J Urol. 2006;176(4 Pt 1):1487–92.
25. Thind P, Lose G, Colstrup H, Andersson KE. The effect of alpha-adrenoceptor stimulation and blockade on the static urethral sphincter function in healthy females. Scand J Urol Nephrol. 1992;26(3):219–25.
26. Reitz A, Haferkamp A, Kyburz T, Knapp PA, Wefer B, Schurch B. The effect of tamsulosin on the resting tone and the contractile behaviour of the female urethra: a functional urodynamic study in healthy women. Eur Urol. 2004;46(2):235–40.
27. Kumar A, Mandhani A, Gogoi S, Srivastava A. Management of functional bladder neck obstruction in women: use of alpha-blockers and pediatric resectoscope for bladder neck incision. J Urol. 1999;162(6):2061–5.
28. Blaivas JG, Flisser A, Tash JA. Treatment of primary bladder neck obstruction in women with transurethral resection of the bladder neck. J Urol. 2004;171(3):1172–5.
29. Peng CH, Kuo HC. Transurethral incision of bladder neck in treatment of bladder neck obstruction in women. Urology. 2005;65(2):275–8.
30. Jin XB, Qu HW, Liu H, Li B, Wang J, Zhang YD. Modified transurethral incision for primary bladder neck obstruction in women: a method to improve voiding function without urinary incontinence. Urology. 2012;79(2):310–3.
31. Zhang P, Wu ZJ, Xu L, Yang Y, Zhang N, Zhang XD. Bladder neck incision for female bladder neck obstruction: long-term outcomes. Urology. 2014;83(4):762–6.
32. Pradhan AA. Botulinum toxin: an emerging therapy in female bladder outlet obstruction. Indian J Urol. 2009;25(3):318–20.
33. Liao YM, Kuo HC. Causes of failed urethral botulinum toxin A treatment for emptying failure. Urology. 2007;70(4):763–6.
34. El-Azab AS, Siegel SW. Sacral neuromodulation for female pelvic floor disorders. Arab J Urol. 2019;17(1):14–22.

Fowler's Syndrome of Recurrent Painless Retention in Women

6

L. N. Dorairajan and Sidhartha Kalra

Learning Objectives

- To discuss the causes of urinary retention in young women.
- To review the typical clinical features associated with Fowler's Syndrome.
- To appreciate the current understanding about etiopathogenesis of this condition.
- To understand how to evaluate a woman suspected to have Fowler's Syndrome.
- To know the management options available to treat a woman with Fowler's Syndrome.

6.1 Introduction

Urinary retention in young women without an organic cause is a rare occurrence and can be a challenging problem to manage. It can be acute-onset sudden retention, with painful inability to pass urine. While chronic urinary retention (CUR) is defined as a significant post void residual urine (PVR) of more than 300 ml after voiding on repeated assessments, though the volume of PVR to define CUR is an arbitrary one and varies with various descriptions. Common clinical manifestations of CUR include frequency, urgency, urge urinary incontinence, nocturia and nocturnal incontinence, often associated on examination, with a palpable but painless bladder [1, 2]. CUR may result in back pressure changes and lead to renal failure. Nevertheless, some patients with CUR may be asymptomatic especially in the initial phase of obstruction and may be diagnosed only incidentally by the presence of a high PVR.

Urinary retention can be either due to bladder outlet obstruction (BOO) or detrusor underactivity (DU). The two may often co-exist. The factors contributing to urinary retention can be anatomical, neurogenic or myogenic. Moreover, some drugs can cause retention as a side effect. Where no organic cause is evident, the retention is deemed as "functional". Most of the time, a clear cause can be demonstrated with routine urological evaluation and genitourinary organ assessment.

Historically, urinary retention in young women with no obvious organic cause was considered secondary to psychogenic illness or an unexplained DUA and required an indwelling catheter or urinary diversion. In 1986, Fowler et al. described a particular pattern of electromyography (EMG) activity recorded using concentric needle electrode in the rhabdosphincter, and associated it with failure of urethral sphincter relaxation in a group of women suffering from unexplained urinary retention [3]. This finding was correlated later with the occurrence of painless urinary retention in polycystic ovarian disease (PCOD) in premenopausal women leading

L. N. Dorairajan (✉) · S. Kalra
Department of Urology, JIPMER, Puducherry, India

N. Khattar et al. (eds.), *Female Bladder Outlet Obstruction and Urethral Reconstruction*,
https://doi.org/10.1007/978-981-15-8521-0_6

to the description of a syndrome, now known as Fowler's syndrome (FS) [4].

Nowadays, such cases of idiopathic urinary retention in young woman have increasingly been recognized by urologists and neurologist. Nevertheless, to label them as FS requires an expert clinical assessment and laboratory correlation. Moreover, FS does not yield to various treatment modalities, including clean intermittent self-catheterization (CISC), which, typically, these patients find very discomforting. Sacral neuromodulation (SNM) has had promising results in carefully selected patients but does have its constraints of cost and malfunctions [5]. This chapter discusses the epidemiology, etiopathogenesis, clinical presentation and management options for FS.

6.2 Defining Fowler's Syndrome

Fowler's syndrome is a painless retention of urine occurring in young women with no obvious organic cause secondary to a poorly relaxing external sphincter activity. This in turn results in inhibition of afferent signals to the bladder leading to a decrease in bladder sensation and detrusor underactivity. Diagnosis is based on clinical, videourodynamic and characteristic electromyography findings of the external urethral sphincter [3, 4]. These are further elaborated in Sects. 6.5 and 6.6.

6.3 Epidemiology

Urinary retention in young women who are otherwise normal is a rare occurrence with limited literature on the true incidence of the problem. Three-hundred cases of acute urinary retention in women were reported over an 11-year period (1996–2007) in a study from Glasgow, UK. Urethral stenosis (diagnosed on cystoscopy) (17%) was the most predominant cause. Urinary tract infection (11%), constipation (7.6%), neurovesical dysfunction (4.7%), gynecological causes (5.3%), postoperative (7%), antidepressant or anticholinergic medications (2.3%) and hematuria from bladder cancer leading to clot retention(4%) were the other causes. Despite 28% patients having no organic cause, only one (0.3%) case was diagnosed as FS, suggesting the rarity of the condition. However, low reporting of this condition might have been due to the difficulty in diagnosis [1]. In a survey conducted among urology consultants in the U.K., unexplained urinary retention was seen in an estimated mean of one woman per year per consultant. It was estimated that a total of 630 patients present annually with urinary retention, which is a small number, indicating the rarity of this disorder in young women [5]. This study included 247 women with unexplained urinary retention referred to a specialized neurourology center over 4 years. The mean age was 35 years in this retrospective study and only 57.5% of those women without a neurological or anatomical cause of voiding LUTS were diagnosed with FS [5]. The diagnosis was made on the basis of a detailed history, maximal urethral closure pressure (MUCP) on urethral pressure profilometry and sphincter volume as measured on ultrasonography with or without electromyography study. While this seemingly high frequency of diagnosis of this rare condition could be due to the fact that the center received patients referred from all over the United Kingdom, it is also possible that the diagnosis is missed by many urologists who might be labelling the condition as dysfunctional voiding without performing detailed investigations to look for this syndrome.

6.4 Pathophysiology of Bladder Dysfunction in Fowler's Syndrome

The etiology of FS is still not very clear. Fowler and her colleagues described an unusual EMG of extrinsic sphincter by using concentric needle electrode examination in young women with idiopathic retention (Fig. 6.1) [3]. Abnormal EMG tracing from the external sphincter had previously been described in various disorders (including multiple sclerosis) and had generically been termed as pseudomyotonia [7]. However,

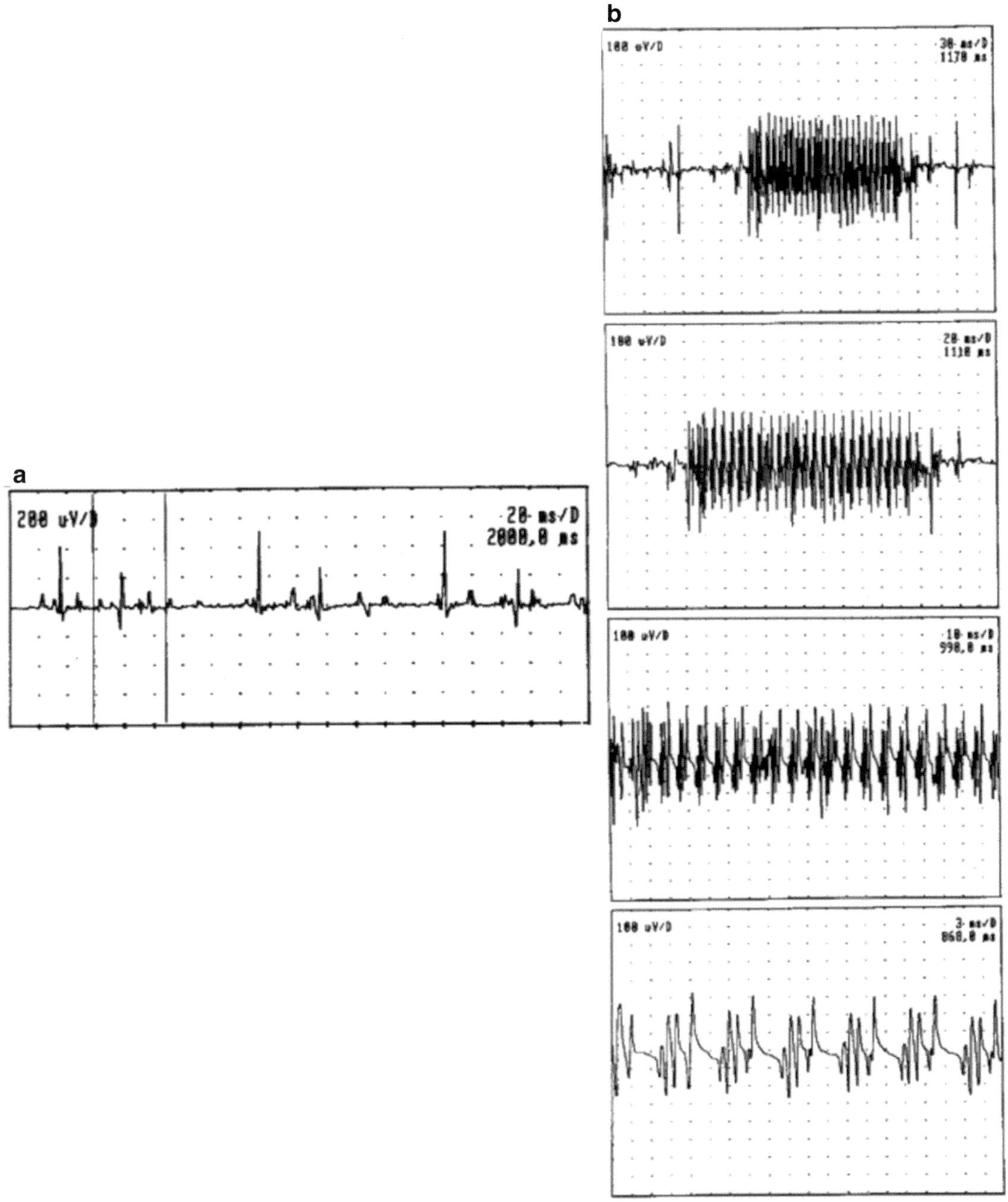

Fig. 6.1 Electromyography recording using concentric needle electrode at striated urethral sphincter. (**a**) Normal resting interference pattern with three or four motor units firing tonically. (**b**) In a woman with Fowler's Syndrome and in urinary retention showing a series of complex repetitive discharges. Note effect of increasingly expanding time base from 30 to 3 ms per division, so that waveform of complexes firing repetitively becomes apparent and forms burst discharge (top) (Reproduced from Swinn MJ, Wiseman OJ, Lowe E, et al. The cause and natural history of isolated urinary retention in young women. J Urol. 2002;167:151 with permission from Wolters Kluwer Health, Inc [6])

what Fowler et al. described was a specific type of hyperactivity comprising complex repetitive discharges and decelerating bursts of the external urethral sphincter (EUS) secondary to the so-called ephaptic intermuscular fibers signal transmission. They suggested that akin to cardiac striated muscle, striated muscle fibers of EUS also activate each other (one to many) through adjoining cell membranes [8, 9]. This is unlike the one to one synaptic transmission at the neuromuscular junction. This results in a vicious cycle that leads to a persistent high tone of the sphincter accompanied by the loss of the ability to relax the sphincter. Also, this long-term hyperactivity of the EUS leads to the hypertrophy of the EUS demonstrable on transvaginal ultrasound by 7.5-Hz probe [10].

This high tone can also be detected in many patients on urethral pressure profilometry (UPP). A high-tone nonrelaxing EUS increases urethral afferent activity, which, in turn, potentiates the spinal pro-continence reflex and inhibits bladder afferent signal from reaching the brain resulting in poor bladder filling sensation and detrusor underactivity (Fig. 6.2). Studies using the neuro-imaging techniques positron emission tomography and functional magnetic resonance imaging have demonstrated an increased activity in the midbrain (periaqueductal grey [PAG]) and limbic cortical regions) with bladder filling in healthy controls, while in women with FS there was no significant midbrain activity observed during bladder filling [12, 13]. These observations thus support the hypothesis of afferent pro-continence reflex mechanism as a probable cause for retention and decreased bladder sensation in FS. But it must be noted that these studies had very small groups of patients. Nevertheless, testing these patients treated with SNM has shown that the activity of PAG and pontine micturition center activity were restored, possibly by suppressing the increased urethral afferent activity via stimulation of S3 nerve root [13]. Other factors such as opiate-based medication can aggravate the void-

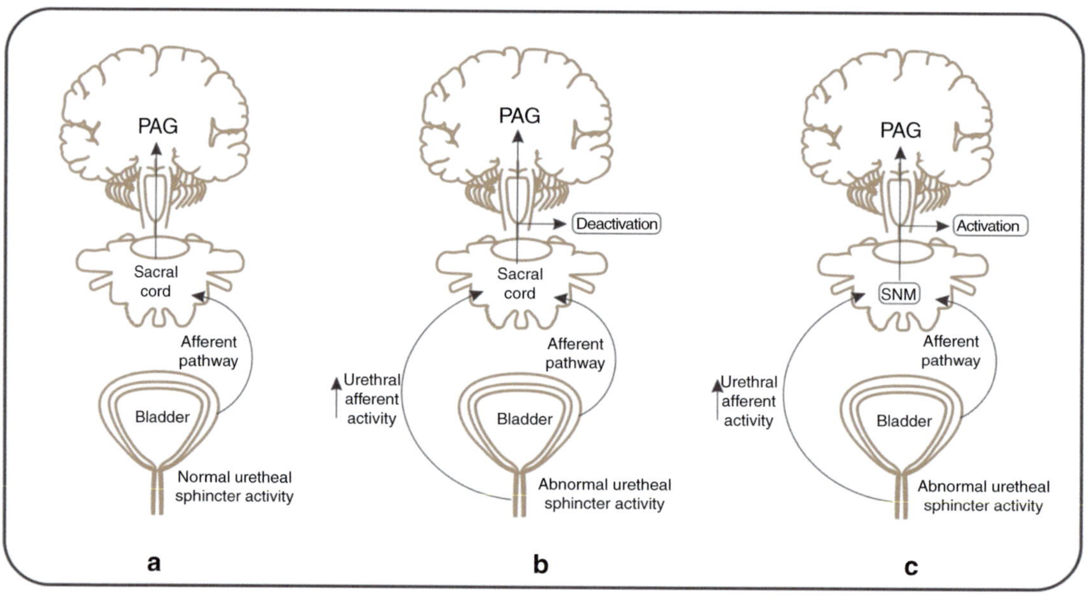

Fig. 6.2 Voiding dysfunction in Fowler's syndrome. (**a**) Normal bladder filling, bladder afferent signaling leads to activation of higher centers (PAG) and normal bladder function. (**b**) In Fowler's syndrome, abnormally strong afferent urethral sphincter activity via sacral cord, leads to inhibition of bladder afferent activity and deactivation of the higher brain centers. **c.** SNM restores bladder afferent transmission (by blocking urethral inhibition) resulting in activation of higher centers and return of bladder function. *PAG* periaqueductal gray, *SNM* sacral neuromodulation (Reproduced with modification from Osman NI, Chapple CR. Fowler's syndrome–a cause of unexplained urinary retention in young women? Nat Rev Urol. 2014;11(02):87 with permission from Springer Nature [11])

ing difficulties in patients suffering from FS, thereby precipitating and increasing the incidence of retention. Exogenous opioids might act through their effects at the sacral cord (Onuf's nucleus), while endogenous opioids possibly act as a neurotransmitter that inhibits detrusor function through a local increase of enkephalin levels in spinal cord [14].

An alternative viewpoint suggested is the presence of hormone-sensitive channelopathy manifesting as localized sphincteric abnormality secondary to relative deficiency of progesterone considering the high association of this disease with PCOD [15, 16]. **But good-quality evidence is lacking to link PCOD with abnormal electromyography of FS** [17]. Whether specific situations, such as general anesthesia, "unmasks" an underlying abnormality, still needs to be proven. Amarenco et al. hypothesized that FS was secondary to an occult generalized dysautonomia in which the only clinical manifestation was voiding dysfunction. They performed five cardiovascular autonomic function tests (CAFTs) that included heart-rate response to deep breathing, cold-pressor response, Valsalva ratio, blood pressure response to standing and sympathetic skin response in ten such women. Six out of ten women had more than two CAFT positive, although none had symptoms of dysautonomia [18]. They concluded that dysautonomia might be the probable cause for voiding dysfunction, similar to autonomic neuropathies like diabetes mellitus or Guillain-Barré syndrome, where voiding problems are seen in 75–100% and 25–28% of patients, respectively [19, 20]. But this conclusion is limited by the fact that this study had a very small number of patients and no control group.

6.5 Clinical Features of Fowler's Syndrome

FS has only been reported in hormonally active women, never in males, with a peak incidence in the third decade of life. A significantly high association with PCOD and endometriosis in up to 50% of the patients has been demonstrated [11]. Typically, these young women present with inability to void and urinary retention with post void residual volumes in excess of a liter of urine, which is disproportionately painless. Some of them may present with voiding lower urinary symptoms associated with urinary frequency and occasional urgency, but incontinence is rarely reported. Straining does not help in emptying and some of these patients intuitively learn to relax their sphincter with marginal benefit [6].

Often a correlation with a triggering event, generally a surgical procedure using regional or general anesthesia, can be found prior to urinary retention. In a study of patients with FS and complete urinary retention, 65% cases had an identifiable triggering event such as gynecological surgery (30%); childbirth (15%), other surgical procedures (including remote sites surgery) (13%) and acute medical conditions (7%) [6]. Whether aesthesia is the cause for such an event still isn't clear. However, it can be a source of medico-legal complaints. Therefore, as there's suspicion of such a possibility, young women with a history of poor voiding or prolonged micturition patterns undergoing surgery should be appropriately counseled before surgery about the possibility of their symptoms getting worse.

Women with FS find self-catheterization for retention often painful, particularly during withdrawal of the catheter, with a sensation of "something gripping." Some of these patients might end up requiring an alternate drainage procedure such as suprapubic catheter [21]. In a recent retrospective review, significantly high association with other co-morbidities, particularly psychological and probable functional disorders, was seen in this group of patients. Whether they are the cause or effect of the problem is still not clear. Data are not suggestive of resolution of these symptoms after a successful neuro-stimulation surgery where the urinary symptoms resolve [21].

Spontaneous recovery of voiding dysfunction is unlikely except in cases where the urinary retention follows childbirth. Nine of 14 such women were found to void spontaneously [6]. Diagnosis of FS in a patient with urinary retention cannot be based only on clinical assessment. A detailed history should be obtained to exclude

Table 6.1 Clinical characteristic of Fowler syndrome

History and clinical examination	• Hormonally active young women • High association with PCOD and endometriosis • Painless retention with large residue in excess of 1 l • Triggering event, e.g. surgery, general anaesthesia, illness • No structural or neurological deficit on examination • Difficulty in self-catheterization
Videourodynamics assessment and urethral pressure profilometry	• Large-capacity bladder • Absent or decreased sensation • Absent or decreased detrusor pressure with low flow • Open bladder neck with midurethral stenosis, with or without posterior urethral dilatation
Concentric needle EMG	• Complex repetitive discharges with decelerating burst
Transvaginal sphincter ultrasonography	• Increased sphincter volume

other possible etiologies, particularly medication history. Antidepressants, sedatives and opiates are well known to cause urinary retention. Discontinuation of these drugs may improve sensations and voiding, in women with unexplained retention [22]. The characteristic features of FS are enumerated in Table 6.1.

6.6 Diagnosis of Fowler's Syndrome

The initial assessment in any young women presenting with urinary retention should focus on good clinical history and thorough lower urinary tract examination, with an assessment of its neural control. Besides the basic routine evaluation, pelvic imaging, usually by ultrasonography, and MRI of the spine and urethrocystoscopy where necessary should be undertaken. Specialized testing with urethral sphincter electromyography (concentric needle), videourodynamic studies, UPP, and transvaginal ultrasonography forms an important tool for diagnosing FS. Diagnostic criteria include at least one reading of bladder volume of 1 l or more, exclusion of other known causes, a high maximum urethral closure pressure on UPP, increased volume of the EUS on ultrasonographic or MRI assessment and, if feasible, a characteristic urethral sphincter EMG.

6.6.1 Videourodynamic Studies (VUDS)

High-quality videourodynamic study holds the key in diagnosing and differentiating various causes of bladder outlet obstruction. Urodynamic studies are generally conducted with a synchronous surface electromyography, which might be of help in diagnosing dysfunctional voiding from other causes such as primary bladder neck obstruction [23]. However, the diagnostic value of surface electromyography in FS is limited. The classical findings noted in a urodynamic study with FS include delayed sensation with a large bladder capacity during filling. The patient is usually unable to void, and there is no rise in detrusor pressure. Sometimes patient voids with poor flow staccato pattern with low-amplitude detrusor contraction, in contrast to the classic high-pressure low-flow pattern seen with other causes of BOO. There is still a paucity of quality videourodynamic data in FS. Common fluoroscopic findings reported are an open bladder neck during voiding and narrowing at the EUS with or without dilation of the proximal urethra.

There are no clear urodynamic criteria defined for diagnosing BOO in women. Most of the women experience difficulty in voiding during a urodynamic assessment. This can sometimes add to the volitional component in interpreting the results [11, 24]. Perhaps a recording of traces over a period of time with natural filling, i.e. ambulatory urodynamics, may play a better role in characterizing the pressure flow dynamics in this group of patients and predict outcome. In some of the studies, there is not always "true" acontractility, but rather detrusor underactivity, which is defined as "a contraction of reduced strength and/or duration resulting in prolonged bladder emptying and/or failure to achieve complete bladder emptying within a normal time-span,", by the International Continence Society [25]. Some studies have shown that patients with detrusor acontractility are less likely to experience successful outcome when treated with SNM than those with detrusor hypocontractility [26].

6.6.2 Concentric Needle Electromyography

EUS normally is in tonic contractile state during rest and relaxes during voiding [27]. Surface (patch) electrodes for EMG is a combined representation of pelvic floor, external anal and urethral sphincter activity. Activity recorded here is not specific for a spontaneous pathological electromyography activity, but rather it is representation of motor unit action potential (it detects presence of activity but not so much the type).On the contrary, concentric needle electromyography of the striated urethral sphincter is more specific for striated external sphincter and has striking diagnostic characteristics for FS [28]. Concentric needle electromyography can be uncomfortable to the patient. Thus, the reactive changes of inactivity due to painful stimuli can be conflicting and it does require specialized equipment and expertise for interpreting accurately.

The abnormal electromyography activity in patients with FS consists of two components—Complex repetitive discharges (CRD) and decelerating bursts (a deceleration of part of the CRD) (Fig. 6.1). CRD sound like helicopters over the audio-amplifier of the EMG machine, while decelerating bursts (DB) are heard as under water whale songs. In one of the studies, EMG analysis showed presence of both CRD with DB in 33 of 57 women (58%) with unexplained urinary retention [4]. These findings only suggest the presence or absence of the abnormality and not the severity or functional impact of the disease. Nevertheless, concentric needle electromyography remains the definitive method of diagnosis [3, 4]. It should be borne in mind that up to 30–53% of healthy asymptomatic women have also been shown to have such abnormal electromyograph activity [29]. These CRDs on single fiber EMG analysis have shown to be of low potential. It is likely that ephaptic transmission between muscle fibers leads to a repetitive, vicious, self-excitation [30]. This abnormal activity is believed to cause involuntary pathological contraction of the EUS. This results in activation of sphincter afferents leading to abnormal voiding. Urinary retention occurs as a secondary effect of this abnormal sphincter contraction and occurs when the inhibitory signals are strong enough. **The finding of CRDs and DB activity in apparently asymptomatic young women, therefore, does not negate the significance of the finding of the EMG activity in explaining urinary retention in a FS** [29]. In clinical practice, concentric needle EMG is not performed except at some focused tertiary-care centers. And most of the women undergo treatment on clinical assessment supported by tests that demonstrate the high-tone nonrelaxing EUS such as VUDS with surface EMG, UPP and transvaginal ultrasonography [10]. And, therefore, **some experts choose to describe this condition as high-tone nonrelaxing sphincter or HTNRS rather than Fowler's syndrome** [31]. This approach can sometimes be inconclusive in suggesting a definitive diagnosis and deciding for definitive management.

6.6.3 Urethral Pressure Profilometry (UPP)

Urethral pressure profilometry (UPP) measures the maximal urethral closure pressure (MUCP), that is difference between the urethral pressure and the intravesical pressure and is an indirect representation of sphincter function. The resting MUCP is typically more than 100 cm of water in women with FS. Wiseman et al. demonstrated a significantly higher MUCP (103 ± 26.4 vs. 76.7 ± 18.4 cm H_2O; $p < 0.001$) in women having FS than in those without any abnormalities [10].

Some researchers suggest that this high MUCP is not specific for FS and is often found in many patients who have dysfunctional voiding [11]. In another retrospective review, no significant difference in MUCP was observed in women with voiding dysfunction having abnormal electromyography versus normal EMG [32]. Also other causes like pelvic floor spasm and extrinsic compression can contribute to high MUCP and should be ruled out. Technical variability and lack of expertise pose a limitation for routinely adapting UPP as a diagnostic tool. The cut-offs for diagnosis of FS using MUCP have not yet been validated. Consequently, UPP is not routinely used in most centers. Further clinical studies are needed to determine its role either in the evaluation of FS or predicting outcomes following sacral neuromodulation.

6.6.4 Transvaginal Sphincter Ultrasonography

EUS volume may be measured using transvaginal ultrasonography with a 7.5-Hz probe. Whether the hypertrophy of EUS seen in patients with FS is a result of overactivity or not is not certain as yet [33]. Wiseman et al. found a significantly higher EUS volume (2.29 ± 0.64 vs. 1.62 ± 0.32 cm^3; $p < 0.001$) in patients with FS [10]. It should be noted that this investigation is operator dependent and no age-specific cut-off values are defined to diagnose high EUS volume. Nevertheless, ultrasonography can serve as an adjunct to other investigations and help in identifying other causes of voiding difficulty such as urethral diverticulum.

6.7 Differentiation from Other Conditions

6.7.1 Other Causes of Urinary Retention in Women

Urinary retention due to anatomical causes are rare in young women. Still, a thorough assessment should be done to rule out extrinsic causes such as urethral diverticula, uterine and cervical fibroids and cysts of the vaginal wall [34]. Other functional causes of urinary retention should be ruled out before diagnosing FS (Table 6.2). These are discussed in greater detail.

6.7.2 Dysfunctional Voiding

Dysfunctional voiding is a learned voiding pattern associated with involuntary intermittent contractions of the striated sphincter and/or pelvic floor muscles during voiding in neurologically normal women leading to intermittent and/or fluctuating flow rate [35].

Approximately 2% of adults referred for urodynamic evaluation have dysfunctional voiding. There is generally a preceding history of a condition such as inflammation, infections such as urethritis, cystitis, and vaginitis, trauma or irritation suffered in childhood or in early adult life [36]. History of psychological trauma or sexual abuse can be a triggering factor for developing such a behaviour [37]. Dysfunctional voiding ending in complete retention (previously called non-neurogenic neurogenic bladder or Hinman syndrome) is very rare. These patients, however, can have upper tract changes and generally the bladder is not atonic in contrast to the findings in FS [36].

Deindl et al. [38] by kinesiological EMG demonstrated that in **dysfunctional voiding there is an abnormal hyperactivity of the urogenital and pelvic diaphragm, including levator ani muscles and external anal sphincter as distinct from FS where there is only isolated EUS involved**. The diagnosis is made using simultaneous videourodynamics and sphincter electromyograph using surface electrodes. On fluoroscopy, a narrowing of the urethra is observed at the level of the striated sphincter with proximal dilatation of the urethra ("spinning-top urethra"). Normal voiding can generally be achieved by behavioral therapy such as pelvic floor muscle relaxation, biofeedback, and cognitive therapy.

Table 6.2 Differential diagnosis of functional urinary retention in women

Clinical diagnosis	Pathogenesis	Videourodynamic characteristic	EMG	Treatment
Fowler syndrome	Poorly relaxing external sphincter with increased urethral afferent signaling leading to DUA	Hyposensory, hypocontractilebladder with absent or low-flow voiding Open bladder neck with midurethral stenosis with or without posterior urethral dilatation.	Increased EUS activity; complex repetitive discharges with decelerating burst	Self-catheterization; SNM Intrasphincteric botulinum toxin
Dysfunctional voiding	Learned behaviour of inability to adequately relax pelvic floor during voiding	Normal sensation with high-pressure low-flow voiding with raised post-void residue Dilated posterior urethra (spinning top)	Increased pelvic floor activity during voiding	Pelvic floor muscle training Biofeedback
Primary bladder neck obstruction	Poor relaxation of bladder neck, smooth muscle hypertrophy	Normal sensory normal capacity bladder High-pressure low-flow voiding With raised PVR Closed bladder neck	Normal	Medical management Bladder neck incision
Idiopathic DUA	Primary failure of detrusor contraction secondary to neurogenic or myogenic failure	Low-pressure low-flow voiding	Normal	Bladder drainage
Chronic intestinal pseudo obstruction	Detrusor failure secondary to visceral neuropathy	Large-capacity hypo-sensory bladder Low-pressure low-flow voiding	Normal	Bladder drainage

6.7.3 Primary Bladder Neck Obstruction

Primary bladder neck obstruction is functional obstruction at the level of bladder neck secondary to smooth muscle hypertrophy or an increased sensitivity of the bladder neck to sympathetic stimulation. Urodynamic studies show a high-pressure low-flow voiding pattern, and there is minimal activity seen on surface electrode electromyography during voiding. Fluoroscopy, during voiding, shows no opening or funneling of the bladder neck [39]. Initial management is to try α-blockers, but this has met with variable success [40]. Transurethral bladder neck incision is an effective treatment for patients failing medical treatment [41].

6.7.4 Idiopathic Detrusor Underactivity

Detrusor underactivity is commonly seen in elderly individuals and can be secondary to neurogenic or myogenic failure. DU without an identifiable cause is rare in young women. Typically, urodynamic studies show a low-pressure, low-flow voiding pattern. There is no effective treatment available at present other than continuous bladder drainage or clean intermittent self-catheterization. Women with FS often report lower-bowel dysfunction and another differential diagnosis is chronic idiopathic pseudo-obstruction, a rare syndrome characterized by chronic bowel obstruction without an identifiable anatomical cause. LUT dysfunction in the form of detrusor hypo-contractility has been reported in up to 10–69% of such patients [42, 43].

6.7.5 Neurogenic Bladder

Neurological causes generally present with identifiable clinical signs and symptoms. Voiding dysfunction is a significant feature in patients suffering from lesions of the conus medullaris or the cauda equina. Retention may also occur following radical pelvic surgery due to surgical damage to the sympathetic ganglia and post-ganglionic fibers. Multiple Sclerosis can lead to urinary retention and these patients will have other symptoms of limb weakness and visual disturbances.

6.8 Treatment Options

Unexplained urinary retention in young women often attracts extensive work up, including invasive investigations, be it under the care of a urologist or of a gynecologist. The primary aim of treatment in these patients is to ensure adequate emptying of the bladder. Clean intermittent self-catheterization, although bothersome, is generally the first option for these patients. Various strategies to relax the sphincter, such as medications and local injection of botulinum toxin, have been tried; the only treatment that has been most effective in restoring voiding is sacral nerve stimulation.

Most of these patients with time start associating their symptoms secondary to psychogenic factors. Whether they are the cause or consequence of this problem is still unclear [6]. Thus, it is important for a treating clinician to have individualized patient approach not only from the point of organic issues but also to deal with the patient psychological state. Efficacy of treatment depends a lot on patient motivation. Given the profound psychological limitations, an honest discussion with the patient right at the onset of treatment regarding the likely outcomes is essential for the success of the treatment.

6.8.1 Bladder Drainage

Clean intermittent self-catheterization for bladder drainage is the primary line of management for urinary retention with frequency of catherization depending upon the degree of incomplete bladder emptying. Women with FS often report difficulties in performing self-catheterization, especially complaining of a gripping sensation while attempting to remove the catheter. In a survey conducted among women with FS, out of 91 patients 69% reported this gripping sensation and discomfort during catherization [6]. Therefore, an experienced health care professional should be involved in teaching CISC to these patients with adequate understanding of the problem. A suprapubic catheter, if needed, is clearly not an ideal definitive treatment option in young women. A continent diversion with a catheterizable stoma, although more invasive, but does not interfere with patient's self-perception of body image or day-to-day activities and may be preferred by such patients [44].

6.8.2 Oral Pharmacotherapy

Currently no pharmacotherapy has been proven to be effective for voiding in FS. A placebo-controlled randomized trial using phosphodiesterase inhibitor (nitric oxide-induced relaxation of the rhabdosphincter) in women with FS didn't show any promising results [45]. There is little evidence to suggest that α-blockers are effective in treating women with voiding dysfunction. Chang et al. have demonstrated an improvement in symptoms in women with voiding dysfunction with tamsulosin [46]. Nevertheless, in clinical practice, these medications have not been found to be beneficial in women with FS. Although oral bethanechol has been tried as a treatment for detrusor acontractility causing retention, there is a lack of evidence for its efficacy in women with FS having sphincteric overactivity as well.

6.8.3 Intrasphincteric Botulinum Toxin Injection

Urethral sphincter botulinum toxin injection has been evaluated in patients with neurogenic sphincter dysfunctions, such as detrusor sphincter dyssynergia due to injury to the spinal cord [47]. The rationale for using botulinum toxin in sphincter hyperactivity and voiding dysfunction is by relaxing the EUS and thereby reducing outflow obstruction and/or reversing the inhibition of detrusor function and improving voiding. There has been some success reported with botulinum toxin injection in women with voiding dysfunction. In a study of 21 patients, both men and women, with neurogenic as well as non-neurogenic voiding dysfunction, 13 women showed improved voiding ability after intrasphincteric injection of 80–100 units of onabotulinum A toxin. Twelve of these patients had detrusor–sphincter dyssynergia, eight cases were of pelvic floor spasticity, and one had detrusor acontractility due to multiple sclerosis [48]. Experience of this therapy in FS is limited. Initially six women with FS were treated with low-dose botulinum toxin (200 units abobotulinumtoxin A) injection into the EUS at the site of the abnormal electromyograph activity. None of the patients showed any symptomatic improvement [49]. Abobotulinumtoxin A (Dysport™) has been used only in the context of clinical trials for the treatment of various types of voiding dysfunctions and is not approved for such uses in either the US or in Europe. For ease of understanding, from the experience gained out of these trials, the dose of abobotulinumtoxin A used is 2.5 times the dose of onabotulinumtoxin A used for these conditions [50]. A recently conducted pilot study with high-dose botulinum toxin (100 units onabotulinum toxin) in ten women with FS demonstrated a significant improvement in voiding symptoms with no serious side effects. In women who had incomplete retention, Qmax of 8.12 ml/s improved to 15.8 ml/s at week 10. Spontaneous voiding resumed in four of the five women and progressive improvement in voiding continued up to week 10. There was a reduction in mean PVR from 260 to 89 ml and the mean static UPP 23 cm H_2O. None of the patients reported stress urinary incontinence and 70% of these women opted for a repeat injection when the effect diminished over time [51]. Patients with detrusor underactivity had higher chances of failure. In comparison to the earlier trial, here a much higher dose of botulinum toxin (100 units of onabotulinum vs. 200 units of abobotulinum A toxin) was used and it is possible that if the toxin dosage is inadequate, the effect may be suboptimal or short lived. There is risk of developing SUI when a larger dose is used and though the incidence reported is low, patients who wish to undergo this treatment should be counseled about this transient risk of SUI. This study suggests that intrasphincteric botulinum toxin injection could become a possible out-patient based alternative in women who find CISC is intolerable and sacral neuromodulation may not be feasible.

6.8.4 Sacral Neuromodulation

The only modality of treatment that has stood the test of time in restoring normal micturition in women with FS is sacral neuromodulation (SNM). This technique involves the modulation of the neural circuit associated with lower urinary tract function by delivering an electric current to stimulate the S3 nerve root, thereby restoring a balance in neural control and the lower urinary tract (LUT) function.

Various viewpoints have evolved in its mechanism in FS from theories like stimulation "re-educates the pelvic floor" to a more viable theory of release of afferent-mediated sphincter inhibition allowing the LUT to be "switched on" again. This is supported by the fact that clinical recovery in bladder sensation and voiding occurs within hours of activation SNM simulator [52]. **However, electromyography and urodynamic studies performed post stimulation have shown that poor relaxation of the EUS persists despite successful voiding and voiding is possibly due to forceful contraction of detrusor** [53].

SNM has a success rate of about 70% for full restoration of spontaneous voiding. Success is usually defined as a more than 50% improvement in various bladder diary measures such as frequency of voids and voided volumes or number of catheterizations and catheter volumes [11, 52]. Datta et al. observed that 42 out of 60 women with urinary retention maintained spontaneous voiding post SNM during follow-up over a mean period of 7 years [54]. In other studies of SNM for nonobstructive retention, van Voskuilen et al. demonstrated 76.2% efficacy at 70.5 months and Elhilali et al. showed an efficacy of 78% at 77 months [55, 56]. A more recent study that followed up patients for an average period of 46.8 months suggests that success rate with SNM was higher in patients with idiopathic retention who were diagnosed to have FS (73%) as compared to those without a diagnosis of FS (58%) [57]. De Ridder and colleagues also observed a better 5-year-outcome with SNM in women with urinary retention having an abnormal sphincter EMG suggestive of FS [58].

The SNM is performed as a two-stage implantation process. In first screening stage, a temporary stimulating electrode is implanted through the S3 foramen under fluoroscopy, as a day-care procedure under local anesthesia. Optimal lead placement is determined by a subjective sensation of "tingling" or "throbbing" in the vaginal/rectal area supported by signs such as anal contraction and ipsilateral hallux flexion. Patient receives electrical stimulation by an external battery and clinical response with voiding diary is assessed for 4–7 days. Implantation of a permanent implantable pulse generator (IPG) in the buttocks is performed if a satisfactory improvement in voiding function is observed. Most of the clinicians prefer implanting permanent lead in the first stage itself so as not to disturb the lead position during second stage, provided patient has good response in the first place [59].

The major limitation of this effective treatment is its high cost (the cost of implant and leads is, at present, approximately £6000) and this is especially an impediment to its wider use in developing countries. Patients should also be counseled regarding failure or need of revision of device before starting SNM. The failure of the permanent implant occurs in about 25% of patients, surgical revision of device is required in about 30–50%, and battery replacement is needed in about 5–7 years. Complications include lead breakage, lead migration, device failure, device infection or pain at the implant site [60].

6.9 Conclusion

Fowler's syndrome is a possible diagnosis in any young woman presenting with unexplained high-volume urinary retention. Diagnosis is aided by specific investigations directed at evaluating the functioning of striated urethral sphincter like MUCP, sphincter volume and sphincter EMG. Treatment options include sacral neuromodulation, and intra-sphincteric botulinum toxin injection with reasonable success rates. Clean intermittent self-catheterization is an option, but many patients find it extremely uncomfortable and that affects their compliance with this treatment.

Clinical Case Scenario

A 22-year-old girl presented with urinary retention 2 weeks after uncomplicated diagnostic laparoscopy. She was being evaluated for dysfunctional menstrual bleeding with suspicion of endometriosis. She initially reported decreased per-day voiding frequency and prolonged voiding duration. Subsequently, she had an episode of urinary tract infection and was not able to void since that. Magnetic resonance imaging (MRI) brain and spine was performed which did not reveal any occult neurological dysfunction. Videourodynamics with surface EMG was performed for better charecterisation of the voiding dysfunction (Fig. 6.3). Pressure-flow study revealed decreased bladder sensations and hypotonic large capacity bladder. She was diagnosed with FS based on her medical history, clinical symptoms and urodynamic findings.

She did not tolerate clean intermittent self-catheterization initially due to pain and was put on continuous catheter drainage, but subsequently she adapted to self-catherization in due course. Later, a S3 neurostimulator device was implanted restoring her ability to void. She

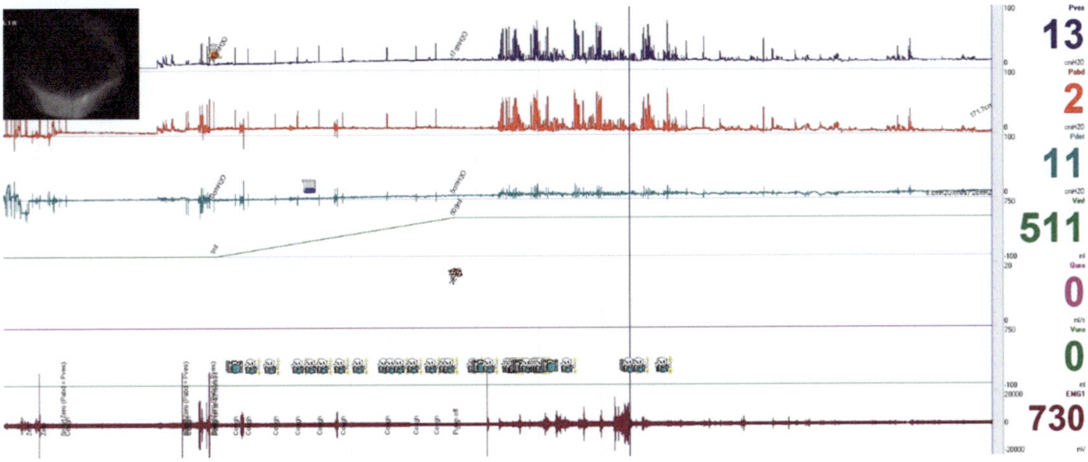

Fig. 6.3 Videourodynamics showing a normally complaint large capacity bladder with impaired contractility and increased surface electromyogram activity during voiding with poor funneling of bladder neck

remains under follow-up for any device- or disease-related sequelae.

Key Learning Points

- Fowler's syndrome is characterized by recurrent unexplained episodes of acute painless urinary retention in young women.
- Unlike dysfunctional voiding, which is a disorder of the pelvic floor muscle, the muscle primarily involved is the rhabdosphincter or the external urinary sphincter muscle.
- The striated sphincter fibers persistently activate each other leading to a high-tone nonrelaxing sphincter, which can be demonstrated during both filling and voiding phase.
- This persistent high tone leads to ultrasonologically demonstrable hypertrophy of the EUS and causes reflex inhibition of detrusor activity during initiation of voiding leading to a finding of detrusor underactivity.
- Typical patterns on EMG with needle electrodes were considered pathognomonic, but their identification in normal women has resulted in loss of their sacrosanct status.
- A trigger factor (most commonly a pelvic surgery) can be identified on history.
- Correlation of clinical features with imaging and videourodynamic studies with EMG forms the basis of diagnosis of this condition.
- Clean intermittent self-catheterization is typically painful in these women.
- Intrasphincteric botulinum toxin injections have been shown to be beneficial in some studies.
- Sacral neuromodulation is curative with acceptable long-term results and is the treatment of choice.

References

1. Ahmad I, Krishna NS, Small DR, Conn IG. Aetiology and management of acute female urinary retention. Br J Med Surg Urol. 2009;2:27–33.
2. Abrams PH, Dunn M, George N. Urodynamic findings in chronic retention of urine and their relevance to results of surgery. BMJ. 1978;2:1258–60.
3. Fowler CJ, Kirby RS. Abnormal electromyographic activity (decelerating burst and complex repetitive discharges) in the striated muscle of the urethral sphincter in 5 women with persisting urinary retention. Br J Urol. 1985;57:67–70.
4. Fowler CJ, Christmas TJ, Chapple CR, Parkhouse HF, Kirby RS, Jacobs HS. Abnormal electromyographic activity of the urethral sphincter, voiding dysfunction, and polycystic ovaries: a new syndrome? BMJ. 1988;297:1436–8.
5. Kavia RB, Datta SN, DasGupta R, Elneil S, Fowler CJ. Urinary retention in women: its causes and management. BJU Int. 2006;97:281–7.
6. Swinn MJ, Wiseman OJ, Lowe E, Fowler CJ. The cause and natural history of isolated urinary retention in young women. J Urol. 2002;167:151–6.

7. Potenzoni D, Juvarra G, Bettoni L, Stagni G. Pseudomyotonia of the striated urethral sphincter. J Urol. 1983;130:512–3.
8. Panicker JN, DasGupta R, Elneil S, Fowler CJ. Urinary retention. In: Fowler CJ, Panicker JN, Emmanuel A, editors. Pelvic organ dysfunction in neurological disease: clinical management and rehabilitation. New York, NY: Cambridge University Press; 2010. p. 293–306.
9. de Groat WC, Fraser MO, Yoshiyama M, Smerin S, Tai C, Chancellor MB, et al. Neural control of the urethra. Scand J Urol Nephrol. 2001;207(Suppl):35–43.
10. Wiseman OJ, Swinn MJ, Brady CM, Fowler CJ. Maximum urethral closure pressure and sphincter volume in women with urinary retention. J Urol. 2002;167:1348–51.
11. Osman NI, Chapple CR. Fowler's syndrome – a cause of unexplained urinary retention in young women? Nat Rev Urol. 2014;11(2):87–98.
12. Kavia R, DasGupta R, Critchley H, Fowler CJ, Griffiths D. A functional magnetic resonance imaging study of the effect of sacral neuromodulation on brain responses in women with Fowler's syndrome. BJU Int. 2010;105:366–72.
13. DasGupta R, Critchley HD, Dolan RJ, Fowler CJ. Changes in brain activity following sacral neuromodulation for urinary retention. J Urol. 2005;174:2268–72.
14. Singh SK, Agarwal MM, Batra YK, Kishore AV, Mandal AK. Effect of lumbar-epidural administration of tramadol on lower urinary tract function. Neurourol Urodyn. 2008;27:65–70.
15. Hanna MG, Wood NW, Kullmann DM. Ion channels and neurological disease: DNA based diagnosis is now possible, and ion channels may be important in common paroxysmal disorders. J Neurol Neurosurg Psychiatry. 1988;65:427–31.
16. Das Gupta R, Fowler CJ. The management of female voiding dysfunction: Fowler's syndrome—a contemporary update. Curr Opin Urol. 2003;13:293–9.
17. Duijkers IJ, Klipping C. Polycystic ovaries, as defined by the 2003 Rotterdam consensus criteria, are found to be very common in young healthy women. Gynecol Endocrinol. 2010;26:152–60.
18. Amarenco G, Raibaut P, Ismael SS, Rene-Corail P, Haab F. Evidence of occult dysautonomia in Fowler's syndrome: alteration of cardiovascular autonomic function tests in female patients presenting with urinary retention. BJU Int. 2006;97:288–91.
19. Buck AC, Reed PI, Siddiq YK, Chisholm GD, Fraser TR. Bladder dysfunction and neuropathy in diabetes. Diabetologia. 1976;12:251–8.
20. Sakakibara R, Hattori T, Kuwabara S, Yamanishi T, Yasuda K. Micturitional disturbance in patients with Guillain-Barre syndrome. J Neurol Neurosurg Psychiatry. 1997;63:649–53.
21. Hoeritzauer I, Stone J, Fowler C, Elneil-Coker S, Carson A, Panicker J. Fowler's syndrome of urinary retention: a retrospective study of co-morbidity. Neurourol Urodyn. 2016;35(5):601–3.
22. Panicker JN, Gamé X, Khan S, Kessler T, Gonzales G, Elneil S, et al. The possible role of opiates in women with chronic urinary retention: observations from a prospective clinical study. J Urol. 2012;188:480–4.
23. Brucker BM, Fong E, Shah S, Kelly C, Rosenblum N, Nitti VW. Urodynamic differences between dysfunctional voiding and primary bladder neck obstruction in women. Urology. 2012 Jul;80(1):55–60.
24. Raz S. Editorial comment on "maximum urethral closure pressure and urinary retention". J Urol. 2002;167:1351.
25. Abrams P, Cardozo L, Fall M, Griffiths D, Rosier P, Ulmsten U, et al. The standardisation of terminology of lower urinary tract function: report from the standardisation sub-committee of the international continence society. Neurourol Urodyn. 2002;21(2):167–78.
26. Drossaerts J, Rademakers K, van Koeveringe G, Van Kerrebroeck P. The value of urodynamic tools to guide patient selection in sacral neuromodulation. World J Urol. 2015;33(11):1889–95.
27. Fowler CJ, Kirby RS, Harrison MJ, Milroy EJ, Turner-Warwick R. Individual motor unit analysis in the diagnosis of disorders of urethral sphincter innervation. J Neurol Neurosurg Psychiatry. 1984;47:637–41.
28. Mahajan ST, Fitzgerald MP, Kenton K, Shott S, Brubaker L. Concentric needle electrodes are superior to perineal surface-patch electrodes for electromyographic documentation of urethral sphincter relaxation during voiding. BJU Int. 2006;97:117–20.
29. Tawadros C, Burnett K, Derbyshire LF, Tawadros T, Clarke NW, Betts CD. External urethral sphincter electromyography in asymptomatic women and the influence of the menstrual cycle. BJU Int. 2015;116(3):423–31.
30. Fowler CJ, Kirby RS, Harrison MJ. Decelerating burst and complex repetitive discharges in the striated muscle of the urethral sphincter, associated with urinary retention in women. J Neurol Neurosurg Psychiatry. 1985;48(10):1004–9.
31. Malde S, Solomon E, Spilotros M, Mukhtar B, Pakzad M, Hamid R, et al. Female bladder outlet obstruction: common symptoms masking an uncommon cause. Low Urin Tract Symptoms. 2019;11:72–7.
32. Kavia RB, Datta SN, Das Gupta R, Elneil S, Fowler CJ. Urinary retention in women: its causes and management. BJU Int. 2006;97:281–7.
33. Noble JG, Dixon PJ, Rickards D, Fowler CJ. Urethral sphincter volumes in women with obstructed voiding and abnormal sphincter electromyographic activity. Br J Urol. 1995;76:741–6.
34. Carlson KV, Fiske J, Nitti VW. Value of routine evaluation of the voiding phase when performing urodynamic testing in women with lower urinary tract symptoms. J Urol. 2000;164:1614–8.
35. Groutz A, Blaivas JG, Pies Sassone AM. Learned voiding dysfunction (non-neurogenic, neuro-

genic bladder) among adults. Neurourol Urodyn. 2001;20:259–68.
36. Carlson KV, Rome S, Nitti VW. Dysfunctional voiding in women. J Urol. 2001;165:143–7.
37. Fan YH, Lin AT, Wu HM, Hong CJ, Chen KK. Psychological profile of female patients with dysfunctional voiding. Urology. 2008;71:625–9.
38. Deindl FM, Vodusek DB, Bischoff C, Hofmann R, Hartung R. Dysfunctional voiding in women: which muscles are responsible? Br J Urol. 1998;82:814–9.
39. Hickling D, Aponte M, Nitti V. Evaluation and management of outlet obstruction in women without anatomical abnormalities on physical exam or cystoscopy. Curr Urol Rep. 2012;13:356–62.
40. Kessler TM, Studer UE, Burkhard FC. The effect of terazosin on functional bladder outlet obstruction in women: a pilot study. J Urol. 2006;176:1487–92.
41. Peng CH, Kuo HC. Transurethral incision of bladder neck in treatment of bladder neck obstruction in women. Urology. 2005;65:275–8.
42. Mousa H, Hyman PE, Cocjin J, Flores AF, Di Lorenzo C. Long-term outcome of congenital intestinal pseudoobstruction. Dig Dis Sci. 2002;47:2298–305.
43. Lapointe SP, Rivet C, Goulet O, Fekete CN, Lortat-Jacob S. Urological manifestations associated with chronic intestinal pseudo-obstructions in children. J Urol. 2002;168:1768–70.
44. Woodhouse CR, Gordon EM. The Mitrofanoff principle for urethral failure. Br J Urol. 1994;73:55–60.
45. Datta SN, Kavia RB, Gonzales G, Fowler CJ. Results of double-blind placebo-controlled crossover study of sildenafil citrate (viagra) in women suffering from obstructed voiding or retention associated with the primary disorder of sphincter relaxation (Fowler's syndrome). Eur Urol. 2007;51:489–95.
46. Chang SJ, Chiang IN, Yu HJ. The effectiveness of tamsulosin in treating women with voiding difficulty. Int J Urol. 2008;15(11):981–5.
47. Dykstra DD, Sidi AA, Scott AB, Pagel JM, Goldish GD. Effects of botulinum a toxin on detrusor-sphincter dyssynergia in spinal cord injury patients. J Urol. 1988;139:919–22.
48. Phelan M, Franks M, Somogyi GT, Yokoyama T, Fraser MO, Lavelle JP, et al. Botulinum toxin urethral sphincter injection to restore bladder emptying in men and women with voiding dysfunction. J Urol. 2001;165:1107–10.
49. Fowler CJ, Betts CD, Swash M, Fowler CG. Botulinum toxin in the treatment of chronic urinary retention in women. Br J Urol. 1992;70:387–9.
50. Peyronnet B, Gamé X, Vurture G, Nitti VW, Brucker BM. Botulinum toxin use in neurourology. Rev Urol. 2018;20(2):84–93.
51. Panicker JN, Seth JH, Khan S, Gonzales G, Haslam C, Kessler TM, et al. Open label study evaluating outpatient urethral sphincter injections of onabotulinum toxin a to treat women with urinary retention due to a primary disorder of sphincter relaxation (Fowler's syndrome). BJU Int. 2016;117(5):809–13.
52. Swinn MJ, Kitchen ND, Goodwin RJ, Fowler CJ. Sacral neuromodulation for women with Fowler's syndrome. Eur Urol. 2000;38:439–43.
53. DasGupta R, Fowler CJ. Urodynamic study of women in urinary retention treated with sacral neuromodulation. J Urol. 2004;171:1161–4.
54. Datta SN, Chaliha C, Singh A, Gonzales G, Mishra VC, Kavia RB, et al. Sacral neurostimulation for urinary retention: 10-year experience from one UK centre. BJU Int. 2008;101(2):192–6.
55. Van Voskuilen AC, Oerlemans DJ, Weil EH, van den Hombergh U, van Kerrebroeck PE. Medium-term experience of sacral neuromodulation by tined lead implantation. BJU Int. 2007;99(1):107–10.
56. Elhilali MM, Khaled SM, Kashiwabara T, Elzayat E, Corcos J. Sacral neuromodulation: long-term experience of one center. Urology. 2005;65(6):1114–7.
57. Peeters K, Sahai A, De Ridder D, Van Der Aa F. Long-term follow-up of sacral neuromodulation for lower urinary tract dysfunction. BJU Int. 2014;113(5):789–94.
58. De Ridder D, Ost D, Bruyninckx F. The presence of Fowler's syndrome predicts successful long-term outcome of sacral nerve stimulation in women with urinary retention. Eur Urol. 2007;51(1):229–33.
59. Janknegt R, Weil E, Eerdmans P. Improving neuromodulation: technique for refractory voiding dysfunctions: two-stage implant. Urology. 1997;49:358–62.
60. Elneil S. Urinary retention in women and sacral neuromodulation. Int Urogynecol J. 2010;21(Suppl 2):475–83.

7 Pelvic Organ Descent as a Cause of Bladder Outlet Obstruction

Arabind Panda and Nikhil Khattar

Learning Objectives

- To appreciate the impact of pelvic organ prolapse on lower urinary tract symptoms and as a cause of bladder outlet obstruction in women.
- To understand the outcome of prolapse reduction with regards to improvement in voiding symptoms.

7.1 Introduction

Pelvic organ prolapse (POP) can be defined as a loss of support of one or more of the pelvic organs leading to protrusion into or outside the vagina [1].

POP includes anterior vaginal prolapse (cystocele), posterior vaginal prolapse (rectocele), apical or uterine prolapse, enterocele and perineal descent. **There is a strong association with parity** (4:1 in women with 1 and 8.4:1 in women with two children compared to non-parous women). Less than 1% of POP occurs in nulliparous women [2]. **Other significant risk factors are age, increased intra-abdominal pressure—constipation, hysterectomy and obesity, connective tissue disorder** (Marfan syndrome, Ehlers Danlos syndrome) [3].

Up to 41% of women between 50 and 79 years have POP. However, in the majority of cases, it remains asymptomatic until it descends till the hymenal ring [4].

Severe degrees of prolapse is believed to be an etiologic factor for both urethral obstruction and stress urinary incontinence. In addition, it may result in several other lower urinary tract symptoms, which may be secondarily related to the obstructive effects of prolapse or may be related to generalised pelvic floor ligament laxity or stretch. This chapter looks at the cause-and-effect relationship of prolapse and lower urinary tract symptoms especially bladder outlet obstruction (BOO).

7.2 Classification of Prolapse

Several classification systems have been described for POP.

Traditionally, systems describe either the structures behind the vaginal wall that are presumed to be prolapsed or define it according to the area of the vaginal wall that is prolapsed (Table 7.1).

The Pelvic Organ Prolapse Quantification (POP-Q) scale has been recently used to standardize the assessment of POP [6]. Six fixed points are measured above or below the hymen

A. Panda (✉)
Urology and Renal Transplantation, Krishna Institute of Medical Sciences, Secunderabad, Telangana, India

N. Khattar
Female Urology, Reconstructive Urology and Neurovesical Dysfunction, Medanta, The Medicity, Gurugram, India

N. Khattar et al. (eds.), *Female Bladder Outlet Obstruction and Urethral Reconstruction*,
https://doi.org/10.1007/978-981-15-8521-0_7

Table 7.1 Traditional systems to describe prolapse

Based on the structures behind the vaginal wall that are presumed to be prolapsed	In terms of the part of the vaginal wall prolapsed	Baden-Walker halfway system [5]
Cystocele/ cystourethrocele	Anterior vaginal wall prolapse	**Grade 0**: Normal position for every site
Rectocele/enterocele	Apical prolapse	**Grade 1**: Descent halfway to the hymen
Uterine prolapse	Cervical prolapse	**Grade 2**: Descent to the hymen
Uterine procedentia	Posterior vaginal wall prolapse	**Grade 3**: Descent halfway past the hymen
	Perineal descent	**Grade 4**: Maximal possible descent for each site

while the patient is straining and relaxed, respectively. The total vaginal length, length to the genital hiatus and the perineal body are noted.

Anterior compartment prolapse with associated SUI can result from damage to the pubocervical fascia and descent of the bladder (cystocele) and bladder neck (SUI). Posterior compartment prolapse is caused by laxity or injury of the rectovaginal septum resulting in protrusion of the rectum (rectocele) or the small bowel (enterocele). Apical compartment prolapse is the descent of the uterus or cervix or the vaginal cuff post hysterectomy. Commonly, POP involves more than one compartment.

7.3 Effects of Pelvic Organ Prolapse on the Bladder and Its Outlet

Bladder outlet obstruction is commonly associated with severe pelvic organ prolapse. The symptoms mostly relate to voiding lower urinary tract symptoms—slow stream, a need to strain in order to void, dribbling with a prolonged flow (Table 7.2). They often need to digitally push the prolapsed part to void well. This points to a causal relation between prolapse and voiding dysfunction. In many women with POP, surgical correction of POP unmasks latent stress urinary incontinence (SUI) and urge leak, which again is an indicator that urethra had been compressed by the existing prolapse, which helped concealing the incontinence [7].

Table 7.2 Common symptoms in pelvic organ prolapse

Urinary	Weak stream/poor flow
	Straining to void
	Sense of incomplete evacuation
	Frequency and urgency
	Manual reduction of the prolapse to void well
Vaginal	Bulge in the perineal area
	Bleeding and ulceration in the protruding part

7.3.1 Pelvic Organ Prolapse and Bladder Outlet Obstruction

In a large population-based study, up to 1/5th of women having stage 2 POP and 1/3 of those with stage 3 or 4 POP had voiding LUTS [8]. A retrospective study assessing the relationship between cystocele and BOO in 200 women found a statistically significant relationship between grade of cystocele and BOO [9]. Romanzi et al. [10] studied this effect in a prospective manner in 60 women and also studied difference in urodynamic parameters after reduction of prolapse either surgically or by a pessary. They noted a **significantly high urodynamic outlet obstruction in women with high-grade cystocele (72%) vs. low-grade cystocele (6%)**. They further demonstrated that **after reduction of prolapse in grade 3–4 cystocele group, 17 out of 18 women showed disappearance of urodynamic BOO**. Seven (39%) of these 18 women also developed SUI after prolapse reduction further confirming a compressive effect of cystocele over the urethra.

Dancz and Özel examined whether descent beyond a specific point in anterior prolapse, measured by Aa and Ba on POP-Q score, causes obstruction. Interestingly, any Aa or Ba value had poor predictive value. **The aetiology of outlet obstruction in POP is likely to be multifactorial and cannot be correlated to POP-Q values alone** [11]. This study did not assess voiding symptoms for posterior compartment prolapse. Occasionally, the symptoms may be due to associated pelvic floor dysfunction or an underactive detrusor. Very severe prolapse can cause ureteric obstruction due to kinking of the distal ureters along with urethral obstruction due to extrinsic compression [12] (Fig. 7.1).

Deitz et al. [13] used translabial ultrasound to quantify prolapse and study the relationship between POP and voiding dysfunction in women with POP and LUTS. The ultrasound was done with a full bladder at rest and also with Valsalva to produce maximum possible descent.

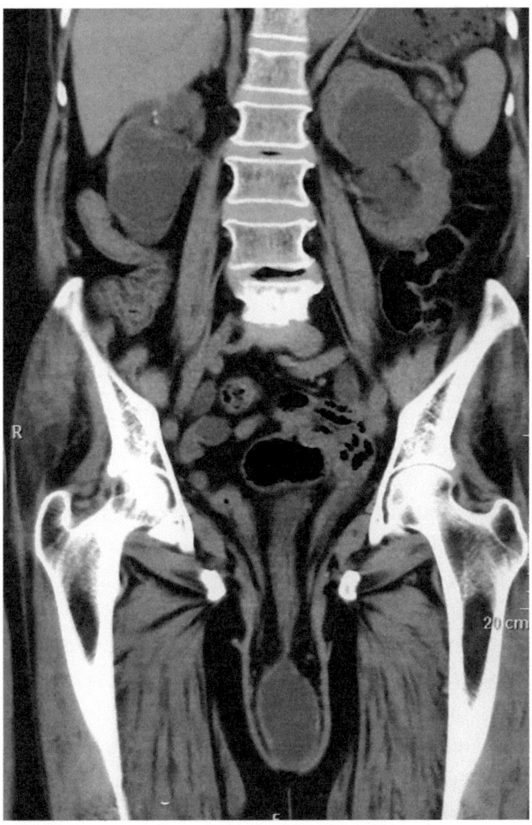

Fig. 7.1 Complete procidentia causing kinking of bilateral ureters with obstructive uropathy. This resolved after hysterectomy and surgical correction of the prolapse

Interestingly, they found presence of an enterocele or a rectocele to be having most consistent negative effect on uroflow parameters, while the apical descent had only a minimal effect, which was not significant. In anterior compartment descent, it was observed that there were two anatomical configurations at neck during valsalva **a.** Anterior prolapse with an open neck with loss of posterior angle of urethra and bladder (retrovesical angle) as is seen as a funnelling during normal voiding **b.** Anterior prolapse with an intact retrovesical angle. It was with type 'b' that the negative effect on flow parameters was significantly associated, while the type 'a' configuration did not negatively impact the flow rates. **This implies that with anterior prolapse, a kinking effect may be the cause of obstruction while with posterior prolapse, compressive effect may be the cause.** This relationship remains to be studied further by other researchers. Whatever be the exact cause of bladder outlet obstruction in prolapse, there is evidence that POP-associated outlet obstruction can cause detrusor remodelling, resulting in overactivity [14].

7.3.2 Pelvic Organ Prolapse and Overactive Bladder

There seems to a correlation between overactive bladder (OAB)/detrusor overactivity (DO) and cystocele. Both POP and OAB are independently common conditions in women, making it difficult to determine a causal association. OAB by definition is an idiopathic condition and all obvious causes should be ruled out. However, it is very common to label a woman with OAB ignoring a mild-to-moderate prolapse [15]. In a review of prevalence of OAB in patients with POP [14], there was a higher prevalence of subjective OAB, but the urodynamic findings of DO varied between studies. The relative risk (RR) of OAB in community setting was reported to be up to 5.8 in women with POP, whereas the RR observed in hospital-based studies was between 1.2 and 3.4. The studies reviewed had conflicting relation between the compartment of prolapse (whether anterior or central) and the OAB symptoms. The incidence of overactive bladder symptoms can be more than 30%. Interestingly, **unlike voiding difficulties, which increase with increasing stage, it was observed that the OAB symptoms were seen more often in lesser degrees of prolapse and urgency and urge incontinence were less likely in higher grades of prolapse.** The review also showed that the OAB symptoms have good likelihood of reduction after correction of the POP by either pessary or surgery. Women in whom there was improvement in flow rates after prolapse reduction and those with bladder trabeculations had more likelihood of improvement in OAB symptoms. **A prospective study specifically looked for resolution of OAB symptoms after prolapse surgery and demonstrated a relief in 60% of patients** [16]. There are several prevalent theories regarding POP-induced detrusor overactivity. De Boer et al. have postulated that obstruction causes the detrusor to become hypertrophic and irritable and the changes make the reflex arc of micturition more sensitive. A large cystocele can cause traction on the urethra opening the bladder neck. Urine entering the urethra can then trigger detrusor contractions [14].

7.3.3 Pelvic Organ Prolapse and Stress Urinary Incontinence

SUI, mostly latent and in a small percentage overt, can be present in up to 80% of cases of moderate-to-severe prolapse (Grade 2–4). It is hypothesized that the apparent continence is due to the kinking or compression of the urethra, which is relieved by prolapse reduction. **Unmasking of occult stress leak after prolapse correction is seen in 36–80% of clinically continent females with high degrees of prolapse** [17].

7.4 The Case for a Pessary Trial

Pessaries are devices, usually made from medical grade silicone, that can be fitted in the vagina to keep the prolapse in its reduced state. **Since the improvement in both voiding difficulties and OAB symptoms after prolapse repair can be predicted after a trial of pessary, it may be prudent to provide the woman with a pessary in the clinic after complete evaluation and re-evaluate after 1 week for resolution of symptoms.** With a pessary trial, occult stress urinary incontinence was revealed in 60–70% females with grade II-IV prolapse who never complained of incontinence [18, 19]. It could also reveal SUI missed after a clinical exam done after prolapse reduction in 19% of patients [18]. The challenge may be experienced in finding a correct pessary fitting for the patient and for the patient to retain the pessary [20].

Ring pessaries are available in different sizes ranging from no. 2–7. The average fit size is 4 or 5 and finding a correct size for a patient may require trying out [21]. Assessing the size of a pessary for patient can be done while performing clinical examination in an empty bladder after manually reducing the prolapse and inserting two fingers in the vaginal cavity with the tip of middle finger in the posterior fornix and index finger against the pubic arch. The distance between the tip of middle finger and index finger where it touches the symphysis pubis gives the approximate size of the ring to be tried. A folded and lubricated ring pessary (which unfolds itself after insertion) of the assessed size is inserted in the vagina after separating the labial folds and placed obliquely between the vaginal wall anteriorly and the posterior fornix (Fig. 7.2). A finger is swept around the ring to check for pressure points and patient is made to cough or Valsalva to ensure that the pessary is not very loose. Test for occult SUI can be done when the bladder is full, but she is made to stay in clinic premises till she passes urine at least once. She can then be called again between 1 and 2 weeks for reassessment of urinary symptoms. A concern has been for the pessary to be a direct cause for causing outlet obstruction, which was dispelled with a prospective study by Romzanzi et al. mentioned earlier [10], where 94% of their patients with urodynamic BOO had an improved free uroflowmetry after pessary reduction demonstrating that a trial with a ring pessary can help in differentiating the symptoms of BOO due to POP from other causes

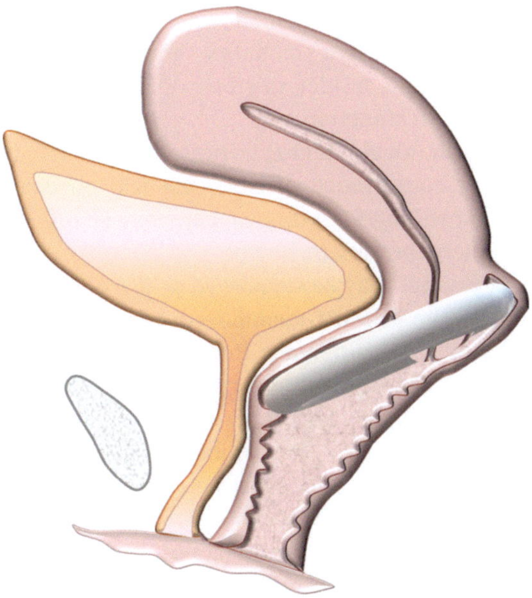

Fig. 7.2 Obliquely placed ring vaginal pessary in place

[10]. It can also help predicting successful voiding in women with POP and retention after prolapse repair with a sensitivity of 89% and specificity of 80% [22]. **Hence, pessary reduction is the best simulation for a surgical repair and can help predict improvement in urinary symptoms before surgery, unmask occult SUI and set patient expectations and thus may help to prognosticate the outcome and counsel accordingly. Moreover, an effective resolution of symptoms establishes a direct relation between POP and symptoms and precludes the need for a further VCUG or UDS studies.**

7.5 Evaluation

7.5.1 History and Physical Examination

Careful history of the lower urinary tract symptoms is elucidated. Any urgency episodes or urge incontinence is recorded after ruling out urinary tract infection. Symptoms suggestive of stress urinary incontinence are particularly enquired. Straining to void, suprapubic pressure to void or improve the urinary stream, if present, is recorded. Bowel symptoms suggestive of constipation are noted if present. Obstetric history, particularly the number of vaginal deliveries, abortions, or a hysterectomy, is recorded as is any history suggestive of any neurological disorder. A bladder diary is recommended if there is significant urgency or urge leak.

Objective evaluation can be done with a Pelvic Floor Distress Inventory (PFDI), using its Urogenital Distress inventory (UDI-6/8) component [23].

A complete general physical examination is performed as pulmonary, renal and endocrinological conditions may be in part responsible for the symptoms and can influence treatment. Dullness on percussion is specifically looked for in the suprapubic area. If the bladder is palpable, this is noted. A pelvic examination in the lithotomy position is necessary to characterize the extent and compartments involved. A speculum (preferably split) is then inserted to visualize the cervix/vaginal cuff and the vaginal length is noted. Apical descent is looked for during the Valsalva manoeuvre. POP-Q staging can be done at this stage. A distended bladder is looked for and palpated through the anterior vaginal wall.

Stress test for stress urinary incontinence is performed with the bladder comfortably full and any involuntary leakage of urine with coughing is recorded. A focused neurological examination for perineal sensations, bulbocavernosal reflex and anal reflex is performed.

If necessary, the prolapse can be re-evaluated in the standing position to note its full extent.

A uroflowmetry is the initial specialized investigation to document a poor flow. An attempt should be made to reduce the POP with a ring pessary and repeat the uroflowmetry (pessary trial). **If the curve of the pre- and post-reduction uroflowmetry appear inconclusive, it might be prudent to do a voiding cystourethrogram and demonstrate the anatomical obstruction of the urethra on lateral films.** The role of urodynamics (UDS) in POP is still evolving. In patient with a high post void residual urine due to detrusor underactivity, outlet obstruction or due to a combination, urodynamics may distinguish underactive detrusor and therefore help in prognostication [24]. Though most patients with POP and high PVR have been observed to void well with prolapse repair alone and continued to have a high PVR if concomitant anti-incontinence surgery was added [25]. Therefore, in these patients, an additional anti-incontinence procedure during POP repair is contraindicated. In women with POP and OAB, pre-operative detrusor overactivity on UDS may not be predictive of post-operative urge incontinence. Preoperative UDS as a tool for postoperative prognostication of UUI is, therefore, not very useful.

An ultrasound of the kidneys, ureters and bladder with post void residual urine is needed to assess for concomitant ureteric obstruction, which can coexist due to kinking of bilateral ureters in severe prolapse. If such an obstruction exists, it is imperative to attempt reduction of the prolapse to normalize the renal function before definitive repair. Occasionally, this may be difficult to do in long standing procidentia.

A complete haemogram and renal function tests should be done in all cases.

7.6 Modalities of Treatment for Pelvic Organ Prolapse

The detailed treatment of prolapse is beyond the scope of this book, a brief outline is presented here.

Pelvic floor muscle therapy (PFMT): conservative measures, including lifestyle modifications and supervised PFMT program, are often offered to women with less severe degrees of prolapse. A systematic review, which included four trials (857 women) comparing PFMT vs. a control group, concluded that PFMT increases the chance of improvement in degree of prolapse by 17% and also led to improvement in bladder symptoms [26]. In a contemporary systematic review assessing the benefits of PFMT vs. controls, which included 13 studies with 2340 patients, also reported improvement in prolapse symptom scores and bladder symptoms. There was no difference demonstrated in need for further treatment in both patient populations [27]. The bladder symptoms studied in RCTs included in these reviews were SUI and urgency incontinence and not voiding dysfunction. PFMT, however, is a noninvasive modality and should be employed in milder degrees of prolapse and voiding dysfunction.

Mechanical devices (pessaries): Patients failing conservative management and not suitable/unwilling for a surgical cure may be offered long-term pessary treatment.

Pessaries may be supportive or space occupying. In the PESSRI-randomized controlled trial, there was no difference in symptom reduction between ring and space-occupying Gelhorn pessaries [28]. In general, ring pessaries are used for relatively lower grades of prolapse, while Gelhorn pessaries are used for severe grades of prolapse. In a prospective study, 94 of 171 non-hysterectomised postmenopausal women with POP grade III–IV were chosen for long-term pessary as their treatment and at a median 27 months of follow up, 80% continued the use. Half of the 20% that discontinued the use, did so in the first week of use [29]. Ninety two percent of 52 patients who reported voiding difficulties and 75% of 44 having urge incontinence at baseline improved within a month of pessary use. Among patients who continued using pessary, 31% experienced adverse events in form of extrusion requiring reinsertion (18%). Some had ulceration (10%) and a few (2.6%) had discomfort with discharge. In another retrospective study reporting prolonged use of pessary in 192 postmenopausal women (age >75 years, $n = 92$) with equal distribution of a ring or a Gelhorn pessary, 65% continued the pessary use at the end of study [30]. The probability of continued pessary use beyond 5 years was 62% in women <75 years and 38% in women >75 years of age. Vaginal erosions were the most common side effect prompting discontinuation.

Careful examination of vaginal mucosa is important before recommending a prolonged pessary use. Women with atrophic mucosa should be prescribed topical oestrogens for at least 2 weeks before pessary use. History of hysterectomy, pelvic reconstructive surgery for prolapse and posterior prolapse are risk factors for failure of the initial insertion [30]. Maintenance and subsequent change can be done by patient herself or by a nurse practitioner at home.

Surgical Management of Prolapse: The surgical options can be categorized as **native tissue repair vs. biological graft or synthetic mesh repair**. The approach may be vaginal or abdominal. The decision of additional hysterectomy vs. uterine preservation (especially applied to apical compartment prolapse) must be considered.

For anterior compartment prolapse, following conclusions were drawn from a metanalysis of 33 randomised studies [31]: The awareness of prolapse, recurrence and reoperation for prolapse is more likely after a native tissue repair than in a mesh repair. Mesh exposure rates however are up to 11% over 3 years. Due to increased morbidity, the use of vaginal mesh repair is not recommended for POP. The awareness of prolapse and recurrence rates after a biodegradable mesh are similar to those of native tissue repair.

For apical compartment prolapse, the options are either a transvaginal procedure (high utero-sacral ligament fixation or sacrospinous ligament fixation) or transabdominal sacrocolpopexy (open or minimally invasive). Sacrocolpopexy is the procedure with best subjective satisfactory results and least awareness, less dyspareunia and lower recurrence rates as compared to transvaginal procedures [31]. The procedure can be well performed through laparoscopic/robotic techniques with comparable efficacy. Transvaginal mesh procedures are not recommended due to higher complication rates.

For posterior compartment prolapse, transvaginal repairs are preferable while avoiding mesh use.

In addition, obliterative procedures like colpocleisis can be offered to old patients with higher degrees of prolapse who are not sexually active and not fit for any other surgery.

7.7 Prophylactic SUI Repair During Transvaginal POP Repair

There is a significant subset of patients who have occult stress incontinence because of either kinking or compression of urethra, and therefore there is an argument for simultaneous anti-incontinence procedure during repair.

Whereas the anterior compartment prolapse repair alone may provide some continence to women with POP and 'symptomatic' SUI (4–8%) [32], the option of a simultaneous anti-incontinence procedure can be offered to these patients as it obviates the need for a future SUI surgery with a number needed to treat (NNT) of 2.5 [33]. Those who do not have demonstrable SUI at presentation ('occult' SUI) do not readily accept a prophylactic procedure. However, a concomitant prophylactic mid-urethral sling surgery reduces the development of objective SUI (5% vs. 40%) and risk of second surgery for SUI (1% vs. 15%) with an NNT of 7 [33]. Hence, a prophylactic simultaneous mid-urethral sling should be offered to these women.

Whenever a simultaneous sling surgery is undertaken, the sling placement should be done with a separate incision from colporrhaphy incision (i.e. the incision should not cross the bladder neck, lest the chances of migration of sling upwards become higher). The rest of the technique of sling placement in POP patients is not different from patients with SUI alone.

To summarize, women with POP can present with both voiding and storage lower urinary tract symptoms, incontinence and bowel symptoms. There is a direct cause-and-effect relationship of POP with both BOO and OAB. Severe degrees of prolapse can cause upper tract obstruction with obstructive uropathy and increased urethral resistance with bladder outlet obstruction. These are reversible with surgical or pessary correction of the prolapse. There is also latent stress incontinence in many patients with high-grade prolapse as compression/kinking of the urethra masks stress leak. Concomitant anti-incontinence procedures in a small subset of patients may be justified. The vast majority of urge leaks resolve after repair of the POP. The role of urodynamics is limited to evaluation of POP with associated stress or mixed incontinence and in women with high PVR. The results should be interpreted with caution.

Key Learning Points

- Pelvic organ prolapse is a significant and common cause of voiding dysfunction and bladder outlet obstruction in women. Incidence of BOO is significantly higher with more severe grades of prolapse.
- There is a direct association between severity of prolapse with prevalence of OAB symptoms.
- Clinical examination and relief of symptoms after a vaginal pessary insertion are the most definitive clues to diagnosis. In inconclusive cases, a video-urodynamics can help in ruling out other causes of voiding dysfunction.
- Prolapse reduction (either surgically or with a pessary) helps in significant relief of obstructive voiding symptoms and, to a lesser extent, the storage symptoms.

Acknowledgement Dr. Rubee Khattar, for providing critical inputs to section on "The Case for a Pessary Trial", Dr. Rishi Nayyar, for contributing with the drawing (Fig. 7.2.)

References

1. Milsom I, Altman D, Lapitan MC, et al. Epidemiology of urinary (UI) and faecal (FI) incontinence and pelvic organ prolapse (POP). In: International Consultation on Incontinence, Abrams P, editor. Incontinence: 4th international consultation on incontinence, 5–8 Jul, 2008. Paris: Editions 21; 2009.
2. Mant J, Painter R, Vessey M. Epidemiology of genital prolapse: observations from the Oxford Family Planning Association Study. Br J Obstet Gynaecol. 1997;104(5):579–85.
3. Ashton-Miller JA, Delancey JOL. On the biomechanics of vaginal birth and common sequelae. Annu Rev Biomed Eng. 2009;11:163–76.
4. Hendrix SL, Clark A, Nygaard I, Aragaki A, Barnabei V, McTiernan A. Pelvic organ prolapse in the women's health initiative: gravity and gravidity. Am J Obstet Gynecol. 2002;186(6):1160–6.
5. Baden WF, Walker T. Surgical repair of vaginal defects. Philadelphia, PA: Lippincott; 1992. p. 294.
6. Bump RC, Mattiasson A, Bø K, Brubaker LP, DeLancey JO, Klarskov P, et al. The standardization of terminology of female pelvic organ prolapse and pelvic floor dysfunction. Am J Obstet Gynecol. 1996;175(1):10–7.
7. Brubaker L, Cundiff GW, Fine P, Nygaard I, Richter HE, Visco AG, et al. Abdominal sacrocolpopexy with Burch colposuspension to reduce urinary stress incontinence. N Engl J Med. 2006;354(15):1557–66.
8. Slieker-ten Hove MCP, Pool-Goudzwaard AL, Eijkemans MJC, Steegers-Theunissen RPM, Burger CW, Vierhout ME. The prevalence of pelvic organ prolapse symptoms and signs and their relation with bladder and bowel disorders in a general female population. Int Urogynecol J Pelvic Floor Dysfunct. 2009;20(9):1037–45.
9. López González PA, López López AI, López Cubillana P, Escudero Bregante F, Doñate Iñiguez G, Ruiz Morcillo JC, et al. Does cystocele have a role in bladder outlet obstruction. Actas Urol Esp. 2010;34(2):189–93.
10. Romanzi LJ, Chaikin DC, Blaivas JG. The effect of genital prolapse on voiding. J Urol. 1999;161(2):581–6.
11. Dancz CE, Ozel B. Is there a pelvic organ prolapse threshold that predicts bladder outflow obstruction? Int Urogynecol J. 2011;22(7):863–8.
12. Gomes CM, Rovner ES, Banner MP, Ramchandani P, Wein AJ. Simultaneous upper and lower urinary tract obstruction associated with severe genital prolapse: diagnosis and evaluation with magnetic resonance imaging. Int Urogynecol J Pelvic Floor Dysfunct. 2001;12(2):144–6.
13. Dietz HP, Haylen BT, Vancaillie TG. Female pelvic organ prolapse and voiding function. Int Urogynecol J. 2002;13(5):284–8.
14. de Boer TA, Salvatore S, Cardozo L, Chapple C, Kelleher C, van Kerrebroeck P, et al. Pelvic organ prolapse and overactive bladder. Neurourol Urodyn. 2010;29(1):30–9.
15. Patil A, Duckett JR. Effect of prolapse repair on voiding and bladder overactivity. Curr Opin Obstet Gynecol. 2010;22(5):399–403.
16. Johnson JR, High RA, Dziadek O, Ocon A, Muir TW, Xu J, et al. Overactive bladder symptoms after pelvic organ prolapse repair. Female Pelvic Med Reconstr Surg. 2019.
17. Chaikin DC, Groutz A, Blaivas JG. Predicting the need for anti-incontinence surgery in continent women undergoing repair of severe urogenital prolapse. J Urol. 2000;163(2):531–4.
18. Chughtai B, Spettel S, Kurman J, De E. Ambulatory pessary trial unmasks occult stress urinary incontinence. Obstet Gynecol Int. 2012;2012:392027.
19. Reena C, Kekre AN, Kekre N. Occult stress incontinence in women with pelvic organ prolapse. Int J Gynecol Obstet. 2007;97(1):31–4.
20. Ballert KN. Urodynamics in pelvic organ prolapse: when are they helpful and how do we use them? Urol Clin North Am. 2014;41(3):409–17, viii.
21. Bordman R, Telner D. Practice tips. Pessary insertion: choosing appropriate patients. Can Fam Physician. 2007;53(3):424–5.
22. Lazarou G, Scotti RJ, Mikhail MS, Zhou HS, Powers K. Pessary reduction and postoperative cure of retention in women with anterior vaginal wall prolapse. Int Urogynecol J Pelvic Floor Dysfunct. 2004;15(3):175–8.

23. Shumaker SA, Wyman JF, Uebersax JS, McClish D, Fantl JA. Health-related quality of life measures for women with urinary incontinence: the Incontinence Impact Questionnaire and the Urogenital Distress Inventory. Continence Program in Women (CPW) Research Group. Qual Life Res. 1994;3(5):291–306.
24. Winters JC, Dmochowski RR, Goldman HB, Herndon CDA, Kobashi KC, Kraus SR, et al. Urodynamic studies in adults: AUA/SUFU guideline. J Urol. 2012;188(6 Suppl):2464–72.
25. Liang C-C, Tseng L-H, Chang S-D, Chang Y-L, Lo T-S. Resolution of elevated postvoid residual volumes after correction of severe pelvic organ prolapse. Int Urogynecol J. 2008;19(9):1261–6.
26. Hagen S, Stark D. Conservative prevention and management of pelvic organ prolapse in women. Cochrane Database Syst Rev. 2011.
27. Li C, Gong Y, Wang B. The efficacy of pelvic floor muscle training for pelvic organ prolapse: a systematic review and meta-analysis. Int Urogynecol J. 2016;27(7):981–92.
28. Cundiff GW, Amundsen CL, Bent AE, Coates KW, Schaffer JI, Strohbehn K, et al. The PESSRI study: symptom relief outcomes of a randomized crossover trial of the ring and Gellhorn pessaries. Am J Obstet Gynecol. 2007;196(4):405.e1–8.
29. Dueñas JL, Miceli A. Effectiveness of a continuous-use ring-shaped vaginal pessary without support for advanced pelvic organ prolapse in postmenopausal women. Int Urogynecol J. 2018;29(11):1629–36.
30. Ramsay S, Tu LM, Tannenbaum C. Natural history of pessary use in women aged 65–74 versus 75 years and older with pelvic organ prolapse: a 12-year study. Int Urogynecol J. 2016;27(8):1201–7.
31. Maher C, Feiner B, Baessler K, Christmann-Schmid C, Haya N, Brown J. Surgery for women with anterior compartment prolapse. Cochrane Database Syst Rev. 2016.
32. Baessler K, Christmann-Schmid C, Maher C, Haya N, Crawford TJ, Brown J. Surgery for women with pelvic organ prolapse with or without stress urinary incontinence. Cochrane Database Syst Rev. 2018.
33. van der Ploeg J, van der Steen A, Zwolsman S, van der Vaart C, Roovers J. Prolapse surgery with or without incontinence procedure: a systematic review and meta-analysis. BJOG Int J Obstet Gynaecol. 2018;125(3):289–97.

Female Urethral Stricture

8

Rishi Nayyar, Devanshu Bansal,
and Bharti Uppal Nayyar

Learning Objectives

- To understand the current perspectives in diagnosis of female urethral stricture.
- To review the current understanding of etiology and presentation of this condition.
- To differentiate urethral stricture from other pathologies with similar presentation and imaging findings.
- To understand the limitations of investigations used for clinical workup of a suspected urethral stricture.
- To know the various management options available and their judicious use for treatment of female urethral stricture.
- To describe the advantages/disadvantages of various surgical approaches for female urethral stricture.

R. Nayyar (✉) · D. Bansal
Department of Urology, All India Institute of Medical Sciences, New Delhi, India

B. U. Nayyar
Department of Obstetrics and Gynecology, All India Institute of Medical Sciences, New Delhi, India

8.1 Introduction

Among the various de-novo causes of bladder outlet obstruction in females, a true urethral stricture is perhaps among the least common causes. Traumatic strictures and occasional near-obliterate strictures of other etiologies are obvious. Instead, it is the more common type of presentation with partial occlusive stricture that gets often confused with some other conditions causing lower urinary tract symptoms (LUTS) in females, because these other forms are much more common in clinical practice than a true stricture.

8.2 Definition and Epidemiology

Female urethral stricture is an uncommon, poorly understood, and perhaps under-reported condition. Around 2.7–8% of all women with voiding complaints are found to have bladder outlet obstruction [1]; and among them, only around 4–18% women are found to have a true urethral stricture [2, 3]. Some proposed causes of rarity of urethral stricture as a cause of bladder outlet obstruction in females are given in Table 8.1.

Definition of female urethral stricture is not well defined and there is no universally acceptable definition of normal urethral caliber as well [4]. Studies in healthy women usually report a

N. Khattar et al. (eds.), *Female Bladder Outlet Obstruction and Urethral Reconstruction*,
https://doi.org/10.1007/978-981-15-8521-0_8

Table 8.1 Proposed causes for lower incidence of urethral stricture in females compared to males

• Shorter length of urethra
• Entire urethral length is viscerally located: less exposed to trauma
• More mobility than male posterior urethra
• No surrounding spongiosa: Thus, no surrounding spongiofibrosis
• No tunica albugenia layer against which fibrosis or lumen can get compressed
• Voiding at lower pressures: Thus, lower reflux into urethral glands
• Difficult diagnosis among various differentials

urethral caliber of 22–30 Fr [5]. **Various authors define stricture as an inability to pass a 12–20 Fr urethral catheter** [3, 5, 6]. Due to lack of consensus on threshold urethral caliber to define urethral stricture, and to avoid inclusion of patients with functional bladder outlet obstruction (BOO), Osman et al. proposed the following definition for female urethral stricture: "A symptomatic, anatomical narrowing of the urethra based on a failure of catheterization, urethral calibration, visual inspection, or endoscopy or radiography" [7]. **The essence of diagnosis of urethral stricture in females is demonstration of an anatomical scarring in the urethra** as the cause of obstruction. Unlike males, entire urethral length in females is located viscerally within the confines of deep pelvis and therefore always running only as a differential diagnosis among a host of other more common problems emanating out of other surrounding anatomical structures, like external or internal sphincter, pelvic floor ring and its tonus, cystocele, urethral diverticulum, and so on. Therefore, mere demonstration of a narrowing with proximal dilatation on contrast imaging is not an infallible way of diagnosis of urethral stricture in females, unlike anterior urethral stricture in males. Retrograde study in females is also not clinically useful with its inherent limitations due to short urethral length [4]. Not only this, absence of spongiosa and therefore spongiofibrosis lets urethra not be affected by dense fibrosis from inflammatory causes despite more prevalence of lower urinary tract infection (UTI) in females. Also, absence of tunica albugenia or prostate, unlike in males, may allow some degree of dilatation before the stricture becomes functionally relevant to cause symptoms of outlet obstruction. For the same reason, it may be difficult to perceive true caliber of female urethra during blind calibration with a catheter or bougie/dilator because absence of a surrounding albugenia-like tough structure allows easy dilatation of such softer strictures during evaluation itself. Notwithstanding, other causes of bladder outlet obstruction like angulation due to a tight pelvic ring or hypertrophied external sphincter may be perceived as a narrowing during calibration. Hence office calibration also is not a foolproof way for diagnosis of a female urethral stricture. Previous authors have also questioned the usefulness of urethral calibration [8]. Diagnosis may be relatively easier in cases with stricture at the meatus like in elderly females with senile vaginitis. The narrowing of the meatus is visible to the naked eye during local examination. Also, the terminal urethra in females has a more fibrotic collagen ring (Lyon's ring) surrounding the urethra rendering it to easier diagnosis during calibration. Uroflowmetry or urodynamics by themselves can only give a physiological diagnosis of outlet obstruction and that is also not standardized for females, as discussed in previous chapters. Voiding patterns in females are very variable due to variability in voiding position like sitting, squatting, or standing; racial differences; age differences; and holding patterns due to non-availability of toilets. Even videourodynamics is not enough to establish a stricture because mere demonstration of an apparent area of obstruction on imaging is not synonymous with female urethral stricture.

8.3 Etio-Pathogenesis

Various common causes of female urethral stricture include trauma, iatrogenic injury, malignancy, radiation, or obstetric injury [2]. Urethritis by itself, although common, has been reported only rarely as a cause of female urethral stricture [7]. King et al. reported gonorrhea and infectious etiology as the most common cause of stricture in females in 1931, even though compared to males, female urethra embryologically represents that part of urethra which is generally not involved in inflammation [9]. With improved management of infections and access to healthcare for females, inflammatory infectious causes of stricture would also have reduced drastically, and it is difficult to find any reported case in contemporary practice, if any.

Obstetric and pelvic trauma usually leads to severe urethral narrowing and may lead to total urethral obliteration or bladder neck destruction. Majority of urethral injury sustained due to pelvic trauma are seen in girls compared to women. Because urethra is caged inside bony pelvis and is relatively mobile, urethral injuries are uncommon and partial injuries may even be missed because it is easy to pass catheter in a shorter and straight urethra. When severe, these injuries are frequently associated with concomitant genital injuries and urethro-vaginal fistulae. Obstetric injury usually involves proximal urethra and occurs due to prolonged labor leading to ischemic pressure necrosis or instrumentation of the urethra against the pubic bone [10, 11].

Predominant causes of urethral stricture in developed countries are iatrogenic, including traumatic urethral catheterization, urethral or vaginal surgery (including urethral diverticulectomy, urethral sling placement) and pelvic irradiation for malignancies (leading to end organ arterial obliteration and subsequent fibrosis) [12]. Long-term indwelling catheterization leads to stricture formation due to pressure necrosis [13].

The causes of urethral stricture are tabulated in Table 8.2. To the best of our knowledge, there is no histopathological study available in literature specifically directed to female urethral stricture disease, indicating a major lacuna in our understanding of urethral inflammation and fibrosis in females.

Table 8.2 Etiology of female urethral stricture

Trauma
Pelvic fracture
Obstetric injury
Iatrogenic
Urethral diverticulectomy
Urethral sling placement
Anterior vaginal surgery
Traumatic/long-term urethral catheterization
Pelvic irradiation
Others
Infection
Urethral malignancy
Idiopathic

8.4 Clinical Features

Urethral stricture may occur in any age group of females and there is no known genetic, racial, or geographical predilection. Previous urethritis, inguinal lymph nodes and history of sexually transmitted diseases may be relevant. **Patients usually present with storage and/or voiding symptoms** including straining to void, poor urinary stream, frequency, urgency, nocturia, and/or sense of incomplete bladder emptying. Patients may also present with painful micturition, urethral pain, recurrent urinary tract infection and in rare cases with uremia due to chronic retention [4, 6]. However, correlation of storage or voiding LUTS with the specific diagnosis of anatomic female urethral stricture is tenuous at best, and using a symptom-based diagnosis has led to unnecessary urethral dilatation of many patients in the past [7]. Because there is no direct correlation between the type of female LUTS and final diagnosis, refractory LUTS of any kind may be an indication for detailed assessment in females for a possible urethral stricture even when it involves more invasive investigations like urethro-cystoscopy and examination under anesthesia. Here a clinical "working diagnosis" assumes significance pending the final diagnosis, and the role of urethral dilatation at this juncture, before a final diagnosis is made, is controversial. It must be emphasized that many pathologies other than stricture may temporarily respond to urethral dilatation making diagnosis based on response to urethral dilatation also a poor method of diagnosis of stricture [14]. At our center, we would generally avoid use of blind dilatation before cystoscopy. Patients with traumatic strictures often present with suprapubic cystostomy in situ after being managed initially for other injuries.

Local examination is an essential component of patient management and should include a focused urological and genital examination. Lichen sclerosis, meatal stenosis, and periurethral abnormalities may be evident on local examination. Vaginal and per speculum examination should be done to assess the status of the vagina and any coexistent genitourinary fistula or pelvic organ prolapse. The quality of local tissues including vaginal mucosa, introital mucosa, and labia minora should also be assessed for possible use in surgical reconstruction of the stricture [14]. Pelvic examination may also be a chance for a screening PAP smear examination for the appropriate age group females.

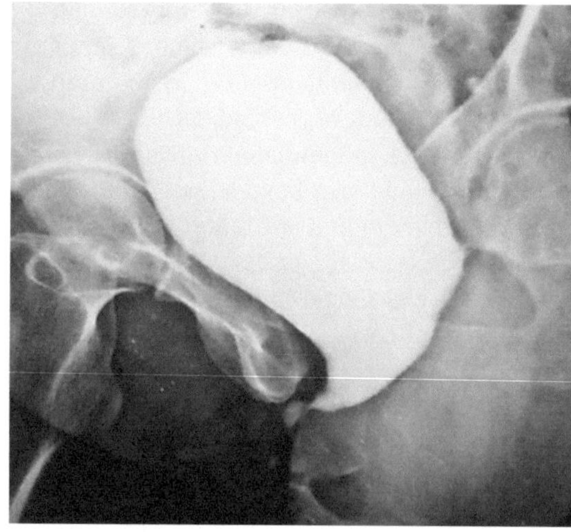

Fig. 8.1 Voiding cystourethrogram in a 29-year-old lady with poor urine flow showing a mid-urethral narrowing with proximal dilatation and back pressure changes in bladder. Post-void residual urine was 130 cc

8.5 Investigations

A high index of suspicion as well as judgment is required for making a diagnosis of female urethral stricture due to variable clinical presentation and lack of a proper cut off threshold of urethral caliber. **Evaluation should include etiology, site, length and density of stricture, pelvic floor muscle strength, vaginal and vulval health, oral health in case oral graft is contemplated, evaluation for sexual function, any pre-existing incontinence, and patient's expectations**.

Initial evaluation should be done using uroflowmetry and post-void residual volume (PVR) estimation. A plateau-shaped curve on uroflowmetry suggests a fixed anatomical obstruction indicating a stricture [15]. Urethral calibration is an easy method to assess the size of the patent urethral lumen. As mentioned previously, a variable threshold of 12–20 Fr urethral caliber has been used by various authors, although majority will agree to a 14 Fr caliber cut-off. This should be standardized for the institution. Patient must be relaxed as young girls are often very anxious during urogenital examination without anesthesia, and this may thus lead to artificially tight urethra even in the absence of a true stricture.

Voiding cysto-urethrography (VCUG) should be obtained in all cases as anatomical configuration of bladder and urethra besides the descent of bladder neck and urethra could provide important clues to diagnosis and areas to focus during endoscopy (Fig. 8.1). **Endoscopic urethral calibration with a pediatric cystoscope or ureteroscope should be considered early** in the diagnostic workup of a patient in whom history, examination and uroflowmetry suggest a differential diagnosis of a stricture. Urethro-cystoscopy helps to directly visualize the stricture. However, length of urethral stricture may be difficult to assess and it may not be possible to insert the scope in severe strictures (Fig. 8.2). Use of a pediatric cystoscope or ureteroscope is a great help in this regard. Otherwise a Compact™ 14 Fr cystoscope which has a shorter bevel (Richard Wolf, Knittlingen, Germany) is a very useful tool (Fig. 8.3). It is an integrated cystourethroscope system with telescope lens, bridge and sheath all in-built in one scope as one piece. It is recommended as the lumen opens at its terminal end and the distention of the urethra is much better, compared to a standard cystoscope with an open ventral area and beak with the subsequent loss of fluid at the open ventral aspect of the scope. A standard cystoscope requires a Nickell's adaptor for fruitful urethroscopy in females. A 0- or 12-degree lens gives the best luminal view. We avoid inserting jelly into the urethra which may

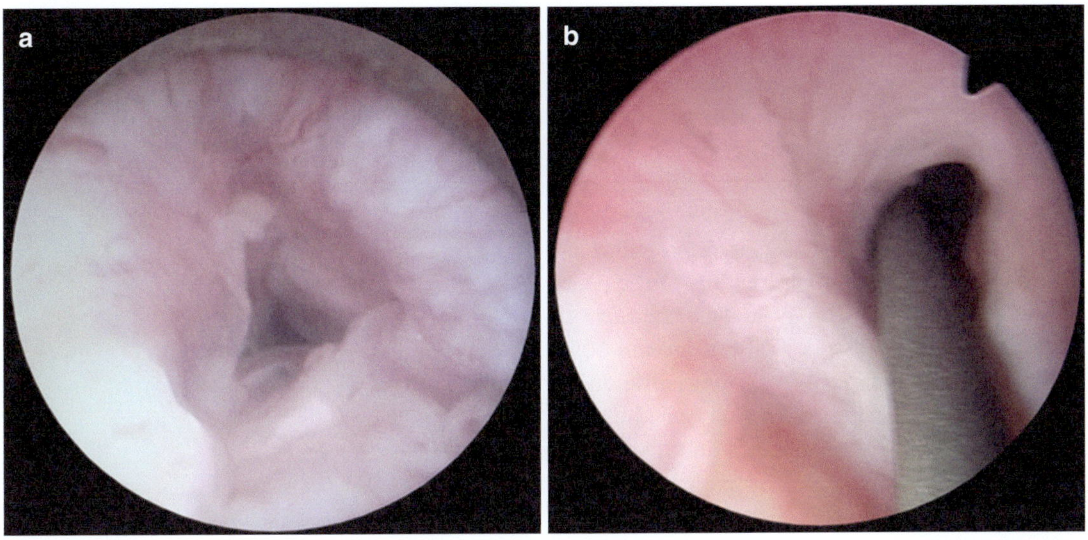

Fig. 8.2 Urethroscopy showing (**a**) Mid-urethral superficial fibrous scarring suggestive of stricture urethra in the same patient as in Fig. 8.1. It was easily dilatable with the endoscope over a guide wire. (**b**) Mid urethral dense stricture not visible on the mucosa but had significant fibrosis underneath and was difficult to dilate even with pediatric cystoscope

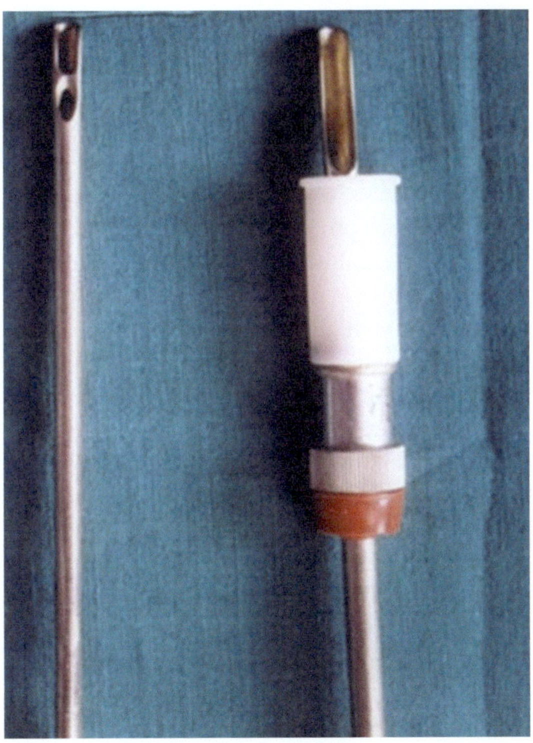

Fig. 8.3 A compact/integrated cystourethroscope with a short bevel and a standard 17 Fr cystoscope with a Nickell's adaptor for female urethroscopy

traumatize the urethra from syringe hub or rapid stretching of urethra. It is used only on the instrument tip before insertion, to provide best unscathed view. Because of its short length, it is difficult to distend the female urethra during urethroscopy for assessment regarding its distensibility. Therefore, bladder should be near full to reduce irrigation fluid moving into the bladder. Short of this, unless the stricture is narrower than the viewing endoscope (pediatric cystoscope, ureteroscope or standard cystoscope), there is every chance that it may be missed even during endoscopy, particularly if it is short and flimsy. **Any parched appearance, associated force required to move in the scope or telescoping of mucosa with the tip of scope should be carefully assessed**. Caution should also be exercised not to take a voluntary squeeze by the patient due to a full bladder for a stricture.

Other relevant investigations include transvaginal ultrasound with insertion of gel in the urethra, which might show proximal urethral dilation with narrowing at stricture site with associated secondary changes like bladder diverticulae and vesicoureteral reflux. However, it has only an experimental role in contemporary practice.

Urodynamics, especially with the use of fluoroscopy, may be helpful in equivocal cases and before surgical intervention. This usually reveals a high-pressure, low-flow pattern. Although urodynamic pressure cut-offs are not consistent across studies [16], a detrusor contraction at maximum flow of more than 25 cm H_2O and peak flow of less than 12 ml/s may suggest obstruction with a sensitivity and specificity of around 60% [17]. Video-urodynamics may be particularly useful and usually demonstrates an open bladder neck with wide proximal urethra and distal narrow area in the urethra [18].

MRI is rarely required and may identify defects in urethral and peri-urethral tissue or urethral tumors. Sagittal T2-weighted images provide the best visualization of tumor extent [19].

8.6 Management

The diagnosis of urethral stricture should not be based on a single investigation as no test has enough sensitivity and specificity to be used in isolation. It should be a corroborative diagnosis from history, examination, and multiple investigation findings including endoscopy.

Primary repair has been advocated in acute urethral trauma if patient's condition is stable [20]. However, a significant proportion of cases end up with delayed repair due to a lack of available expertise or severe associated injuries requiring more urgent attention. Detailed discussion about primary female urethral trauma is outside the scope of this chapter and book.

Varied minimally invasive and open surgical options are available for management of female urethral stricture (Tables 8.3 and 8.4). However, these options are supported by limited literature in the form of mostly case series and retrospective case reviews. Consequently, variable success rates of various procedures are reported in literature and none can be advocated over one another for its efficacy. A recent anatomical study indicates a relative higher nerve density in posterior urethra than anterior, more so in proximal urethra [21]. Distal urethra showed significantly more large vessels compared with the proximal posterior urethra. How such anatomical observations can be applied clinically to various available approaches is a work in progress.

Table 8.3 Minimally invasive management options for female urethral stricture

Urethral dilation
Optical internal urethrotomy
Core through (cut-to-the-light procedure)

Table 8.4 Open surgical management options for female urethral stricture

Distal urethral stricture
Heineke-Mikulicz meatoplasty
Distal-Mid-Proximal urethral stricture
Flap urethroplasty
Anterior vaginal wall flap (Blandy-like flap)
Vestibular flap (Montorsi flap)
Lateral vaginal wall flap (Orandi-like flap)
Free graft urethroplasty
Technique
Dorsal/Anterior onlay
Ventral/Posterior onlay
Dorsal inlay
Ventral inlay
Double face graft
Tissue
Vaginal mucosa
Introital labial mucosa
Oral buccal, labial or lingual mucosa
Tubed flap or graft urethroplasty
End to end anastomotic urethroplasty
Transecting
Non-transecting
Proximal urethral/bladder neck stricture
Anterior bladder tubed flap (Tanagho flap)
Tanagho flap
Reverse Tanagho (Nayyar) flap

Given the short length of female urethra and poorly understood sphincteric mechanisms, continence has always remained a concern for any female urethral reconstruction. However, all available literature suggests that unless the entire length of urethra requires repair, continence is generally not an issue with continence results of more than 90% across all series and types of repairs for short strictures [7]. However, for cases with complete urethral loss, it is our belief that unless the pelvic muscle strength is strong, it is very difficult to assure continence and consent must be obtained in this regard. At our center, we generally add a pubovaginal autologous sling procedure in cases involving both bladder neck and mid urethral complex.

Overall, **the goals of management in cases of female urethral stricture are alleviation of symptoms; prevention of complications like upper tract damage, infections, or stones; and preserve urogenital function in terms of continence and sexual function**. Pharmacotherapy has no role in management.

8.6.1 Urethral Dilation and Optical Internal Urethrotomy

Urethral dilation is usually the first-line option used for management of female urethral stricture [22]. It is an office-based procedure and is technically easy to perform. However, as discussed earlier blind dilatation should be avoided before diagnosis in our view. Also, it is important to understand that although urethral dilation may be used for initial management of stricture, **recurrence rates are high and long-term success rate may be as low as 47%** or even lower on long-term follow-up. Success rate of dilation further deteriorates in patients with history of previous urethral dilation [7]. Furthermore, recurrent stricture in this setting may be more fibrotic and may adversely affect the success of open surgical repair [23].

There is limited data to support use of optical internal urethrotomy, and it is usually used to treat mid urethral strictures. This may be done with the use of cold knife or holmium laser. The stricture is usually incised at 3 and 9 o'clock positions, although some authors give an additional incision at 12 o'clock [24]. In cases of severe short segment mid-proximal urethral strictures with indwelling suprapubic catheter, a cut to the light procedure may be performed as a minimally invasive treatment [25].

Overall, literature to support long-term success of minimally invasive treatment options is limited and is considered inferior to open surgical repair. Therefore, in cases of dense urethral stricture, a low threshold should be kept to offer open surgical repair.

8.6.2 Open Surgical Management

A multitude of open surgical options are available for female urethral stricture management. The reported **success rates of open surgical management are usually high, with overall success rates ranging from 91% to 94%** [7]. The various open surgical options are listed in Table 8.4. A complete obliteration necessitates either a cut to light/core through procedure in cases of very short stricture or a tubed flap or graft procedure. In most cases, however, a substitution augmentation procedure is done. Here, it should also be emphasized that most procedures for female urethroplasty have been named in literature according to taxonomy of urethroplasty in males. Thus, the true "ventral" urethral side in anatomical position has been wrongly labeled as "dorsal" when describing the urethroplasty procedures in females.

Further stepwise details about individual techniques are discussed in subsequent chapters. The key technical points to remember that are common to all kinds of open surgical repair of urethral stricture are listed in Table 8.5. Ascertaining proximal extent of stricture is difficult during these surgeries and is based mostly on visual cues during surgery corroborated with pre-operative imaging. The fibrosis is generally not expansive and very difficult to palpate. Nonetheless, the callus/fibrotic tissue must be adequately excised particularly in post-traumatic cases undergoing tubed flap/graft urethroplasty. Post-menopausal females or cases with atrophic/senile vaginitis may benefit from a short-course local estrogen therapy. It may help improving local vascularity, and tissue elasticity with improved healing [4].

Since flap repairs bring a vascularized tissue for reconstruction, it may be assumed that they would have better success rates. However, case series of both type of repairs report a high success rate of 80–90% in literature [2, 5–7, 10, 15, 26] with limited complications. Therefore, **based**

Table 8.5 Key points for surgical repair of female urethral stricture

Pre-operative [4]
Absence of vaginal infection
Sterile urine culture
Use of vaginal estrogens (if indicated)
Adequate gap from last urethral dilation (usually 3 months)
Intra-operative [2, 4]
Use of urethral guidewire to avoid creation of false passage
Absorbable suture material
Careful dissection of involved structures
Adequate mobilization of periurethral and vaginal tissue
Use of well vascularized flaps
Non-overlapping tension-free repair
Adequate bladder drainage
Well-vascularized bed for grafts with quilting
Use of interposition flaps (e.g., Martius flap) as needed (ventral procedures)
Careful preservation of clitoral neurovascular tissue (dorsal procedures)

on current evidence no technique can be recommended over another for any stricture type. Nonetheless, individualized patient management is suggested. **A post-traumatic case with poor base for graft uptake may benefit with a vascularized tissue transfer** like a bladder flap rather than a graft procedure. On the other hand, a short mid-urethral stricture could do well with any technique the surgeon is comfortable with and least morbid for the patient. **Buccal graft may be preferred in young females, lichen sclerosus or senile vaginitis** to avoid taking vaginal graft or sexual issues. Otherwise, vaginal graft suffices well in females with roomy and healthy vagina. Vaginal mucosa is clinically similar to buccal mucosa in its properties with respect to wetness, elasticity, and take at recipient site. It also has highly vascular arborization plexus in sublamina, though direct comparative histopathological studies against buccal mucosa are lacking. Distal vaginal mucosa is more rugose and thicker compared to mid and proximal vagina, and therefore less suitable for graft uptake. Inner skin/mucosa of labia minora can be used both as free graft [27] or flap based [28] on peri-urethral/paravaginal fat or labial fat pad. It is thin and much easily harvested without much donor site morbidity. However, it should be avoided in cases with lichen sclerosus or atrophicus. Local application of estrogens for 3 months improves the vascularity and thickness of introital and vaginal mucosa, but in our opinion, it may be better to use buccal mucosa in such cases than depend upon pharmacological treatment for improvement of tissues. Irrespective, local estrogens may still be used for general vaginal health.

As regards the choice of approach, there is again insufficient evidence in literature to make any kind of recommendation. There are proposed advantages to both dorsal and ventral approaches as described in Table 8.6. As a matter of principle, we generally avoid vaginal manipulation, unless necessitated because of other factors. Therefore, dorsal approach is our first choice. Because the urethra is primarily supplied by longitudinal branches of inferior vesical artery, the vascularity of urethra is generally not of concern with its mobilization by any of the approaches. A double-faced graft may also be placed by either approach, if required [29].

Inlay graft placement techniques have been described with the intention to avoid urethral mobilization and hence avoid urethral devascularization. However, the anatomic descriptions of

Table 8.6 Possible advantages of dorsal or ventral approaches for female urethral stricture repair

Dorsal approach	Ventral approach
Sturdy, vascular and immobile tissue bed	Easier approach with more space to operate
No hypospadiac meatus	Vaginal vascularized flap can be taken
Urine flow directed anteriorly, avoids vaginal pooling and post-void dribbling	Incontinence procedures can be easily added, if required
Posterior urethral tissue plane remains untouched for any subsequent surgery, if required	No injury to clitoral corporal bodies
Less chances of urethro-vaginal fistula or diverticulum formation	No injury to clitoral neuro-vascular bundle
Does not require steep Trendelenburg positioning	Less chances of injuring pubourethral ligaments and sphincteric complex

female urethral vascular supply to support such hypothesis are distinctly lacking. Nevertheless, using the principle of Asopa's inlay technique of male urethral stricture repair, inlay graft placement has been described both by ventral or dorsal approaches [30]. A ventral or dorsal inlay from inside the urethra is also feasible, made easier by use of a nasal speculum to increase endoluminal space for making incision and taking sutures [31, 32]. Such an approach entails least mobilization and disconnection of urethra from its surrounding adventitia. However, there are no comparative studies to conclude which of the techniques (stretching the urethra for working endo-luminally versus a clean-cut urethrotomy from outside) results in less tissue injury or provides better results.

End to end anastomotic urethroplasty has been described for short segment obliterate mid or proximal strictures [25], but it would tend to cause urethral shortening. Additionally, it inherently requires mobilization of urethra at both ends with excision of obliterate segment. Results in such a scenario are heavily dependent upon the vascularity of distal urethra from surrounding tissues (distal anterior vaginal wall and introital branches of internal pudendal artery supplying the meatus) which may not be sufficiently quantifiable to predict results of surgery. We have performed buccal mucosal tubed graft and bladder mucosal tubed graft in such scenarios with good results and follow-up of more than 2 years in each [33–35]. Continence procedure need not be added if bladder neck is intact.

Strictures involving bladder neck like post-traumatic pelvic fracture associated injuries or severe obstetric injuries are a specific subset requiring more elaborate surgical repair. Incontinence is also a particular concern that must be discussed with the patient in preoperative workup. A supra-pubic approach and Tanagho's bladder flap has been described earlier with acceptable results for continence and voiding [36]. The results become poorer with increasing length of the flap to bridge the gap [37, 38]. We have described a bladder flap technique in this setting, wherein an anterior bladder flap is flipped downward to create neourethra. The continence results with this technique have been very encouraging so far without use of any additional anti-continence procedure [39]. Labia minora pedicled flap or vaginal pedicled flaps are other options in such cases. Though these options use transvaginal approach, unlike Tanagho's repair (which uses the detrusor fibres near the bladder neck) they do not provide any continence mechanism. Therefore, they require a concomitant sling procedure for satisfactory results [37].

Because most female urethral strictures are short in length and do not accompany dense or deep spongiofibrosis, we believe almost all open repairs are likely to provide suitable results. It is upon us as surgeons to master one technique and be aware about all others and their principles to an extent to be able to provide best care to our patients.

8.7 Follow-Up and Management of Recurrent Stricture After Previous Urethroplasty

There is no set protocol defining how to follow-up the cases after a urethroplasty procedure. **A uroflowmetry and PVR should be done in all at 3 months or earlier if symptoms recur**. A VCUG or urethroscopy after 3 months also helps in confirming the repair. Most practitioners generally rely upon a urethroscopy. Hampson et al. defined stricture recurrence in their multi-institutional retrospective series as failure to pass a 17 Fr scope [40]. They reported a stricture recurrence rate of 23% (9/39 cases) with mean time to recurrence of 14 months. Five cases recurred within 9 months, three after 24 months while time to failure was not reported for one. It is prudent to reconfirm the stricture as the cause of symptoms before any repeat procedure is contemplated. In this regard, urethroscopy and demonstration of anatomical fibrotic narrowing again serves as best judge for the surgeon. Failures after dorsal graft urethroplasty have generally been managed with urethral dilatations. A vascularized vaginal or labial skin flap may be chosen, particularly if ischemia and poor graft uptake is deemed as cause of failure [40]. A ventral onlay or inlay procedure may also be an option. A re-do dorsal graft approach though feasible [40] should be used only with caution for higher chances of failure.

Salvage procedure like continent stoma may rarely be required for those with multiple failed repairs and are not able to do self-calibration/dilation, do not want a urine bag, and desire to maintain continence [35].

8.8 Future Directions

Lacunae exist in our knowledge in every aspect of urethral stricture and bladder outlet obstruction in females. Therefore, future research needs to be focused on all these aspects. Animal models of female rodents are available and used for study of bladder outlet obstruction. However not much is specifically available with respect to urethral stricture disease. Focused anatomical studies are needed to provide a pathophysiological basis for causation, treatment, and prognostication of female urethral stricture disease. Use of histopathology in every case undergoing female urethroplasty may be a next step to correlate management with disease processes. On the clinical aspects, comparisons of various techniques and graft materials is the logical next step for studies. Patient-reported outcome measures in terms of impact on voiding, continence, and sexual function should also be assessed for better acceptance among surgeons and patients alike. Fetal amnion is commonly used in gynecological practice for McIndoe vaginoplasty. Its role in female urethral stricture repair, however, remains unexplored and may be considered. But before all that one must make a conscious effort of moving away from practice of blind urethral dilatation in women presenting with voiding difficulty simply because it is considered an easy office procedure with little side effects.

Clinical Case Discussion

A 38-year-old lady presented with prolonged time for micturition, poor stream, and frequency for the last 8 months. She had three children, all supervised normal vaginal deliveries. Last child birth was 4 years ago. She was sexually active with no history of trauma, sexually transmitted disease, or catheterization. There were no known co-morbidities or any neurological disease. She had no constipation or recurrent urinary infections. She had undergone urethral calibration and dilation four times over 8 months, with relief lasting hardly 7–10 days each time. Local genital examination was normal. Urine routine showed two or three pus cells. A uroflow (Fig. 8.4) showed peak flow of 18.8 ml/s but waving peak, average flow of 6.3 ml/s and void duration of 1 min 32 s for a void volume of 500 cc. Post-void volume was nil. A voiding cystourethrogram was done, catheterization for which was difficult and was done using 5 Fr feeding tube. Endoscopic examination with 11 Fr pediatric cystoscope showed tight narrowing just beneath the meatus in the distal-mid urethra. A diagnosis of urethral stricture was thus made using a combination of all findings. Dorsal graft urethroplasty was done with good relief of symptoms at 6 months.

Key Learning Points

- Female urethral stricture is an uncommon cause of bladder outlet obstruction in females. Its evaluation and management are still evolving. The literature is sparse and incoherent given the relative rarity of disease and discrepancies in its definition and description.
- Diagnosis is dependent upon demonstration of anatomical fibrotic narrowing along with functional obstruction. Alternative diagnosis like dysfunctional voiding, external sphincter dysynergia, and Fowler's syndrome must be carefully searched for.
- Except for direct visualization on urethroscopy, no single non-invasive investigation has high sensitivity and specificity for diagnosis of female urethral stricture.
- A multitude of therapeutic options are available for female urethral stricture, including minimally invasive or substitution urethroplasty procedures.
- Repeated dilatation has poor long-term success rate.
- Urethroplasty should be considered early, particularly if a second dilatation is unsuccessful.

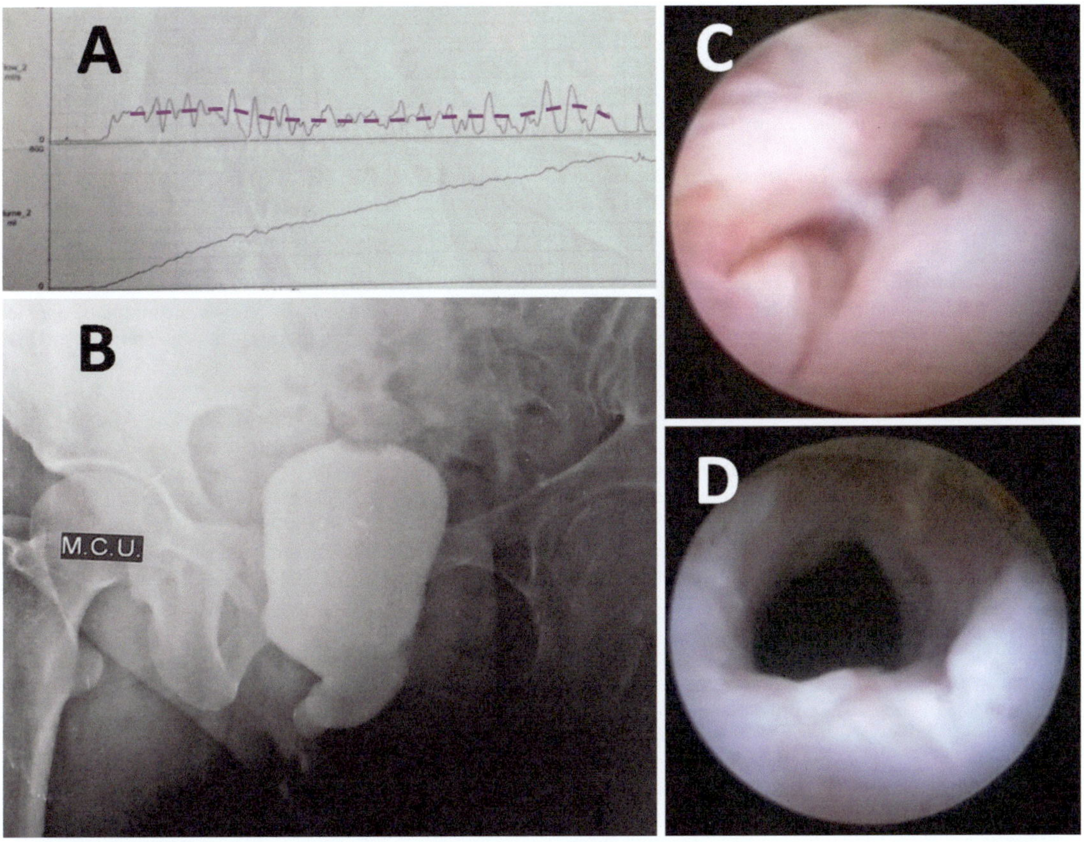

Fig. 8.4 Investigation findings in a case of urethral stricture. (**a**) Uroflowmetry showing a prolonged flow with waving peaks. Averaged out flow (dashed purple line) giving a box-pattern (static flow) kind of appearance of flow curve. (**b**) Voiding cystourethrography showing dilated proximal and mid urethra with distal stricture. (**c**) Urethroscopy with pediatric scope confirmed tight fibrotic stricture just underneath the meatus for about 5 mm. (**d**) Proximal urethra was very dilated

- Success rates >90% can be achieved at short-to-medium follow-up with urethroplasty.
- Not enough evidence to recommend one urethroplasty technique or approach over another.
- The risk of incontinence appears low after urethroplasty.

References

1. Carr LK, Webster GD. Bladder outlet obstruction in women. Urol Clin North Am. 1996;23(3):385–92.
2. Faiena I, Koprowski C, Tunuguntla H. Female urethral reconstruction. J Urol. 2016;195(3):557–67.
3. Hoag N, Chee J. Surgical management of female urethral strictures. Transl Androl Urol. 2017;6(S2):S76–80.
4. Waterloos M, Verla W. Female urethroplasty: a practical guide emphasizing diagnosis and surgical treatment of female urethral stricture disease. Biomed Res Int. 2019;2019:1–13.
5. Osman NI, Chapple CR. Contemporary surgical management of female urethral stricture disease. Curr Opin Urol. 2015;25(4):341–5.
6. Gormley EA. Vaginal flap urethroplasty for female urethral stricture disease. Neurourol Urodyn. 2010;29(S1):S42–5.
7. Osman NI, Mangera A, Chapple CR. A systematic review of surgical techniques used in the treatment of female urethral stricture. Eur Urol. 2013;64(6):965–73.
8. Gleason DM, Bottaccini MR, Lattimer JK. What does the bougie a boule calibrate? J Urol. 1969;101(1):114–6.
9. King MW. Stricture of the female urethra. Am J Surg. 1931;13(2):251–5.

10. Flisser AJ, Blaivas JG. Outcome of urethral reconstructive surgery in a series of 74 women. J Urol. 2003;169(6):2246–9.
11. Roenneburg ML, Wheeless CR. Traumatic absence of the proximal urethra. Am J Obstet Gynecol. 2005;193(6):2169–72.
12. Blaivas JG, Santos JA, Tsui JF, Deibert CM, Rutman MP, Purohit RS, et al. Management of urethral stricture in women. J Urol. 2012;188(5):1778–82.
13. Andrews HO, Shah PJ. Surgical management of urethral damage in neurologically impaired female patients with chronic indwelling catheters. Br J Urol. 1998;82(6):820–4.
14. Ackerman AL, Blaivas J, Anger JT. Female urethral reconstruction. Curr Bladder Dysfunct Rep. 2010;5(4):225–32.
15. Mukhtar BMB, Spilotros M, Malde S, Greenwell TJ. Ventral-onlay buccal mucosa graft substitution urethroplasty for urethral stricture in women. BJU Int. 2017;120(5):710–6.
16. Kuo H-C. Urodynamic parameters for the diagnosis of bladder outlet obstruction in women. Urol Int. 2004;72(1):46–51.
17. Defreitas GA, Zimmern PE, Lemack GE, Shariat SF. Refining diagnosis of anatomic female bladder outlet obstruction: comparison of pressure-flow study parameters in clinically obstructed women with those of normal controls. Urology. 2004;64(4):675–9.
18. Rosenblum N, Nitti VW. Post-urethral suspension obstruction. Curr Opin Urol. 2001;11(4):411–6.
19. Kawashima A, Sandler CM, Wasserman NF, LeRoy AJ, King BF, Goldman SM. Imaging of urethral disease: a pictorial review. Radiographics. 2004;24(Suppl_1):S195–216.
20. Patel DN, Fok CS, Webster GD, Anger JT. Female urethral injuries associated with pelvic fracture: a systematic review of the literature. BJU Int. 2017;120(6):766–73.
21. Mazloomdoost D, Westermann LB, Mutema G, Crisp CC, Kleeman SD, Pauls RN. Histologic anatomy of the anterior vagina and urethra. Female Pelvic Med Reconstr Surg. 2017;23(5):329–35.
22. Keegan KA, Nanigian DK, Stone AR. Female urethral stricture disease. Curr Urol Rep. 2008;9(5):419–23.
23. Smith AL, Ferlise VJ, Rovner ES. Female urethral strictures: successful management with long-term clean intermittent catheterization after urethral dilatation. BJU Int. 2006;98(1):96–9.
24. Rosenblum N, Nitti VW. Female urethral reconstruction. Urol Clin North Am. 2011;38(1):55–64.
25. Hemal AK, Dorairajan LN, Gupta NP. Posttraumatic complete and partial loss of urethra with pelvic fracture in girls: an appraisal of management. J Urol. 2000;163(1):282–7.
26. Petrou SP, Rogers AE, Parker AS, Green KM, McRoberts JW. Dorsal vaginal graft urethroplasty for female urethral stricture disease. BJU Int. 2012;110(11) Pt C:E1090–5.
27. Rehder P, Glodny B, Pichler R, Exeli L, Kerschbaumer A, Mitterberger MJ. Dorsal urethroplasty with labia minora skin graft for female urethral strictures. BJU Int. 2010;106(8):1211–4.
28. Tao TT, Xu QK, Hu Q, Huang XJ, Chen J, Wang WZ, Lv BD, Duan Y. Novel surgical technique for female distal urethral stricture disease: an evaluation of efficacy and safety compared with urethral dilatation. Int J Clin Exp Med. 2018;11(11):12002–7.
29. Joshi PM, Kulkarni SB. A new technique of double-face buccal graft urethroplasty for female urethral strictures. Turk J Urol. 2019;46(2):165–8.
30. Önol FF, Önol ŞY, Tahra A, Boylu U. Ventral inlay labia minora graft urethroplasty for the management of female urethral strictures. Urology. 2014;83(2):460–4.
31. Hoag N, Gani J, Chee J. Vaginal-sparing ventral buccal mucosal graft urethroplasty for female urethral stricture: a novel modification of surgical technique. Investig Clin Urol. 2016;57(4):298–302.
32. Nayak P, Mandal S, Das M. Ventral-inlay buccal mucosal graft urethroplasty for female urethral stricture. Indian J Urol. 2019;35(4):273–7.
33. Singh RK, Kaushal D, Khattar N, Nayyar R, Manasa T, Sood R. Pediatric pelvic fracture urethral distraction defect causing complete urethrovaginal avulsion. Indian J Urol. 2018;34(1):76–8.
34. Bansal D, Nayyar R, Singh P, Jain S. Individualized management of obliterative urethral stricture in females – five patients five management strategies. Indian J Urol. 2019;35(Suppl 1):S8.
35. Nayyar R, Bansal D, Singh P, Jain S, Seth A. Individualized Management of Obliterative Urethral Stricture in Females – Four Patients Four Management Strategies. J Clin Urol. 2020; 13(4): 261–66.
36. Tanagho EA. Bladder neck reconstruction for total urinary incontinence: 10 years experience. J Urol. 1981;125(3):321–6.
37. Radwan MH, Abou Farha MO, Soliman MG, et al. Outcome of female urethral reconstruction: a 12-year experience. World J Urol. 2013;31:991–5.
38. Blaivas JG. Vaginal flap urethral reconstruction: an alternative to the bladder flap neourethra. J Urol. 1989;141:542–5.
39. Nayyar R, Jain S, Sharma K, Pethe S, Sharma P. A novel anterior bladder tube for traumatic bladder neck contracture in females: initial results. Urology. 2020;139:201–06.
40. Hampson LA, Myers JB, Vanni AJ, Virasoro R, Smith TG 3rd, Capiel L, Chandrapal J, Voelzke BB. Dorsal buccal graft urethroplasty in female urethral stricture disease: a multicenter experience. Transl Androl Urol. 2019 Mar;8(Suppl 1):S6–S12.

Bladder Outlet Obstruction After Sling Surgery for Stress Urinary Incontinence

9

Sanjay Sinha

Learning Objectives

- Understanding of epidemiology and etiology of postoperative voiding dysfunction.
- Recognition and diagnostic evaluation; limitations of diagnostic testing.
- Awareness of various management options and their implications.
- Outcome of intervention and implications for counseling.

9.1 Introduction

Voiding dysfunction following sling surgery for stress urinary incontinence is not uncommon and can be associated with significant morbidity. It remains the commonest indication for salvage procedures. The presentation can be varied ranging from persistent immediate postoperative retention to more subtle presentations such as intractable storage symptoms or discomfort. Voiding dysfunction may also occur concomitant with other complications such as urethral sling exposure. In the absence of high-quality evidence and established criteria for defining female bladder outlet obstruction, there is lack of consensus regarding key aspects of diagnosis and management. This chapter examines the presentation, diagnosis and management of voiding dysfunction following sling surgery for stress urinary incontinence sling.

S. Sinha (✉)
Apollo Hospitals, Hyderabad, India

9.2 Scope of the Problem

Early postoperative obstruction has been reported to occur in 1.9–19.7% of women following a midurethral sling [1]. This wide range reflects not just differences in technique but also differences in the way retention has been defined by authors. A recent Cochrane review found no difference in the voiding dysfunction rate between autologous pubovaginal slings and midurethral slings but the numbers were small and studies not designed for addressing this question [2]. Voiding dysfunction was less likely to occur in women undergoing a transobturator tape as compared with a retropubic tape (37 studies, 6200 participants, OR 0.53; 95% CI: 0.43, 0.65) [3]. Within the sub-groups of different approaches, it was less likely with a down-to-up approach to retropubic tapes as compared with top-down (5 studies, 631 participants, OR 0.40; 95% CI: 0.18, 0.90) and more likely with an inside-out approach to transobturator tapes as compared with an outside-in (8 studies, 1121 participants, OR 1.74; 95% CI: 1.06, 2.88) [3].

In a large randomized trial comparing traditional sling with the Burch colposuspension, voiding dysfunction was more common in the sling group (14% vs. 2% at 24 months, $p < 0.001$)

N. Khattar et al. (eds.), *Female Bladder Outlet Obstruction and Urethral Reconstruction*,
https://doi.org/10.1007/978-981-15-8521-0_9

with all re-do surgeries to address voiding dysfunction in the sling group. Of note, the sling group reported superior efficacy on both subjective and objective parameters [4]. In the large randomized trial comparing retropubic tapes with transobturator tapes, voiding dysfunction needing intervention was noted only in the former (2.7% vs. 0% at 12 months, $p = 0.004$) [5].

9.3 Presentation

In its most profound form, obstruction results in intractable symptomatic retention necessitating placement of a catheter or the need for clean intermittent catheterization. Other presentations include voiding symptoms, elevated residuals, or discomfort during voiding. Of note, patients with obstruction may present exclusively with storage symptoms of urinary frequency and urgency. Women may also present with recurrent urinary tract infection presumably owing to altered voiding dynamics. Voiding dysfunction is classified as complication type 4B in the IUGA-ICS complications terminology document [6].

Given the varied presentation, most guidelines recommend elective evaluation of voiding in all patients undergoing stress incontinence surgery regardless of symptoms. The American Urological Association (AUA) guideline recommends an early postoperative assessment that includes questions with regard to "significant voiding problems, pain, or other unanticipated events" and recommends that all patients should undergo repeat assessment for voiding and storage lower urinary tract symptoms (LUTS), pain or other unanticipated symptoms by 6 months along with measurement of residual urine [7].

In 12% of patients the presentation is delayed and insidious. The diagnosis can be challenging in some of these patients with a varying period of conservative management based on the dominant symptom before a decision is made that the sling is probably obstructive [8].

There are no established preoperative markers of voiding dysfunction following stress incontinence surgery. **Various studies have identified preoperative clinical hesitancy** [9], **valsalva voiding** [10] **or poor flow with low detrusor pressures** [11] **as predictors of postoperative voiding dysfunction.** Of note, these markers identify a sub-set of patients with impaired detrusor contractility or voiding. Other than these patient factors, surgeon-related factors are presumably important with higher voiding dysfunction rates expected with low-volume centers or less experienced surgeons (Table 9.1). **The commonest mistake novice surgeons make is placing the sling too tight!**

9.4 Evaluation

The key to identifying post-sling obstruction is a high index of suspicion for the condition. A detailed clinical assessment (Table 9.2) must include scrutiny of the previous operative notes with regard to the type of surgery, nature of material, steps of technique, any specific problems encountered and the postoperative course. Often but not always, a long-term voiding dysfunction may be heralded by initial voiding difficulty on catheter removal. The ease of clarifying the cause of a patient's symptoms is directly proportional to the availability of documentation prior to the index surgery. Availability of preoperative symptom details (such as history of hesitancy or voiding difficulty), patient-reported outcome measures, post-void residual assessment, and uroflow tracings or urodynamics test results can provide a valuable baseline for comparison.

In the absence of well-defined criteria for bladder outlet obstruction in women no single parameter is completely reliable in making a diagnosis. The classical features of obstruction

Table 9.1 Etiology of voiding dysfunction following stress incontinence surgery

1. Sling too tight
2. Underactive detrusor
3. Mis-placed sling or sutures
4. Tape retraction or shrinkage
5. Uncorrected or de novo anterior compartment prolapse
6. Sling erosion into the urethra with mechanical obstruction

Table 9.2 Clinical evaluation of suspected voiding dysfunction following stress incontinence surgery

History
Urinary tract: details of storage and voiding symptoms, urinary infections
Pre-existing or de novo history of any genitourinary, gastrointestinal, neurological, or gynecological symptoms. Details regarding previous surgery
Examination
Genitourinary: meatus, labia and vagina, bladder, kidneys; previous surgical wound sites for any exposure of synthetics, induration, tight bands, tenderness, induration or inflammation
Digital rectal examination
Focussed Neurological system: specific attention to anal sphincter tone, bulbo-cavernosus reflex, perianal sensation, gait, spine
Investigations
Bladder diary, urine examination, blood glucose. USG KUB with prevoid and post-void bladder volume, uroflowmetry transvaginal ultrasonography to assess the previous surgical site including location of tapes or slings, invasive urodynamics or videourodynamics, micturating cystourethrogram (if video- urodynamics is not available) MRI of the spine (if indicated)

comprise a history of voiding difficulty or retention, elevated residuals, abnormal slow flow, and urodynamic bladder outlet obstruction with coordinated sphincters. However, many women present with more subtle features. Urodynamic bladder outlet obstruction criteria are not universally agreed upon. Blaivas and Groutz defined obstruction as tube-free MFR < 12 mL/s with $P_{det.Qmax} > 20$ cm H_2O, radiographic obstruction despite a sustained contraction of >20 cm H_2O or urinary retention and/or inability to void at urodynamics despite a sustained detrusor contraction of >20 cm H_2O [12]. Nitti suggested using video-urodynamics evidence without a strict application of pressure-flow criteria [13]. These definitions disregard detrusor underactivity, which, although critical to the discussion, remains even less well understood. Figure 9.1 depicts some classical presentations in women with post-sling voiding difficulty ranging from outright obstruction to complete acontractility.

In the postoperative setting a documented change in voiding dynamics might be more valuable than actual recorded pressure-flow. For the woman depicted in Fig. 9.1b, the availability of a preoperative urodynamics trace could be invaluable in taking a decision to takedown the sling. The odds of successful redo surgery might be better if the preoperative trace shows a substantially better void, even in a setting of impaired detrusor function. **Distortion of the urethra noted at contrast imaging (on video-urodynamics or micturating cystourethrogram) may show that the tape is too taut or in an inappropriate position.** Curling of the tape and too close a proximity to the urethra (<3 mm from the longitudinal smooth muscle of the urethra) have been described as markers for tape-associated obstruction on transvaginal ultrasonography [14]. In some patients, however, there might be no imaging or urodynamic evidence and the only clue to obstruction might lie in the temporal association of new-onset voiding difficulty following sling surgery. For the woman depicted in Fig. 9.1c, it might have been reasonable to consider surgical takedown had she presented in the immediate postoperative period especially if she had no preoperative symptomatic voiding difficulty. Careful counseling regarding the uncertainties regarding restoration of spontaneous voiding and the possibility of recurrent incontinence would be mandatory. Indeed, only about one-third of patients will show incontrovertible features of urodynamic obstruction [15].

Cystoscopy can be useful in these women for identifying obvious mechanical obstruction as well as tape exposure that might be associated especially in the urethra. The "snap phenomenon" on passing a Hegar dilator through the urethra has been described as a feature of mechanical obstruction [14].

9.5 Management

The management of bladder outlet obstruction following sling surgery is often determined by the time at which the problem presents and the following discussion is stratified accordingly while recognizing that not all presentations will fit in neatly with this format (Fig. 9.2).

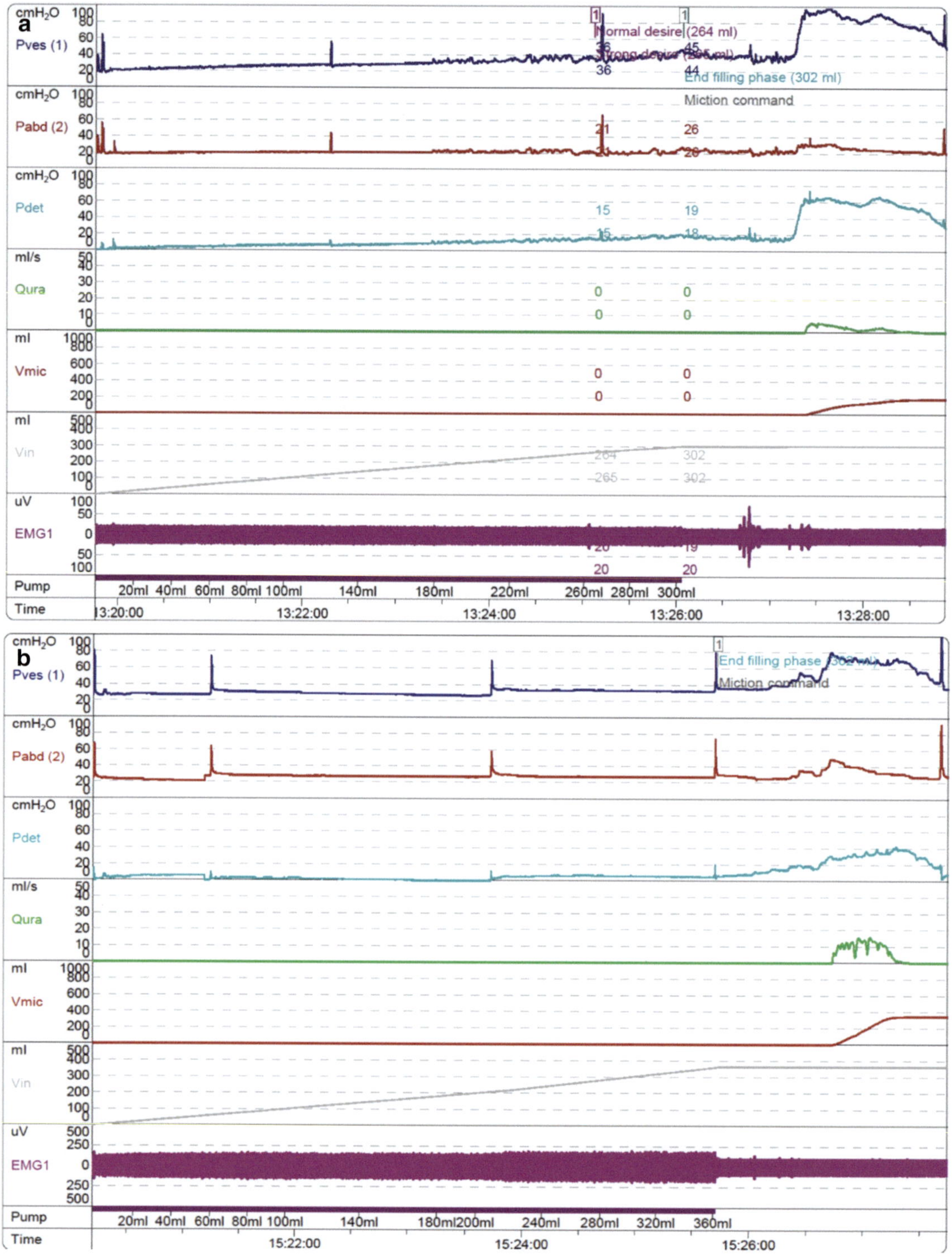

Fig. 9.1 Urodynamic patterns in women with post-sling voiding dysfunction. (**a**) Classical urodynamic obstruction. In a setting of voiding difficulty, this tracing is pathognomonic of obstruction ($P_{det}Q_{max}$ 60 cm H_2O, MFR 5 ml/s). (**b**) Voiding difficulty following midurethral sling. The urodynamics shows underactivity with possible obstruction ($P_{det}Q_{max}$ 35 cm H_2O, MFR 9 ml/s). Preoperative urodynamics for comparison would be invaluable in such a patient. (**c**) Acontractility in a woman presenting with insidious onset voiding difficulty after transobturator tape 7 years ago culminating in retention. This woman has an acontractile bladder and take-down surgery is unlikely to help her

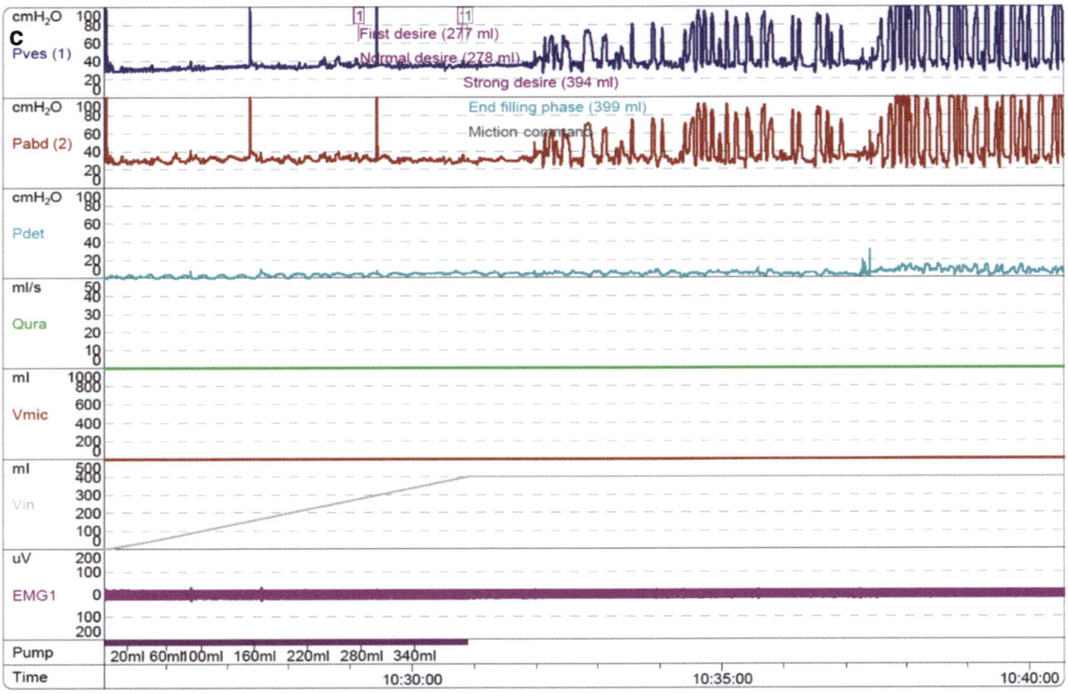

Fig. 9.1 (continued)

9.5.1 Immediate Postoperative Retention

Retention following sling surgery is not uncommon and there is consensus in literature that corrective action is usually not indicated at this point unless there is reason to believe that there was a technical issue at surgery. Typically, the patient is re-catheterized and given another trial after a week. Immediate postoperative retention might be consequent to a variety of issues unrelated to technical aspects of surgery or voiding function such as pain, adverse effects of anesthesia, or impacted stools. There might also be reversible surgical problems such as a wound hematoma. Patients with unresolved retention at the second voiding trial around one week postoperatively are at higher odds of long-term voiding dysfunction even if they ultimately manage to void. Further course of action is dependent on several issues that must include a consideration of the type of surgery, the preoperative voiding function, any intraoperative clues, and, importantly, patient choice. A longer period of waiting is usually considered appropriate for women who have undergone an autologous sling as compared with those undergoing a synthetic midurethral sling.

For women presenting with retention following a synthetic midurethral sling, **one must consider the option of loosening the tape early in the postoperative period, typically within 2 weeks**. In a series of 33 women out of 921 (3.5%) operated in whom retention developed in the immediate postoperative period, 27 women were able to void spontaneously once the sling was released. Early intervention may avoid residual storage symptoms that might persist following voiding dysfunction and reduce the bother to patients [16, 17]. The intervention was not associated with recurrent stress incontinence in any of these 27 women.

Loosening of the sling is easier for patients with an autologous sling or for a mid-urethral sling that has a tensioning suture running through it (allowing a more even distribution of the force). Loosening of the sling should be carried out by re-opening the vaginal incision, identifying the sling, placing an operative instrument carefully

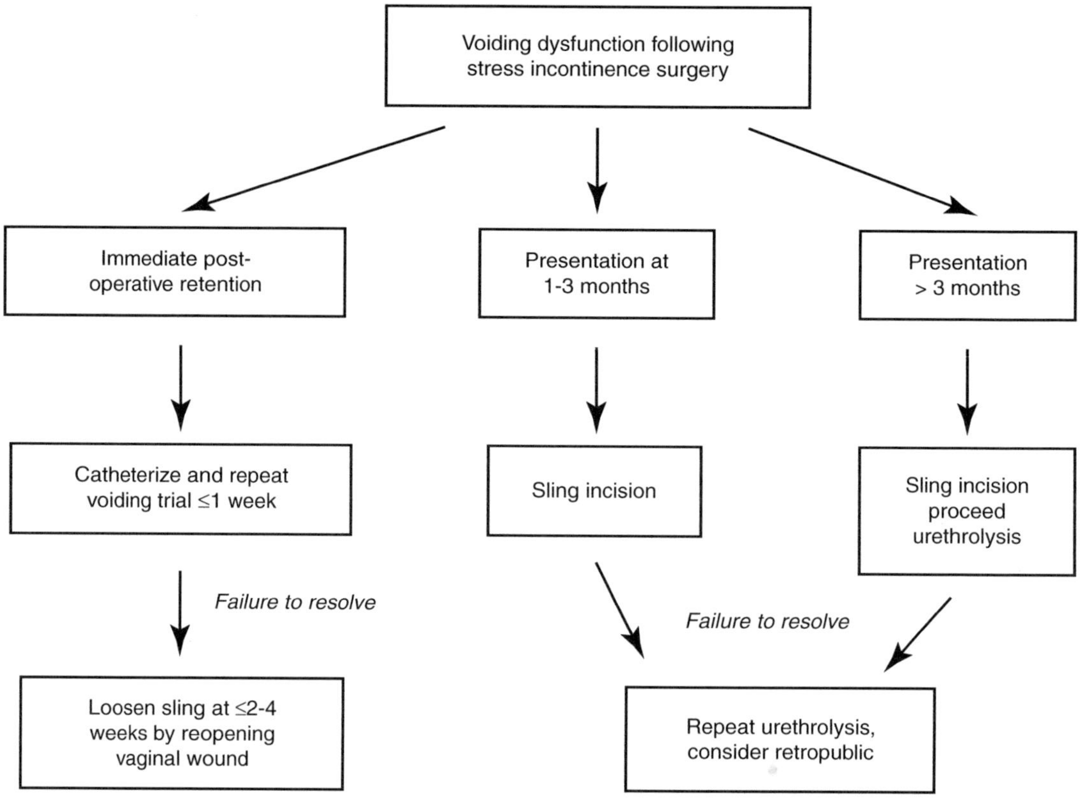

Fig. 9.2 Algorithm for treatment of postoperative voiding dysfunction following stress incontinence surgery

between the urethra and the sling, and giving a gentle, controlled tug. The tug should allow the creation of space (5 mm in the above-discussed series) between the tape and urethra.

Dilatation of the urethra or use of a urethral dilator to push down a synthetic tape manually without re-opening the surgical wound is seldom effective and is not recommended [18]. Such manipulations run the risk of urethral trauma or scarring with exacerbation of obstruction and might increase the odds of urethral erosion. However, in contrast, careful dilatation or a downward urethral tug may be effective and safe following an autologous sling up to 6 weeks following the original surgery [19]. Division of the sling should be avoided within the first 2 weeks in view of a higher possibility of recurrent stress incontinence.

When early intervention is not chosen, it is preferable to initiate clean intermittent self-catheterization. There are several benefits to this policy. It allows patients to carry on with their usual activities or profession, avoids the ill-effects of an indwelling catheter on the urinary tract, is more physiological, enables easy repeated voiding trials, and is better for patient psyche. It has also been reported that a substantial proportion of women who initiate intermittent catheterization will be able to void spontaneously subsequently [17]. The alternative is an indwelling catheter.

9.5.2 Presentation in the First 3 Months

Most patients with persistent retention will opt to undergo further treatment to resolve the problem. Some patients who are able to void on catheter removal initially might present within the first 3 months with voiding difficulty or retention. **At this point tape mobilization is usually ineffec-**

tive due to the associated fibrosis and a formal sling takedown is required. This is typically achieved by re-opening the vaginal wound, dissecting the sling, carefully getting around the sling to allow the placement of an instrument between the sling and urethra or a tape around the sling with careful division of the sling under vision [20]. The importance of identifying and taking 360-degree control of the sling cannot be overemphasized. Sectioning the taut sling without taking complete control is fraught with danger of injury or misidentification of structures and must never be performed. **Sectioning of the sling is accompanied by recoil as the cut ends of the sling retract a little. This intraoperative feeling of recoil must be actively sought and reassures the operator that urethrolysis is unnecessary**.

9.5.3 Presentation Beyond 3 Months

With time, the sling tends to get fixed by fibrotic reaction and **mere sectioning of the sling is usually not enough although this is the first step in the takedown. There is lack of a feeling of recoil and this indicates the need for formal urethrolysis**. While three techniques of urethrolysis are described in literature, the *vaginal*, *suprameatal* and *retropubic* approaches, in patients undergoing urethrolysis for obstruction following mid-urethral sling, the vaginal approach is the commonest. The urethra must be freed from the entire suburethral component of the sling by careful dissection. Dissection is determined by the extent of the fibrosis with the occasional need for extensive dissection. In patients who fail urethrolysis, repeat urethrolysis can be effective. The retropubic approach is usually reserved for repeat urethrolysis or for voiding dysfunction following Burch Colposuspension or Marshall Marchetti Krantz procedure [21].

9.5.4 Complex Presentations

Sling obstruction may be accompanied by other complications, typically sling erosion or exposure within the urethra [20]. This is almost exclusively limited to synthetic mid-urethral slings since erosion of an autologous sling is rare [22]. It might be possible to manage select patients with a limited urethral exposure by endourological technique [23]. This can be achieved by endoscopic removal using mechanical scissors or laser energy. Removal of the edges of the tape and intramural portion can be challenging. Most patients require formal operative removal of the sling to achieve the twin objectives of removing the exposed portion of the sling as well as resolving obstruction.

Sling removal can be achieved by two techniques depending on how the urethra is handled. Traditionally, the urethra is opened to dissect the sling followed by layered urethral closure usually with a Martius labial fat pad interposition before closure of the vaginal wall. A urethra-sparing approach has also been described [24, 25]. Urethra sparing approaches are applicable only when the sling has eroded completely and is lying within the urethra with ventral healing. Suture tagging of the tape and careful extraction by sliding the tape out help to identify the urethral opening allowing accurate repair of the wall on both sides (Fig. 9.3). In some patients, a circumferential incision around the sling on either side of the urethra may be required to enable extraction without formally opening the urethra.

9.6 Outcome of Sling Revision Surgery

Most but not all patients will experience restoration of voiding following revision surgery. In a textbook review, sling incisions were noted to have a success rate of 84–100% [19]. In a large institutional series of 44 women who underwent surgery for voiding dysfunction, voiding dysfunction resolved in about 75% of women. Storage symptoms tended to persist while recurrent stress incontinence was noted in 41%. In this series of patients, 14 patients had a surgical takedown while 20 and 10 patients had vaginal and retropubic urethrolysis respectively [26]. In another review of 198 patients 98% voided fol-

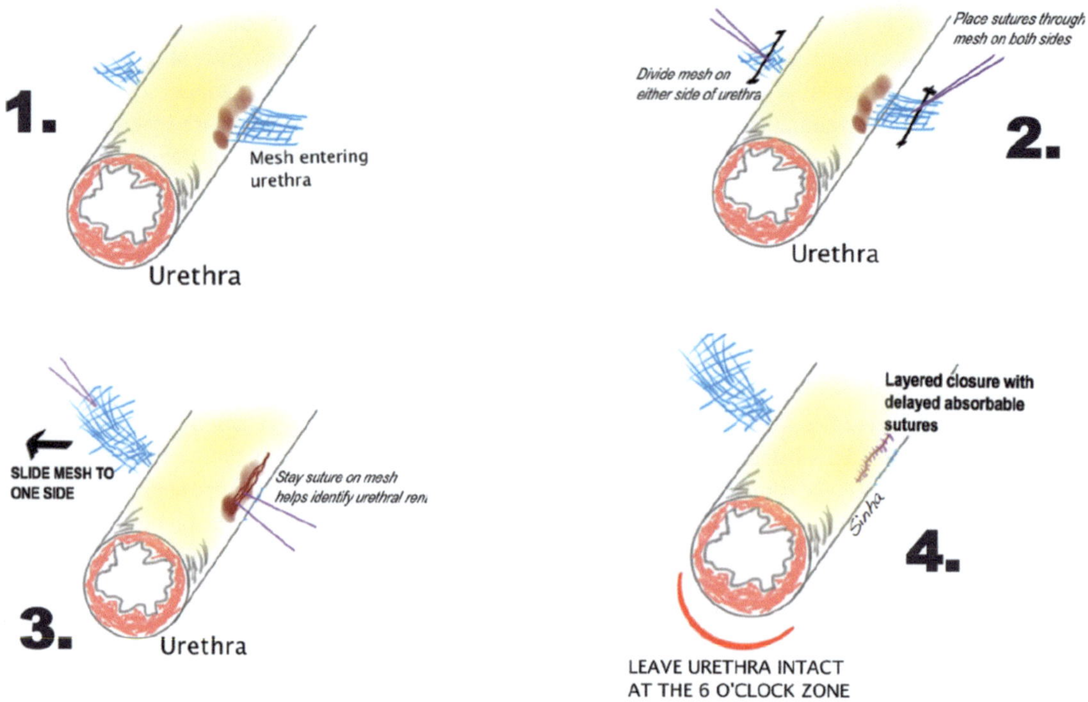

Fig. 9.3 Technique of removal of sling (urethra-sparing approach)

lowing sling incision with a recurrent stress incontinence rate of 60% [14]. In patients requiring a repeat urethrolysis, most of them show resolution of voiding dysfunction with 22 of 24 patients (92%) voiding successfully in one series. Such surgery can be challenging and is best carried out at select centers [21].

The evidence in this regard is not robust and outcomes are dependent, among other factors, on associated voiding dysfunction and the extent of surgical dissection. Patients who were voiding spontaneously prior to surgery and those with low pre-operative post-void residuals tend to do better.

Clinical Case Discussion

A 47-year-old woman presented 2 years after a retropubic tension-free vaginal tape surgery for stress urinary incontinence. The details of preoperative evaluation and intraoperative findings were not available. She had severe voiding difficulty with marked need to strain, marked frequency, and vaginal pain all for the last 8 months. She had undergone hysterectomy 5 years ago. There were no symptoms pertaining to the gastrointestinal or neurological system. Abdominal examination was unremarkable. Vaginal mucosa was healthy and there was no prolapse. There was palpable induration in the area of the sling but no sling exposure in the vagina. There was no demonstrable incontinence. Earlier attempts at catheterization had failed on two occasions elsewhere with complete inability to place a urethral catheter.

Ultrasonography showed normal kidneys with a pre-void bladder volume of 280 ml and a post-void residual of 60 ml. Uroflow was very slow and prolonged with a maximum flow rate of 2 ml/s. Attempted calibration in the outpatient failed with obstruction encountered within the urethra about 1.5 cm from the meatus. The meatus was normal. Cystoscopy was undertaken under general anesthesia and showed near-total occlusion of the urethra with large bulk 3-quadrant mesh exposure in the urethra. There was barely space for the introduction of a glidewire over which a 6F tube could be negotiated into the bladder (Fig. 9.4).

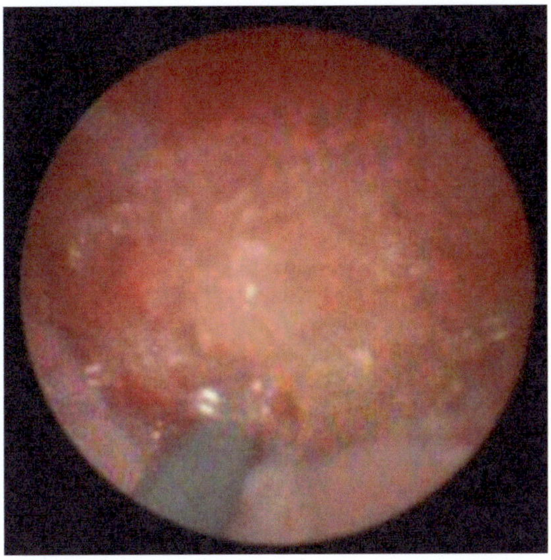

Fig. 9.4 Near-total occlusion of the urethra following a retropubic tape. Cystoscopy at 2 years following failure to place a urethral catheter. There was barely space for placement of a glidewire

Detailed discussions regarding the implication of surgical removal of the eroded mesh were undertaken with the patient in multiple counseling sessions. This included the plan for removal of only the vaginal component of the mesh, the possibility of developing a urethrovaginal fistula or recurrent incontinence, and the possible need for revision surgery. Surgery was carried out from the vaginal approach with identification and removal of the vaginal component (Fig. 9.5). A layered closure with interposition of Martius labial fat pad was performed with an uneventful recovery. She developed recurrent stress urinary incontinence and requires 1 pad/day but is currently uninterested in any interventions. Her voiding difficulty and pain have completely resolved.

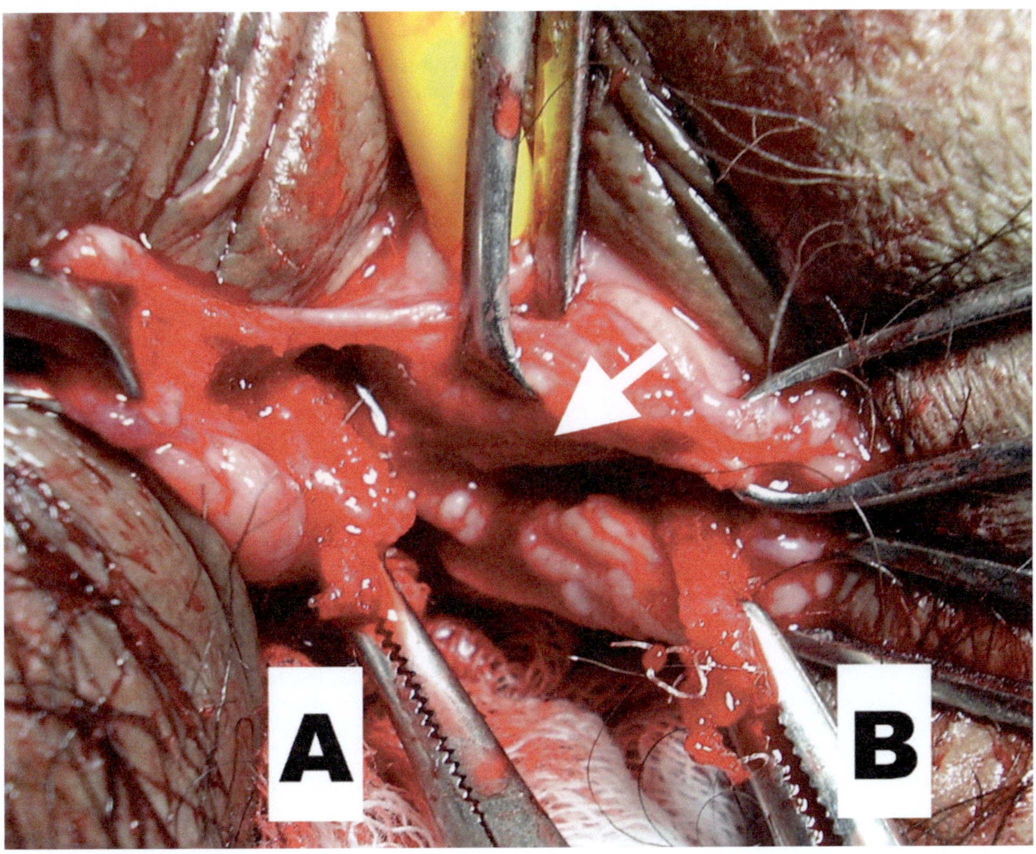

Fig. 9.5 Removal of the vaginal component of mid-urethral sling for large bulk urethral erosion with occlusion. Note the wide-open urethra (white arrow) and the two cut ends of the mesh (A and B)

Key Learning Points

- Post-sling obstruction may present as urinary retention after catheter removal in its severe form or as postoperative voiding dysfunction that may continue to bother patient.
- High index of suspicion with comparison from baseline and chronology of symptoms helps in arriving at a diagnosis. A video-urodynamic study may confirm obstruction. Transvaginal ultrasonography can identify abnormally placed sling.
- The management depends on the timing of presentation after surgery and severity of obstruction.
- Sling loosening can be effective in the first 2 weeks after surgery. Loosening alone might not be enough after 2 weeks, necessitating sling division or takedown.
- A formal urethrolysis may be required beyond 3 months.
- Revision surgery for voiding dysfunction carries morbidity, including the risk of recurrent stress incontinence, and detailed preoperative counseling is recommended.
- Risk of recurrence of incontinence may be there especially with early takedown before fibrosis has set in.

References

1. Daneshgari F, Kong W, Swartz M. Complications of mid urethral slings: important outcomes for future clinical trials. J Urol. 2008;180:1890–7.
2. Rehman H, Bezerra CA, Bruschini H, Cody JD, Aluko P. Traditional suburethral sling operations for urinary incontinence in women. Cochrane Database Syst Rev. 2017;7:CD001754.
3. Ford AA, Rogerson L, Cody JD, Aluko P, Ogah JA. Mid-urethral sling operations for stress urinary incontinence in women. Cochrane Database Syst Rev. 2017;7:CD006375.
4. Albo ME, Richter HE, Brubaker L, Norton P, Kraus SR, Zimmern PE, et al. Burch colposuspension versus fascial sling to reduce urinary stress incontinence. N Engl J Med. 2007;356:2143–55.
5. Richter HE, Albo ME, Zyczynski HM, et al. Retropubic versus transobturator midurethral slings for stress incontinence. N Engl J Med. 2010;362:2066–76.
6. Haylen BT, Freeman RM, Swift SE, Cosson M, Davila GW, Deprest J, et al. An International Urogynecological Association (IUGA)/International Continence Society (ICS) joint terminology and classification of the complications related directly to the insertion of prostheses (meshes, implants, tapes) and grafts in female pelvic floor surgery. Neurourol Urodyn. 2011;30(1):2–12.
7. Kobashi KC, Albo ME, Dmochowski RR, Ginsberg DA, Goldman HB, Gomelsky A, et al. Surgical treatment of female stress urinary incontinence: AUA/SUFU guideline. J Urol. 2017;198:875–83.
8. Carr LK, Webster GD. Voiding dysfunction following incontinence surgery: diagnosis and treatment with retropubic or vaginal urethrolysis. J Urol. 1997;157:821–3.
9. Sanses TV, Brubaker L, Xu Y, Kraus SR, Lowder JL, Lemack GE, et al. Preoperative hesitating urinary stream is associated with postoperative voiding dysfunction and surgical failure following Burch colposuspension or pubovaginal rectus fascial sling surgery. Int Urogynecol J. 2011;22:713–9.
10. Wheeler TL, Richter HE, Greer WJ, Bowling CB, Redden DT, Varner RE. Predictors of success with postoperative voiding trials after a mid urethral sling procedure. J Urol. 2008;179:600–4.
11. Miller EA, Amundsen CL, Toh KL, Flynn BJ, Webster GD. Preoperative urodynamic evaluation may predict voiding dysfunction in women undergoing pubovaginal sling. J Urol. 2003;169:2234–7.
12. Groutz A, Blaivas JG, Chaikin DC. Bladder outlet obstruction in women: definition and characteristics. Neurourol Urodyn. 2000;19:213–20.
13. Nitti VW, Tu LM, Gitlin J. Diagnosing bladder outlet obstruction in women. J Urol. 1999;161:1535–40.
14. Viereck V, Rautenberg O, Kociszewski J, Grothey S, Welter J, Eberhard J. Midurethral sling incision: indications and outcomes. Int Urogynecol J. 2013;24:645–53.
15. Patel BN, Kobashi KC, Staskin D. Iatrogenic obstruction after sling surgery. Nat Rev Urol. 2012;9:429–34.
16. Price N, Slack A, Khong SY, Currie I, Jackson S. The benefit of early mobilisation of tension-free vaginal tape in the treatment of post-operative voiding dysfunction. Int Urogynecol J Pelvic Floor Dysfunct. 2009;20:855–8.
17. Bazi T, Kerkhof MH, Takahashi SI, Abdel-Fattah M, IUGA Research and Development Committee. Management of post-midurethral sling voiding dysfunction. International Urogynecological Association Research and Development Committee opinion. Int Urogynecol J. 2018;29:23–8.
18. Sokol AI, Jelovsek JE, Walters M, Paraiso MFR, Barber MD. Incidence and predictors of prolonged urinary retentionafter TVT with and without concurrent prolapse surgery. Am J Obstet Gynecol. 2005;192:1537–43.
19. Dmochowski RR, Osborn DJ, Reynolds WS. Slings: autologous, biologic, synthetic, and midurethral. In: Wein AJ, Kavoussi LR, Partin AW, Peters CA, editors. Campbell-Walsh urology. 11th ed. Philadelphia, PA: Elsevier; 2016. p. 1987–2038.

20. Gomes CM, Carvalho FL, Bellucci CHS, et al. Update on complications of synthetic suburethral slings. Int Braz J Urol. 2017;43:822–34.
21. Scarpero HM, Dmochowski RR, Nitti VW. Repeat urethrolysis after failed urethrolysis for iatrogenic obstruction. J Urol. 2003;169(3):1013–6.
22. Webster TM, Gerridzen RG. Gone in 24 hours: the feasibility of performing pubovaginal sling surgery with an overnight hospital stay. Can J Urol. 2003;10:1905–9.
23. Sergouniotis F, Jarlshammar B, Larsson PG. Urethral complications after tension-free vaginal tape procedures: a surgical management case series. World J Nephrol. 2015;4:396–405.
24. Velemir L, Amblard J, Jacquetin B, et al. Urethral erosion after suburethral synthetic slings: risk factors, diagnosis, and functional outcome after surgical management. Int Urogynecol J. 2008;19:999–1006.
25. Marks B, Goldman H. Controversies in the management of mesh-based complications. Urol Clin North Am. 2012;39:419–28.
26. Segal J, Steele A, Vassallo B, Kleeman S, Silva AW, Pauls R, et al. Various surgical approaches to treat voiding dysfunction following anti-incontinence surgery. Int Urogynecol J Pelvic Floor Dysfunct. 2006;17:372–7.

Working Algorithm for Female Lower Urinary Tract Symptoms

10

Rishi Nayyar, Nikhil Khattar, and Arabind Panda

Learning Objectives

- To bring the understanding of previous chapters into a clinical perspective to allow developing a rational working algorithm for female LUTS.
- To develop a rational sequence for investigation and management of voiding dysfunction.

Female voiding issues are a manifestation of plethora of poorly understood disease processes that have been categorized and named based on symptom profile, urodynamic finding, radiological imaging, or sometimes a presumptive pathogenetic process. However, the exact pathogenesis, etiology, risk factors, natural history, and therapeutic management of all these disorders are still to be deciphered and leaves lot of lacunae in our understanding of these disorders. Moreover, there is considerable overlap of the symptoms of storage and voiding disorders in women. With many systemic diseases also manifesting through similar symptoms, the clinician has to appropriately investigate the patient and collate all available evidence to reach a proper diagnosis and plan management accordingly. This is important to alleviate symptoms and improve quality of life, to prevent progression of disease, and, if possible, to provide a cure. Individual disease processes that may result in BOO have been dealt with in earlier chapters. In this chapter, **a practical approach to management of female lower urinary tract symptoms (LUTS) is presented with focus on voiding dysfunction and bladder outlet obstruction (BOO)**. The development of such an algorithm is important to

1. To generate awareness about the evidence-based management of female LUTS that is otherwise inadequately covered in general gynecology or urology training.
2. To standardize the management of female LUTS and rationalize the sequencing of investigations ordered for it.
3. To minimize treatment-related adverse effects.

Voiding dysfunction may be considered as an all-encompassing term including any kind of voiding problem arising due to systemic or local causes affecting anatomical or physiological function of bladder, sphincter, or urethra or their neurological control (Fig. 10.1). It may not always be possible to differentiate specific disease process based only on history at first visit, but it serves well to differentiate known systemic

R. Nayyar (✉)
Department of Urology, All India Institute of Medical Sciences, New Delhi, India

N. Khattar
Female Urology, Reconstructive Urology and Neurovesical Dysfunction, Medanta, The Medicity, Gurugram, India

A. Panda
Urology and Renal Transplantation, Krishna Institute of Medical Sciences, Secunderabad, Telangana, India

N. Khattar et al. (eds.), *Female Bladder Outlet Obstruction and Urethral Reconstruction*,
https://doi.org/10.1007/978-981-15-8521-0_10

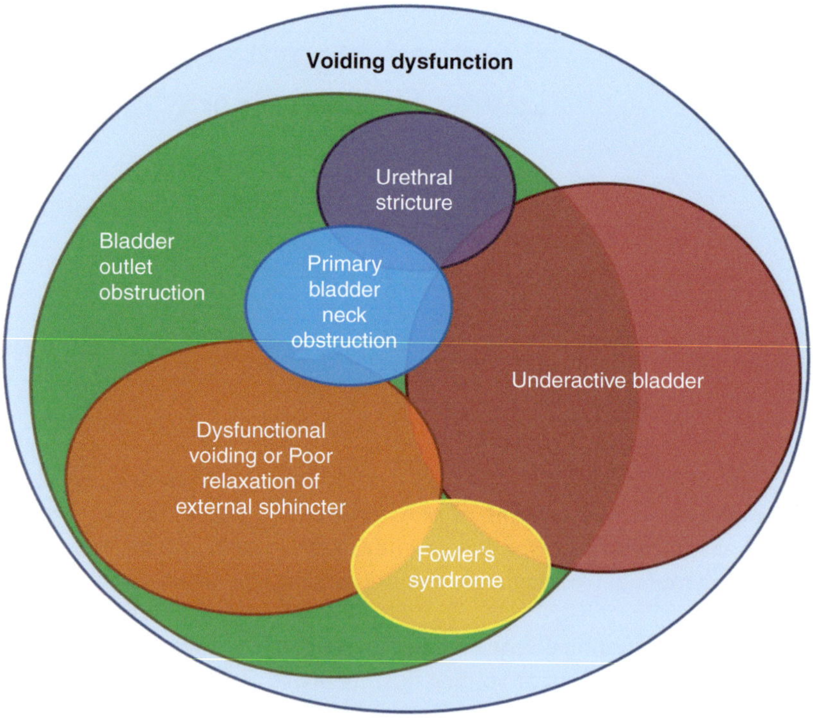

Fig. 10.1 Schematic representation to display the inter-relation among various diagnostic terms used in the context of female voiding dysfunction

diseases; establish the severity of symptoms and impact on quality of life through various scoring symptoms; gauge and moderate the expectations of patients; or start empirical treatment, if any, based on presumed working diagnosis. In general, **voiding dysfunction should be looked for only if symptoms have been consistently present for more than 4 weeks** (expert opinion). It may be reiterated here that as per ICS (International Continence Society) definition, voiding dysfunction is described as an abnormally slow and/or incomplete micturition, based on abnormally slow urine flow rates and or abnormally high post-void residuals, ideally on repeated measurement to confirm abnormality [1]. We suggest **a *Q* max of <15 ml/s or a repeated abnormal uroflow pattern and/or a high post-void residue (PVR) on ultrasound (100 ml or more).** It is clear from this definition that diagnosis of voiding dysfunction cannot be inferred from voiding symptoms directly, and voiding dysfunction in a female should not be labeled so till investigations have been carried out, sometimes including invasive investigations as well [2]. Many cases presenting only with storage type of LUTS also have voiding dysfunction as an underlying cause. Therefore, it is important to keep a high index of suspicion and do above-minimum investigations in all females presenting with any kind of LUTS, recurrent UTI, or bladder pain-like symptoms to the clinic (Fig. 10.2).

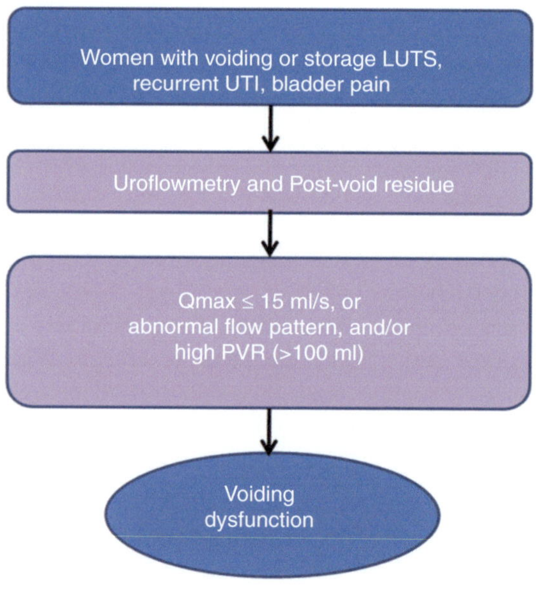

Fig. 10.2 Simple flowchart showing when to suspect voiding dysfunction and when to diagnose a patient as having voiding dysfunction

Many studies have shown that out of all cases diagnosed as voiding dysfunction most patients present with combined storage and voiding LUTS (~60–70%) or isolated storage LUTS (~30–40%). Isolated voiding symptoms alone are uncommon in this setting [3].

A brief overview of storage and voiding urinary symptoms is given in Fig. 10.3. It is the clinician's job to understand the patient's description of her symptoms and fit them into a particular type of storage or voiding dysfunction. However as discussed earlier, it is just a step forward in management and the sensitivity, specificity, or predictive value of any presenting symptom (LUTS) for diagnosis of voiding dysfunction is quite low [4, 5].

10.1 Algorithm for Evaluation of Female LUTS at First Visit

When a patient presents for the first time, **a detailed documentation of type of LUTS, symptom scoring and quality of life or bother assessment must be done**. In addition, the history and examination are directed toward identifying any systemic, or co-existent (neurological, gynecological, psychological, gastrointestinal, endocrinological) disease that may directly impact and present with LUTS (Fig. 10.4). **Uroflowmetry and PVR assessment should be ordered for all** besides a urine routine/culture examination.

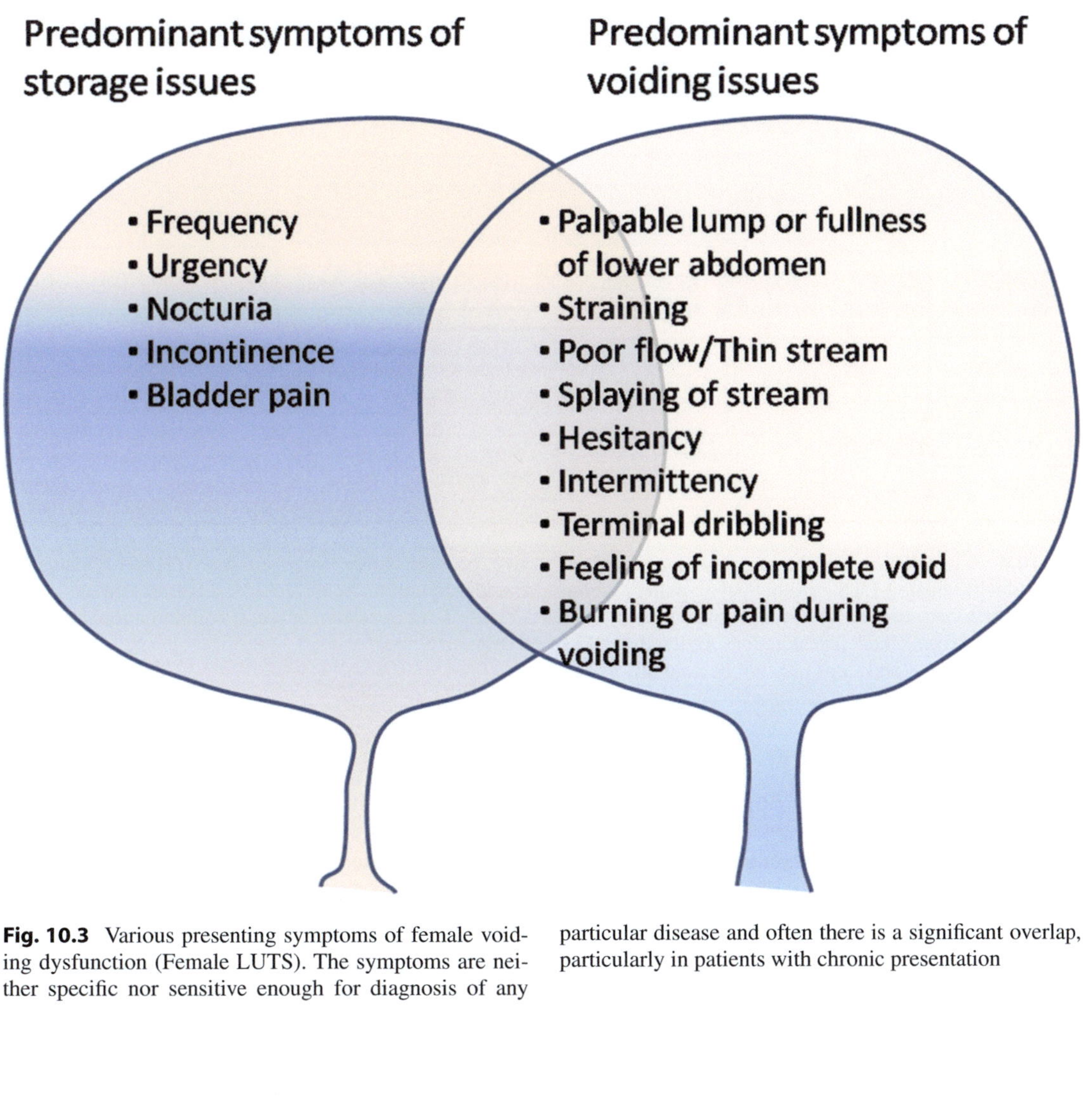

Fig. 10.3 Various presenting symptoms of female voiding dysfunction (Female LUTS). The symptoms are neither specific nor sensitive enough for diagnosis of any particular disease and often there is a significant overlap, particularly in patients with chronic presentation

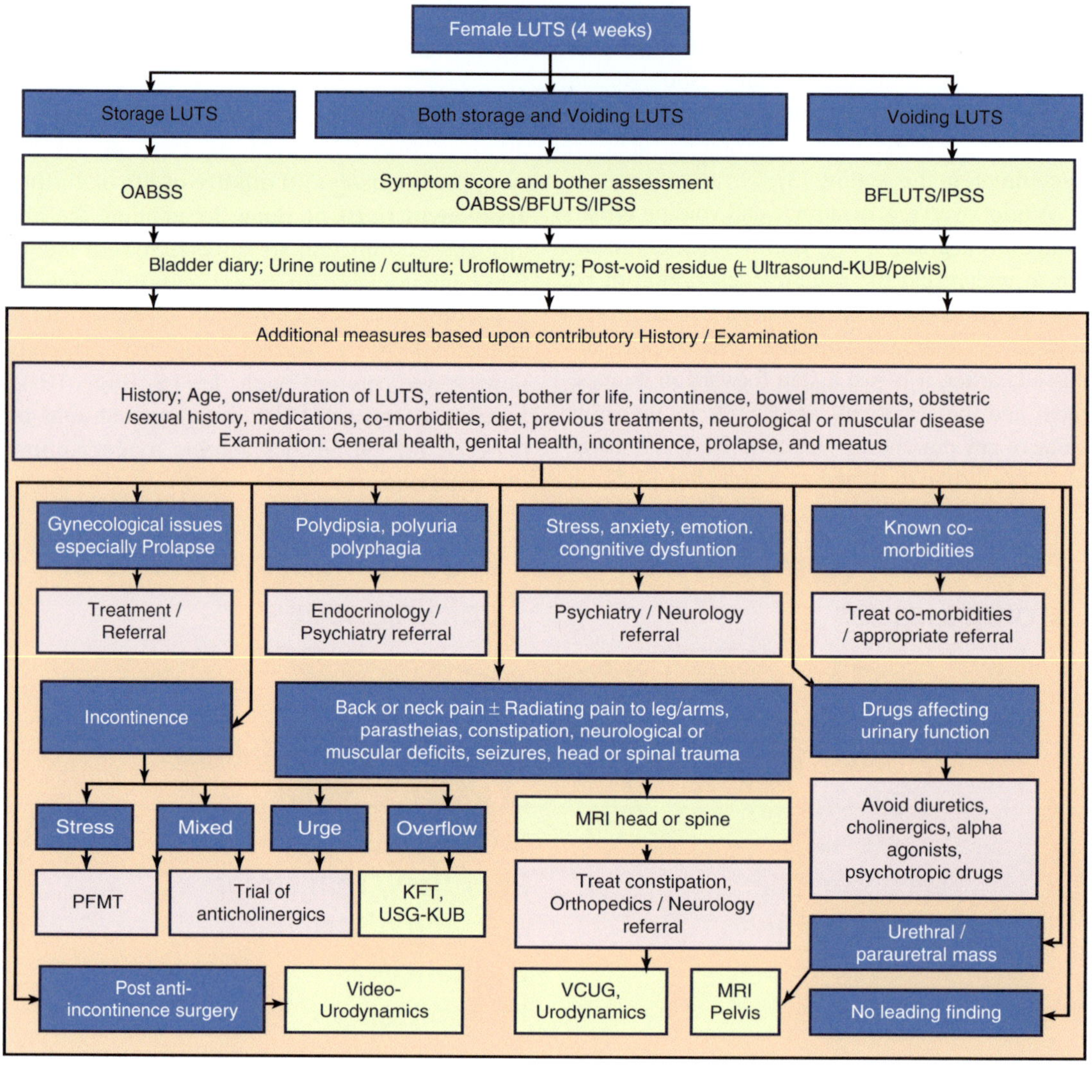

Fig. 10.4 Algorithmic clinical management protocol for evaluation of female LUTS (without pelvic pain or hematuria) at first visit, indicating findings (blue boxes), steps taken (pink boxes), and investigations ordered (yellow boxes). All findings and steps may not be mutually exclusive of each other (orange box) (*OABSS* Overactive Bladder Symptom Score, *BFLUTS* Bristol Female Lower Urinary Tract Symptom Score, *IPSS* International Prostate Symptom Score)

Women who present with LUTS should be examined in a dorsal position to look for pelvic organ prolapse (POP). Higher degrees of prolapse is more commonly associated with voiding dysfunction and BOO [6]. Overactive bladder (OAB) may also be commonly associated with POP. A trial of pessary effectively reduces the prolapse and gives an opportunity to re-evaluate the symptoms in 1–2 weeks. Improvement in symptoms and flow parameters can directly establish a causal relationship and further investigations add little [6]. A surgical repair or a long-term pessary use can be offered. OAB symptoms also get relieved with prolapse reduction in up to 60% of patients [7].

More specific and higher investigations may be in order for a few like the ones who have obvious neurological disease, previous anti-incontinence surgery, or paraurethral mass. In all these situations treatment of primary inciting cause either takes precedence or must be continued simultaneously. For those who have long-standing symptoms, palpable bladder, or features of uremia, an ultrasonogram of the kidney, ureter, and bladder region (KUB) and renal function assessment are necessary. Ultrasonogram of pelvis may also be in order based upon gynecological examination findings.

For cases presenting with LUTS post anti-incontinence surgery, or with acute on chronic retention, or for those on self-intermittent catheterization for voiding, one may directly proceed for voiding cystourethrography (VCUG) and urodynamic studies (UDS). Cases presenting with urinary retention on catheter have an obvious upfront diagnosis of voiding dysfunction.

10.2 Algorithm for Evaluation of Voiding Dysfunction in Subsequent Visits

As discussed earlier, **all patients with any abnormal uroflow pattern, or peak flow <15 ml/s or high PVR (>100 ml), come under the ambit of voiding dysfunction** for further evaluation and management. In clinical practice, it makes sense to get ultrasound KUB also done early on during management, predominantly to assess for prevoid fill volume of bladder and rarely anatomical issues like bladder diverticulum or stones. Often it is very practical to combine ultrasound KUB and pelvis when ultrasound is ordered for a PVR assessment. A trial of alpha blockers may be considered for those who don't have very high PVR (>300 ml) or a static (box-like) flow pattern on uroflowmetry. This is based on the premise that functional obstructions far outnumber urethral stricture disease among women and a large proportion (50–60%) of these may respond reasonably well [8, 9]. Moreover, alpha blockers have also shown acceptable adverse event profile when used in males over long term. Pelvic floor muscle rehabilitation with focus on relaxation exercises should be instituted based on the same premise.

For cases with static flow pattern, **an office urethral calibration helps to select patients who may benefit with urethrocystoscopy upfront**. Office urethral calibration with a soft catheter (18 Fr) may similarly help in those who fail a trial of alpha blockers. A VCUG and UDS would still be required to corroborate anatomical findings with their functional value. Cases with very large PVR (>300 ml) or voiding efficiency of less than 50% and straining pattern on uroflow, have high chances of having underactive bladder [10] and may therefore proceed for UDS directly. However, in most clinical situations and in principle, a VCUG study should precede UDS to depict any reflux, diverticulum, and so on that may impact the interpretation of UDS. Here it may be emphasized that in females there are no definitive radiological markers to identify parts of urethra on VCUG. Therefore, **it is a good practice to place a radiopaque marker at the meatus to better identify course and length of urethra on the X-ray image**. Otherwise it becomes difficult to identify where the urethra ends and hence the site of obstruction may be misinterpreted. Also, **it's a good practice to obtain both side oblique images not to miss any small bladder or urethral diverticulum**. Prolapse is also better depicted on oblique and lateral images. Women who present with any kind of LUTS after an anti-incontinence surgery of any type should preferably be evaluated with video-UDS directly. The temporal relationship of a preceding surgery improves the yield of video-UDS and provides an objective evidence to decide for best course of action. Figure 10.5 gives a simplistic algorithmic overview of management of LUTS and voiding dysfunction in women.

Urodynamic studies form the central pillar for defining the type of voiding dysfunction in combination with VCUG. As the pressure flow cut-offs are still evolving and nomograms need validation, presently the video-urodynamic criteria for considering a diagnosis of BOO or underactive detrusor in the female [11–13] are:

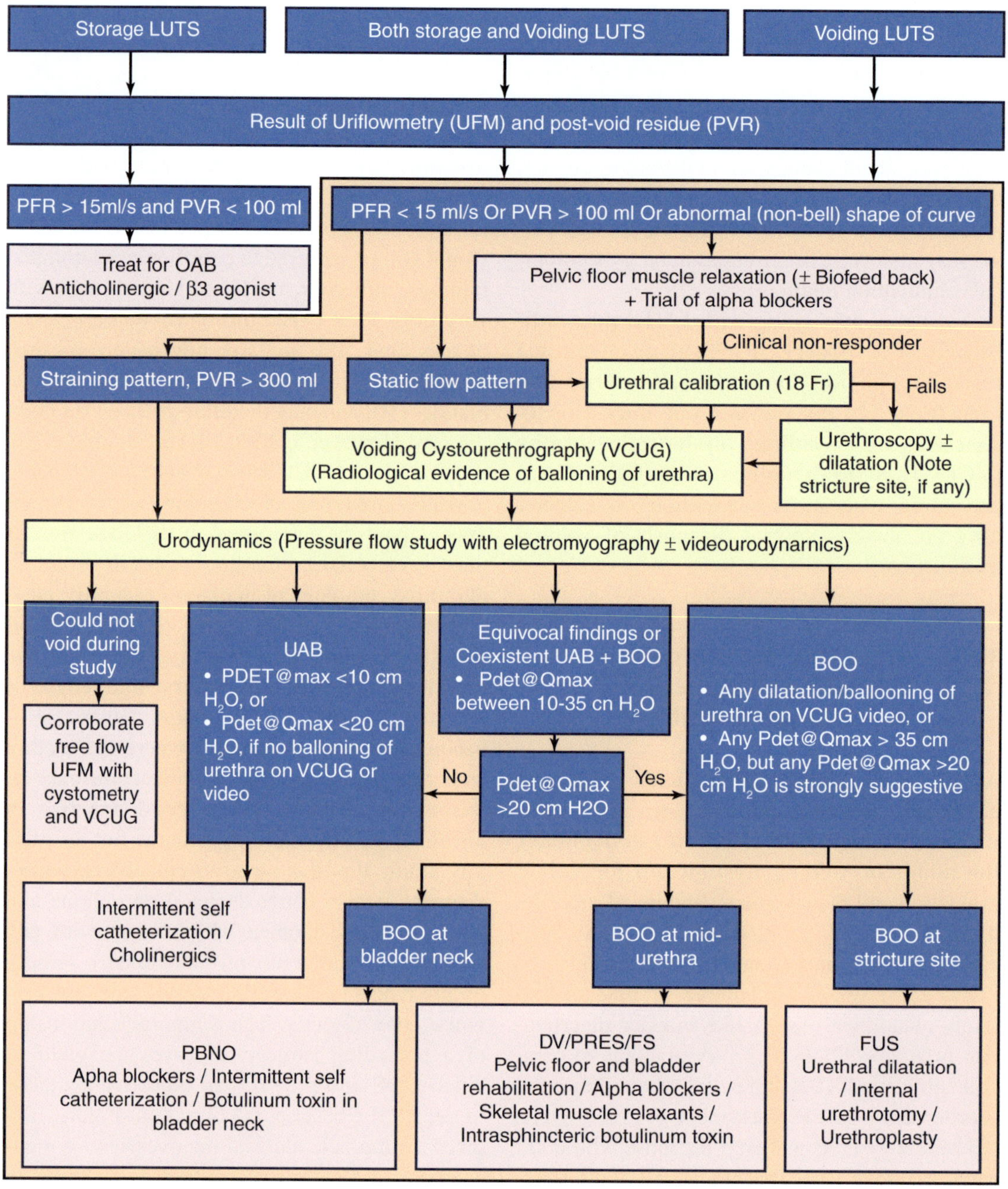

Fig. 10.5 Algorithmic clinical management protocol for evaluation of female LUTS after basic investigational work-up has been done. The findings are indicated in blue boxes, steps taken in pink boxes, and investigations ordered in yellow boxes. Orange box indicates the ambit of voiding dysfunction (*PFR* peak flow rate, *OAB* overactive bladder, *UAB* underactive bladder, *UFM* uroflowmetry, *PBNO* primary bladder neck obstruction, *DV* dysfunctional voiding, *PRES* poor relaxation of external sphincter, *FS* Fowler's syndrome, *FUS* female urethral stricture)

1. **Any dilatation/ballooning in the urethra on Video films/VCUG irrespective of the Pdet@Qmax should be considered as BOO.**
2. **Any Pdet@Qmax > 20 cm of H_2O suggests a strong possibility of BOO** and a value >35–40 virtually confirms BOO in a female.
3. Consider Detrusor underactivity if Pdet@Qmax is <20 cm H_2O. Any value <10 cm H_2O virtually confirms an underactive detrusor.
4. Pdet@Qmax between 10 and 35 cm H_2O can have coexisting BOO and underactivity and reliance should be placed on urethral image suggesting any dilatation during voiding.

For cases where the UDS findings are not very specific and the diagnosis of BOO or underactive bladder (UAB) is not apparent, it may help to repeat the study in same sitting. Similarly, for patients who have underactive detrusor on UDS, a repeat study (may be in same sitting) with balloon of a Foley's catheter blocking the bladder neck may help differentiate those with true detrusor underactivity from those who inherently void only by pelvic floor/sphincter relaxation or abdominal contraction. Isovolumetric contraction measurements of the detrusor may also provide a better estimation of bladder contractility [14, 15]. Overfilling of bladder, non-reduction of prolapse, caliber of catheter, impacted fecaliths, alpha blockers or agonists, and so on may also impact the voiding parameters and should be kept in mind when interpreting the UDS findings. Furthermore, it should be realized that overactivity and underactivity may coexist in the same patient. Overactivity refers to contractions during storage phase while underactivity by its origin refers to voiding phase. In fact, patients with detrusor hyperreflexia with impaired contractility (DHIC) are not uncommon in clinical practice [13]. Overall, UDS findings are not binding on the clinical diagnosis, particularly in a scenario when the results of UDS are equivocal.

The role of electromyography (EMG) is also contributory at best and should not be given an overarching significance. This is because EMG inherently has the least validity and reliability among all UDS tests. This means that EMG trace doesn't always represent true sphincteric activity and is corrupted with action potentials from voluntary pelvic floor, anal or urethral sphincteric activity. Reliability is also low because the placements of leads, type of leads, and many other similar factors have an immense bearing on the type of EMG trace.

The role of pelvic ultrasound or MRI in the management of BOO in women is not yet clearly defined. Measurement of anterior or posterior urethrovesical angle; angle of urethral axis; bladder neck descent; urethral or bladder neck thickness; thickness of pelvic diaphragm; sphincteric thickness; bladder wall thickness; bladder wall ischemia; and change in all these measurements during straining or voiding are all important clinical assessments that are being studied as the evidence support in management of BOO in women is building up [16–18]. In this regard, **the role of transvaginal, transperineal, transrectal ultrasound, and static or dynamic pelvic MRI presently remains investigational**.

Role of urethrocystoscopy is also not very obvious in the scheme of things. The prime reason for endoscopy is to evaluate for anatomical obstruction, predominantly FUS, which is otherwise rare. To improve the pick-up rate and positive predictive value of endoscopy we recommend use of urethral calibration with an 18 Fr soft catheter or a fixed/static flow pattern on UFM to select cases for it. It should be done with an integrated cystoscope sheath (14 Fr) or a pediatric cystoscope (11 Fr). A special effort should be made to inspect urethra completely to diagnose anatomical narrowings before entering the bladder. **It is preferable to perform endoscopy under sedation/anesthesia to avoid the effect of pelvic floor spasm confounding the findings**. For obvious anatomical strictures, a dilatation or definitive reconstruction can be done at the same sitting depending on the case scenario. There is no role for cystoscopy in women with functional obstruction unless the intention is to operate for a functional bladder neck obstruction or intrasphincteric botulinum toxin for dysfunctional voiding (DV)/Fowler's syndrome.

10.3 Follow-Up of Patients with Voiding Dysfunction

Individual follow-up protocol for patients will depend upon their individual diagnosis, severity of symptoms, and baseline back pressure changes or loss of renal function. **In general, a UDS study may be repeated after 3–6 months** to ascertain the impact of treatment and improvement of flow dynamics. For those who don't benefit, UDS may be repeated as clinically indicated or at onset of new symptoms or complications. Once the disease process has stabilized, the frequency of UDS is reduced.

Key Learning Points

- A voiding dysfunction should be suspected in any woman with LUTS (irrespective of storage or voiding symptoms) of more than 4 weeks' duration or recurrent UTI.
- Voiding dysfunction presenting only as voiding symptoms is uncommon.
- A uroflowmetry and PVR should be obtained in all women presenting with LUTS.
- Externally obvious causes like pelvic organ prolapse or periurethral pathologies should be excluded by thorough examination. An office urethral calibration may help detect luminal narrowing.
- A video-urodynamic study (or UDS + VCUG) is the best way to characterize a voiding dysfunction.

Case Discussion

A 65-year-old lady presented with severe voiding LUTS in form of slow stream and prolonged time to empty. The symptoms were progressive over 20 years. Her ultrasonogram revealed a thick-walled bladder with high residual urine of 190 cc and normal upper tracts. On examination she had anterior compartment pelvic organ prolapse reaching above the introitus, the meatus was normal. The symptoms and high residuals disproportionate to grade 1 prolapse, a calibration with 18 Fr was smooth. She did not respond to a trial of alpha-blockers and underwent further evaluation. Voiding films in anteroposterior showed a mild bladder descent, but lateral films confirmed a poorly opening bladder neck (Fig. 10.6a, b). Her urodynamic study revealed a poorly compliant bladder (end filling pressure 80 cm H_2O and very high voiding pressures, i.e., Pdet@Qmax 180 cm H_2O, *Q* max 2 ml/s) (Fig. 10.6c). A final diagnosis of PBNO was made and she was sub-

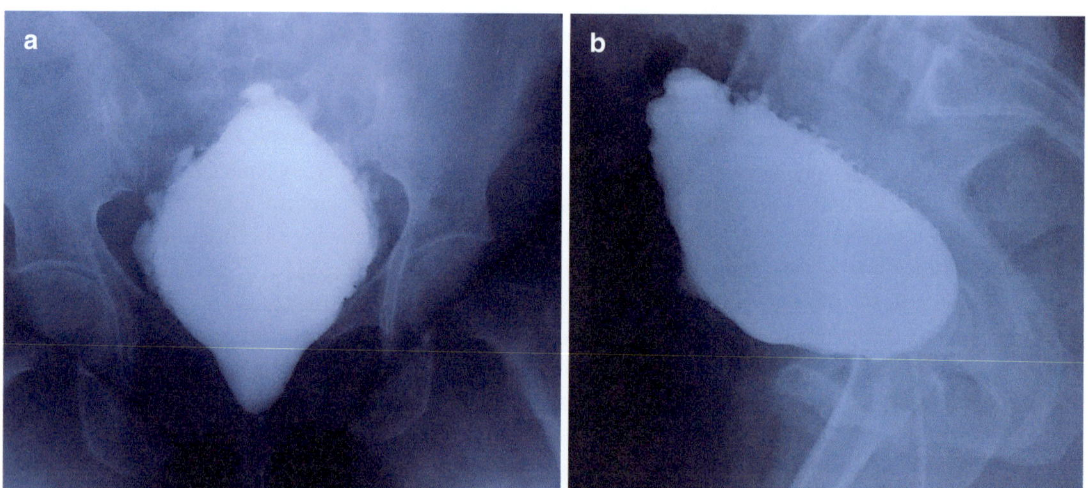

Fig. 10.6 VCUG: (**a**) anteroposterior film showing bladder neck descent during attempted voiding and (**b**) lateral film showing poor opening of neck. (**c**) UDS revealed poorly compliant bladder and urodynamic BOO with Pdet@Qmax of 180 cm H_2O and *Q* max of 2 ml/s. She was diagnosed with PBNO and subjected to (**d**) bladder neck resection, which relieved her symptoms

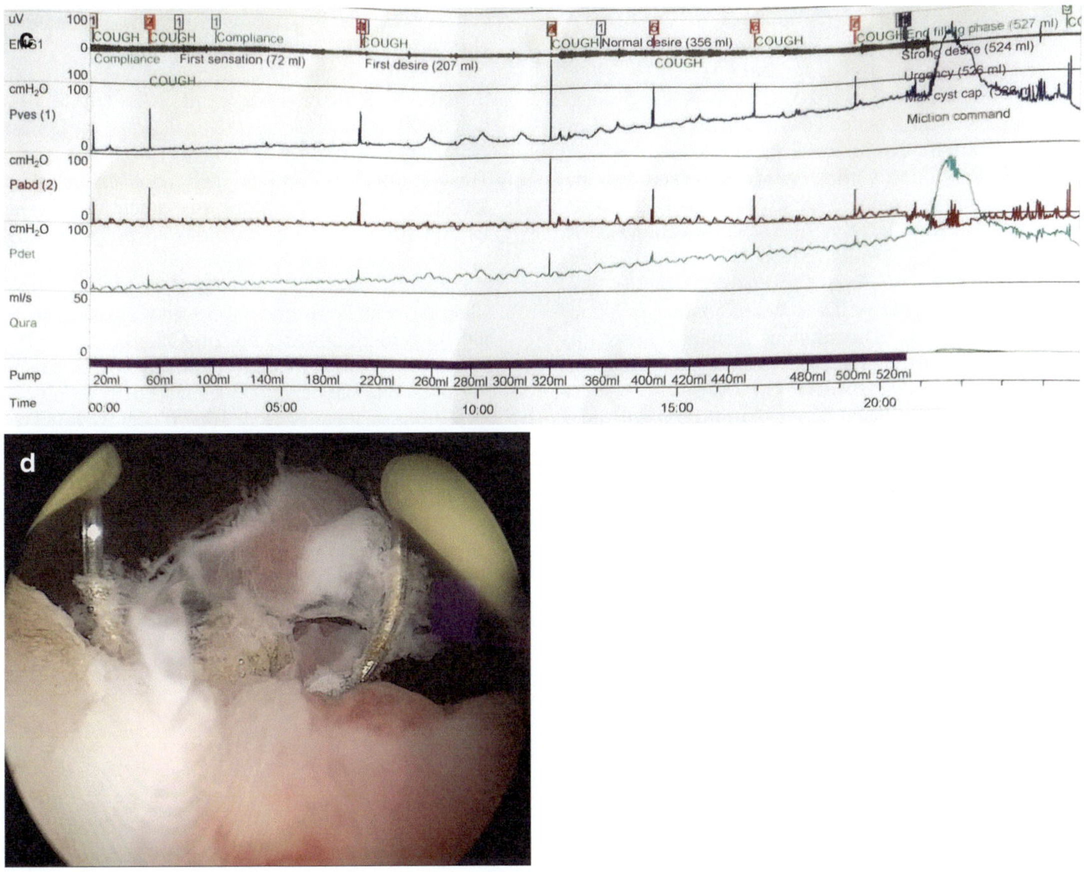

Fig. 10.6 (continued)

jected to bladder neck resection (Fig. 10.6d), which relieved her symptoms.

References

1. https://www.ics.org/glossary/diagnosis/voidingdysfunctionfemale.
2. Abdel Raheem A, Madersbacher H. Voiding dysfunction in women: how to manage it correctly. Arab J Urol. 2013;11(4):319–30.
3. Chuang F-C, Huang K-H, Kuo H-C. Lower urinary tract symptoms and video-urodynamic characteristics of women with clinically unsuspected bladder outlet obstruction. Low Urin Tract Symptoms. 2013;5(1):23–7.
4. Al-Shahrani M, Lovatsis D. Do subjective symptoms of obstructive voiding correlate with post-void residual urine volume in women? Int Urogynecol J Pelvic Floor Dysfunct. 2005;16(1):12–4; discussion 14.
5. Lowenstein L, Anderson C, Kenton K, Dooley Y, Brubaker L. Obstructive voiding symptoms are not predictive of elevated postvoid residual urine volumes. Int Urogynecol J Pelvic Floor Dysfunct. 2008;19(6):801–4.
6. Romanzi LJ, Chaikin DC, Blaivas JG. The effect of genital prolapse on voiding. J Urol. 1999;161(2):581–6.
7. Johnson JR, High RA, Dziadek O, Ocon A, Muir TW, Xu J, Antosh DD. Overactive bladder symptoms after pelvic organ prolapse repair. Female Pelvic Med Reconstr Surg. 2019.
8. Lo T-S. Alpha blockers in the clinical treatment of female lower urinary tract dysfunction. Incont Pelvic Floor Dysfunct. 2010;4(3):69–71.
9. Kim DK, Lee JY, Jung JH, Kim JH, Hah YS, Hong CH, et al. Alpha-1 adrenergic receptor blockers for the treatment of lower urinary tract symptoms in women: a systematic review and meta-analysis. Int Neurourol J. 2019;23(1):56–68.

10. Colaco M, Osman NI, Karakeçi A, Artibani W, Andersson K-E, Badlani GH. Current concepts of the acontractile bladder. BJU Int. 2018;122(2):195–202.
11. Lin C-D, Kuo H-C, SS-D Y. Diagnosis and management of bladder outlet obstruction in women. Low Urin Tract Symptoms. 2016;8(1):30–7.
12. Nitti VW, Tu LM, Gitlin J. Diagnosing bladder outlet obstruction in women. J Urol. 1999;161(5):1535–40.
13. Cohn JA, Brown ET, Kaufman MR, Dmochowski RR, Reynolds WS. Underactive bladder in women: is there any evidence? Curr Opin Urol. 2016;26(4):309–14.
14. Fry CH, Gammie A, Drake MJ, Abrams P, Kitney DG, Vahabi B. Estimation of bladder contractility from intravesical pressure-volume measurements. Neurourol Urodyn. 2017;36(4):1009–14.
15. Tan TL, Bergmann MA, Griffiths D, Resnick NM. Stop test or pressure-flow study? Measuring detrusor contractility in older females. Neurourol Urodyn. 2004;23(3):184–9.
16. Iacobellis F, Reginelli A, Berritto D, Gagliardi G, Laporta A, Brillantino A, et al. Pelvic floor dysfunctions: how to image patients? Jpn J Radiol. 2020;38(1):47–63.
17. Tunn R, Petri E. Introital and transvaginal ultrasound as the main tool in the assessment of urogenital and pelvic floor dysfunction: an imaging panel and practical approach. Ultrasound Obstet Gynecol. 2003;22(2):205–13.
18. Chan L. Pelvic ultrasound in the assessment of female voiding dysfunction. In: Chan L, Tse V, The S, Stewart P, editors. Pelvic floor ultrasound. Cham: Springer International Publishing; 2015. p. 63–76. http://link.springer.com/10.1007/978-3-319-04310-4_5. Accessed 4 Jun 2020.

Part II

Treatment Modalities for Female Bladder Outlet Obstruction and Urethral Reconstruction

11 Pharmacotherapy for Bladder Outlet Obstruction in Females

Mayank Mohan Agarwal

Learning Objectives After reading this chapter the reader will be able to:

- Understand the pharmacology of lower urinary tract (LUT) relevant to pharmacotherapy for lower urinary tract symptoms (LUTS).
- Learn about efficacy and adverse effects of pharmacotherapeutic targets and agents acting on different levels of LUT, i.e., detrusor, bladder neck, external sphincter/pelvic floor.
- Learn about the current evidence and limitation of their use in LUTS in women.

11.1 Introduction

Lower urinary tract (LUT) is richly innervated by autonomic (parasympathetic and sympathetic) as well as somatic nervous system [1]. There are complex arrays of interaction at cerebral cortex, brainstem, spinal cord, and peripheral levels for a smooth storage and voiding function of LUT. Neuronal and neuromuscular interactions happen via neurotransmitters (NT); therefore, an understanding of these neurotransmitters and their known (or potential, as the case may be) functions goes a long way in lucid understanding of pharmacotherapy for lower urinary tract dysfunction.

Peripheral pathways include cholinergic (acetylcholine through muscarinic and nicotinic receptors), adrenergic (norepinephrine through adrenergic receptors) and nonadrenergic-noncholinergic (NANC) pathways. Several NANC neurotransmitters have been studied and contribute variably to LUT function, e.g., nitric oxide, adenosine triphosphate, neuropeptides, vasoactive intestinal peptide, neuropeptide Y, tachykinins, serotonin, prostanoids and rho-kinase [2]. In the central pathways, several amino acids/their derivatives are important neurotransmitters. Glutamate is a major excitatory neurotransmitter; whereas, glycine and gamma-aminobutyric acid (GABA) are major inhibitory ones. The latter two inhibit the micturition reflex at supraspinal and spinal sites and show synergism at places [1].

The voiding dysfunction is majorly divided into storage and voiding function. This chapter aims to describe the pharmacotherapy for voiding dysfunction.

Pharmacotherapeutic agents for voiding dysfunction can be classified into three major categories:

1. Increasing bladder contractility.
2. Decreasing smooth sphincter resistance.
3. Decreased skeletal sphincter resistance.

M. M. Agarwal (✉)
Urology and Kidney Transplant Surgery, Medanta Hospital, Lucknow, Uttar Pradesh, India

N. Khattar et al. (eds.), *Female Bladder Outlet Obstruction and Urethral Reconstruction*, https://doi.org/10.1007/978-981-15-8521-0_11

11.2 Agents Increasing Bladder Contractility

1. *Parasympathomimetic*—**Bethanechol is the only agent in this category which is available for clinical use; however, the efficacy is highly questionable**. Pharmacologically, it selectively stimulates muscarinic cholinergic receptors, sparing nicotinic receptors, thereby increasing bladder sensitivity and contractility. There have been reports of increasing urethral resistance as well, thereby contradicting its bladder effect. In one study, no symptom improvement was seen with use of bethanechol (20 mg tds), while a significant improvement was seen when concomitant alpha-blockers were used [3]. Most studies which have shown efficacy have used subcutaneous route of administration (5–20 mg/day) and oral doses less than 200 mg have found little urodynamic efficacy [4, 5]. Intact neuronal circuits are considered to be essential for its function, while it may have no effect if the muscle itself is poorly responsive.

   Its adverse effects are predominantly due to cholinomimetic effects, such as flushing, sweating, diarrhea, abdominal cramps, miosis, hypersalivation, bronchospasm, and, in severe case, acute circulatory arrest.
2. *Miscellaneous*—Prostaglandins and thromboxane A2 have been shown to be present in human bladder. Studies have shown that intravesical instillation of PGE2 (the most abundant prostaglandin in bladder) results in acute emptying of bladder and triggers sustained improvement in long-term emptying, the mechanism of which is not well known [6]. However, in absence of consistent data and high-quality evidence, its clinical application is limited [7].

   Other studied agents, none of which is clinically used for the purpose, are prokinetics (metoclopramide, cizapride), opioid receptor antagonist (naloxone), and alpha-adrenergic receptor blockers [8].

11.3 Agents Decreasing Smooth Sphincter Resistance

Similar to men, women have internal sphincter at bladder neck composed of smooth muscles. Even though density of α-1A adrenergic receptors is less in women than men, these are sufficiently abundant and therefore natural pharmacotherapeutic targets. In fact, in a study of the effect of tamsulosin on resting urethral tone in female volunteers, Reitz et al. showed a significant reduction along the entire length of urethra [9].

α-1 adrenergic receptor blockers have been of proven efficacy and in use for men since long time. Earlier agents were α-1 non-subtype selective (e.g., prazosin, terazosin, doxazosin) and therefore were associated with cardiovascular adverse events (pertaining to α-1B receptors), particularly postural hypotension/dizziness, mandating dose titration. In fact, these medications were commonly used for hypertensive prostatic obstruction patients for dual purpose. With α-1A/D subtype selective agents such as tamsulosin, silodosin, and naftopidil, dose titration is not required.

1. *Tamsulosin*—Tamsulosin is relatively an α-1A receptor selective agent with affinity to α-1A being 10 times that to α-1B [10].

   It is the most extensively studied agent, in both men and women. The quality and quantity of data on efficacy of tamsulosin for women with voiding dysfunction are not as robust as in men; nevertheless, the published trials do report **significant and consistent improvement of LUTS in these women with a response rate ranging from 35% to 84%** [11]. Pummangura et al. [12] enrolled 140 women with voiding dysfunction and found that tamsulosin 0.2 mg improved International prostate symptoms score (IPSS) significantly over placebo (mean diff 6.1 points over placebo). In an uncontrolled prospective study, Lee et al. [13] enrolled 106 women with voiding dysfunction and categorized them based on urodynamic assessment. Seventy-six had urodynamically proven BOO (based on Blaivas-Groutz nomogram). Mean reduction in IPSS (23.9 ± 6.09 to 16.1 ± 8.17) and PVR (69.13 ± 85.45 to 39.88 ± 48.39 mL) and improvement in maximum flow rates (10.15 ± 2.79 to 13.47 ± 5.65 mL/s) were observed. Improvements in patients with no to mild obstruction and those with moderate to severe obstruction were statistically not different.

Oral absorption of the drug is excellent in fasting conditions (over 90%) and peak concentration reaches in 4–5 h. Elimination half-life is approximately 9–15 h and a steady state is achieved in 5 days of daily dosing. The drug is extensively metabolized in liver by cytochrome p450 enzymes. The daily dose is 0.2–0.4 mg/day, and no dose adjustment is required in patients with chronic kidney disease and mild-to-moderate liver dysfunction. It is not eliminated by dialysis because of high protein binding. There is no safety data available for pregnant and lactating women; based on animal experiments, it is classified as category B in pregnancy.

2. *Terazosin*

   Terazosin is an α-1 receptor selective (non-subtype selective) agent with equivalent affinity to α-1A, B and D subtype.

   In small single arm prospective studies and a small randomized controlled trial (RCT), response rate of 50–80% has been reported in terms of improvement in LUTS and urodynamic parameters [14–16].

   Oral absorption of the drug is excellent (>90%) and bypassing first pass metabolism in liver it rapidly reaches its peak in 1–2 h of intake. It is extensively metabolized in liver by hydrolysis; mean elimination half-life is about 12 h. Since it affects α-1B as much as α-1A, resulting vasodilatation may lead to profound postural hypotension. Therefore, it is started at a small dose of 1 mg/day and progressively escalated to 4–5 mg/day over 1–2 weeks. It is not eliminated by dialysis because of high protein binding. There are no studies on safety in pregnancy, lactation and on teratogenicity.

3. *Alfuzosin*

   Alfuzosin is an α-1 receptor selective (non-subtype selective) agent with equivalent affinity to α-1A, B and D subtype. Despite being subtype nonspecific, it has shown remarkable organ selectivity in isolated human prostate tissue compared to terazosin and doxazosin (141 vs. 19 and 51, respectively) [17].

   Two small prospective single arm studies (total $n = 59$) showed improvement of LUTS without change in urethral resistance (one study), in 2/3rd patients with primary bladder neck obstruction (PBNO) [18, 19]. However, in a moderate-sized RCT the efficacy was found to be equivalent to placebo, questioning its role in this setting [20].

   In view of its tissue selectivity and availability of sustained release preparation, its vascular side effects are markedly reduced compared to other α-1 blockers, obviating the need for dose titration.

4. *Silodosin*

   Silodosin is a highly selective α-1A adrenoceptor antagonist with affinity to α-1A 583 times that of α-1B, making it extremely safe with respect to cardiovascular side effects [21].

   High-quality evidence proves efficacy of silodosin in men with bladder neck obstruction and prostatic obstruction both clinically and urodynamically [22, 23]. Even though no clinical study is available for its role in women with voiding dysfunction, it is widely used clinically (off-label).

   Silodosin is absorbed rapidly (t_{max} 2.6 ± 0.9 h) after oral administration with oral bioavailability of appx 30–40%. It is extensively metabolized in liver by cytochrome P450 and has an elimination $t½$ of 13.3 ± 8.07 h for standard dose of 8 mg/day. The dose should be reduced to 4 mg/day in moderate renal and hepatic failure patients and has not been studied in those with severe disease [24].

   Common adverse effects (>10% incidence) of non-subtype α-1 adrenoceptor blockers terazosin and doxazosin are postural dizziness, asthenia, fatigue, rhinitis, and headache.

These effects are progressively less common in tamsulosin, alfuzosin, and silodosin. Dry ejaculation is very common in silodosin (22–30%) and tamsulosin (6–11%); obviously, these are irrelevant for women [25]. Rarely, stress incontinence has been reported in women [13].

11.4 Agents Decreasing Skeletal Sphincter Resistance

As described in Chap. 4, dysfunctional voiding or high-tone pelvic floor dysfunction is fairly common in women and the treatment approach is multipronged, encompassing pelvic floor relaxation exercises, biofeedback, treatment of constipation, pharmacotherapy, and other measures.

Skeletal muscle relaxants (SMR) are a heterogenous group of medications which are used for neurogenic/non-neurogenic spastic muscular conditions with or without pain. Several agents are available, most of which, except for dantrolene, are centrally acting and many have still obscure mode of action [2]. Some examples are baclofen, tizanidine, tolperisone, chlorzoxazone, carisoprodol, benzodiazepines and gabapentenoids. The role of skeletal muscle relaxant in the management of DV is plausible and, in the absence of a pelvic floor-specific agent, studies have evaluated agents from the above list, i.e., baclofen, diazepam, and tizanidine.

11.4.1 Diazepam

Diazepam is a benzodiazepine derivative which binds to $GABA_A$receptors in CNS and PNS facilitating GABA's inhibitory actions on muscle tone and reflex contractions. It has been studied in women with "high-tone pelvic disorders" with variable results. Oral administration has high propensity for adverse effects and addiction; this has led researchers to study the intravaginal route since the systemic absorption is minimal.

The primary outcome studied has been pain due to spams or constipation; DV has not been studied as such. As a part of multimodal therapy including PFMT and trigger point injection, it showed promise; whereas, in two placebo-controlled RCTs no significant pain reduction was observed after vaginal pessary treatment [26–28].

11.4.2 Baclofen

Baclofen, a GABA derivative, is a centrally acting agonist of $GABA_B$ receptors. It inhibits both monosynaptic and polysynaptic reflexes at spinal level. Through unknown mechanisms it may also have supraspinal effects. GABA-ergic interneurons in sacral spinal cord are responsible for relaxation of EUS during micturition. Therefore, baclofen has been used in relieving dyssynergia in patients with spinal cord injury.

It has been studied in women with dysfunctional voiding in RCT at doses of 5–10 mg t.i.d and found to be moderately useful in terms of improved bladder capacity, flow rates, and EMG relaxation [29, 30]. In view of promising results in these small trials, it is commonly prescribed in dysfunctional voiding in all age groups. However, in the absence of a large body of evidence and long-term data it is an off-label indication only.

It is rapidly absorbed after oral administration with bioavailability 70–80% and reaching peak in 2–4 h. Only 15% is metabolized by liver and over 70% of the active drug is eliminated unchanged in the urine. The half-life of baclofen is approximately 3–4 h. Dosages in pelvic floor dysfunction are not clearly defined; nevertheless, in spastic conditions, it is typically initiated at 5 mg t.i.d and escalated, as required, every 3 days to desired dose (typically 30–75 mg/day). Dose reduction is recommended in renal and hepatic dysfunction. It is not recommended in pregnancy; although safety in pediatric population is not well established, it seems to be reasonably tolerated in children [31].

Adverse effect profile is significant—hypotonia, drowsiness, confusion, nausea (>10%); cognitive impairment, dizziness, speech disturbance, depression, seizure, constipation, asthenia, peripheral edema (1–10%), and many more.

Sudden withdrawal after chronic intake has been associated with serious side effects, e.g., autonomic dysfunction, confusion, seizures, spasticity, psychosis, and even rhabdomyolysis. Therefore, it must be tapered off if required to be discontinued [32].

11.4.3 Tizanidine

Tizanidine is a centrally acting presynaptic α_{2A} and α_{2C} adrenoceptor agonist which works by inhibiting neurotransmitter release from noradrenergic nerves with resultant reduction in facilitation of spinal motor neurons [33]. It has skeletal muscle relaxing and antinociceptive properties. It is chemically related to clonidine; however, its blood pressure–lowering potency is 1/10–1/50th that of latter.

In several RCTs and meta-analyses, tizanidine has been found to be similar in efficacy compared to baclofen in spastic syndromes [33–36]. However, so far there is only one study on its role in dysfunctional voiding. In an open-label RCT El-Hefnawy et al. compared the efficacy of tizanidine and doxazosin in 40 children with DV [37]. Tizanidine group registered reduction in urgency episodes, day time incontinence, and nocturnal enuresis, compared to doxazosin which registered reduction in urge episodes only.

It is rapidly and well absorbed orally (~95%; t_{max} 1.5 h); however, due to first pass metabolism in liver, its oral bioavailability is ~40%. It is metabolized by liver cytochrome P450 enzymes; elimination $t\frac{1}{2}$ is ~2.5 h.

Dosages in pelvic floor dysfunction are not defined; nevertheless, in spastic conditions, it is typically initiated at 2 mg t.i.d and escalated, as required, every 1–4 days to desired dose (max dose 36 mg/day). Dose reduction is recommended in renal and hepatic dysfunction. It is not recommended in pregnancy; although safety in pediatric population is not well established, it seems to be reasonably tolerated in children [38].

Adverse effect profile is significant and somewhat different from baclofen. Dry mouth, somnolence (possibly due to insomnia), dizziness, and asthenia are most common (>10%). A reversible elevation of liver enzymes following tizanidine treatment has been reported in ~5% of patients [33]. It must be tapered off if it needs to be discontinued.

11.4.4 Onabotulinum toxin A

Onabotulinum toxin A (OBoNT) is a neurotoxin produced by *Clostridium botulinum*. SNARE proteins are a large protein complex which mediate intracellular vesicle fusion. Botulinum neurotoxin (BoNT) cleaves SNAP-25 (synaptosome associated protein 25 kDa) rendering SNARE complex (soluble *N*-ethylmaleimide sensitive factor attachment protein receptor) inactive, thereby preventing Ach and other neurotransmitter containing vesicles from exocytosis. Functionally, this inhibits release of Ach and other neurotransmitters from neuromuscular junction paralyzing the muscle.

BoNT was first used in 1980 for strabismus. Since then it has been widely used for several spastic muscle disorders (muscle dystonia, multiple sclerosis, spinal cord injury, chronic migraine, etc.), smooth muscle hyperactive disorders (detrusor overactivity, benign prostate hyperplasia, Hirschsprung disease, chronic anal fissures, Raynaud's phenomena, etc.), chronic pain disorders (tension headache, migraine, neuropathic pain, etc.), hyper-sweating and hyper-salivary disorders, and in cosmetics.

BoNT has been used for men and women with dysfunctional voiding and neurogenic detrusor-sphincter dyssynergia for over three decades [39]. However, in want of high-quality long-term trials, it is not US FDA–approved for these indications, and the usage remains off-label. In a large series of men (n = 48) and women (n = 55) with neurogenic (n = 51) and nonneurogenic (n = 52) external sphincter dysfunction, Kuo et al. reported excellent (38.8%) and moderate (45.7%) improvement in symptoms and urodynamic findings similarly in neurogenic and non-neurogenic conditions [40].

Fifty to 100 units of OBoNT are injected directly into the sphincter muscle either urethroscopically or transperineally. Total dose is diluted in 4–5 mL normal saline and injected at 4 or 5 places (1 mL each).

Adverse effect profile is very safe for sphincter injection. Effects of BoNT per se are minimal; temporary flu-like symptoms and muscle weakness have been reported. More commonly, adverse effects are related to procedure, e.g., hematuria, urinary tract infection, and dysuria. Median lethal dose (LD50) of intravenous injection in monkeys is 39 U/kg; based on this, LD50 for a 70 kg human would be 3000 units. There is insufficient knowledge of complete dose response curve in humans; a ceiling dose of 360 units and minimum 12 weeks' interval is recommended [41].

In conclusion, voiding dysfunction in women is a unique diagnostic and therapeutic challenge. *In view of lack of strong body of evidence, recommendations cannot be made and most pharmacological treatments are off-label.* Nevertheless, clinical studies have shown subjective as well as objective improvement with pharmacotherapeutic agents described above. Therefore, a clinician and patient may discuss risks and benefits of the agent and take a well-informed individualized decision. Needless to say, high-quality RCTs are welcome in this orphaned area to be able to make further recommendations.

11.5 How I Do It

Alpha-1A adrenoceptor blocker (tamsulosin or silodosin) are used as initial empirical treatment in all women who present with voiding symptoms and in whom initial evaluation (history, physical examination, PVR, uroflowmetry, urine routine examination) is suggestive of voiding dysfunction. In the presence of favorable subjective and objective response (most importantly PVR), the therapy is continued long term with periodic reassessment.

As a routine patients are taught pelvic floor strengthening-cum-relaxation exercises and encouraged to practice those. Counseling about the proper voiding position and management of constipation (if any) is done simultaneously. If there is no response to the initial treatment with alpha-blocker and pelvic floor muscle exercises (PFME), a comprehensive urodynamic study consisting of pressure-flow study and micturating cystography with/without EMG with/without urethral pressure profilometry is performed. Further treatment is based on findings of the study. Addition of a skeletal muscle relaxant (most commonly tizanidine) to the above regimen in patients diagnosed with external sphincter/pelvic floor dysfunction is desirable. It is imperative to educate patients regarding pathophysiology and chronicity of the disease, and expected treatment goals. Pelvic floor exercises, treatment of constipation, and the correct position of voiding are re-emphasized. Botox into external sphincter and sacral neuromodulation (InterStim) are the next-line of treatment. The rare patient with urodynamically proven refractory bladder neck obstruction can be offered bladder neck incision.

Key Learning Points

- Alpha adrenergic blockers help reduce resting urethral tone over the entire length of urethra and provide an effective and safe pharmacotherapeutic option for initial empirical treatment of voiding dysfunction, particularly for functional obstructions like PBNO and DV.
- Skeletal muscle relaxants have a plausible role in DV but so far very few studies have shown promising results. Individualized decision making is recommended.
- Intra-sphincteric botulinum toxin is effective in select patients with DV.
- Most pharmacotherapeutic agents for voiding dysfunction in women are only for off-label use pending better quality evidence.

References

1. Miyazato M, Yoshimura N, Nishijima S, Sugaya K. Roles of glycinergic and gamma-aminobutyricergic mechanisms in the micturition reflex in rats. LUTS Low Urin Tract Symptoms. 2009;1(S1):S70–3.
2. Canda AE, Cinar MG, Turna B, Sahin MO. Pharmacologic targets on the female urethra. Urol Int. 2008;80(4):341–54.

3. Yamanishi T, Yasuda K, Kamai T, et al. Combination of a cholinergic drug and an α-blocker is more effective than monotherapy for the treatment of voiding difficulty in patients with underactive detrusor. Int J Urol. 2004;11(2):88–96.
4. De Wachter S, Van Meel TD, Wyndaele JJ. Study of the afferent nervous system and its evaluation in women with impaired detrusor contractility treated with bethanechol. Urology. 2003;62(1):54–8.
5. Finkbeiner AE. Is bethanechol chloride clinically effective in promoting bladder emptying? A literature review. J Urol. 1985;134(3):443–9.
6. Andersson KE, Wein AJ. Pharmacology of the lower urinary tract: basis for current and future treatments of urinary incontinence. Pharmacol Rev. 2004;56(4):581–631.
7. Hindley RG, Brierly RD, Thomas PJ. Prostaglandin E2 and bethanechol in combination for treating detrusor underactivity. BJU Int. 2004;93(1):89–92.
8. Andersson K-E, Wein AJ. Pharmacologic management of lower urinary tract storage and emptying failure. In: Wein AJ, Kavoussi LR, Partin AW, Peters CA, editors. Campbell-Walsh urology. 11th ed. Philadelphia: Elsevier; 2016. p. 1967–2002.e14.
9. Reitz A, Haferkamp A, Kyburz T, Knapp PA, Wefer B, Schurch B. The effect of tamsulosin on the resting tone and the contractile behaviour of the female urethra: a functional urodynamic study in healthy women. Eur Urol. 2004;46(2):235–40.
10. Schwinn DA, Price DT, Narayan P. α1-adrenoceptor subtype selectivity and lower urinary tract symptoms. Mayo Clin Proc. 2004;79(11):1423–34.
11. Meyer LE, Brown JN. Tamsulosin for voiding dysfunction in women. Int Urol Nephrol. 2012;44(6):1649–56.
12. Pummangura N, Kochakarn W. Efficacy of tamsulosin in the treatment of lower urinary tract symptoms (LUTS) in women. Asian J Surg. 2007;30(2):131–7.
13. Lee KS, Han DH, Lee YS, et al. Efficacy and safety of tamsulosin for the treatment of non-neurogenic voiding dysfunction in females: a 8-week prospective study. J Korean Med Sci. 2010;25(1):117–22.
14. Low BY, Liong ML, Yuen KH, et al. Terazosin therapy for patients with female lower urinary tract symptoms: a randomized, double-blind, placebo controlled trial. J Urol. 2008;179(4):1461–9.
15. Kessler TM, Studer UE, Burkhard FC. The effect of terazosin on functional bladder outlet obstruction in women: a pilot study. J Urol. 2006;176(4):1487–92.
16. Kumar A, Mandhani A, Gogoi S, Srivastava A. Management of functional bladder neck obstruction in women: use of A-blockers and pediatric resectoscope for bladder neck incision. J Urol. 1999;162(6):2061–5.
17. Wilde MI, Fitton A, McTavish D. Alfuzosin: a review of its pharmacodynamic and pharmacokinetic properties, and therapeutic potential in benign prostatic hyperplasia. Drugs. 1993;45(3):410–29.
18. D'Armiento M, Damiano R, De Sio M, Perdonà S, Santonastaso C, Mattace RD. Ruolo dell'alfuzosina nei disturbi di vuotamento funzionali nella donna [Role of alfuzosin in the treatment of functional voiding disorders in women]. Arch Ital Urol Androl. 1997;69(Suppl 1):43–5.
19. Athanasopoulos A, Gyftopoulos K, Giannitsas K, Perimenis P. Effect of alfuzosin on female primary bladder neck obstruction. Int Urogynecol J. 2009;20(2):217–22.
20. Lee YS, Lee KS, Choo MS, et al. Efficacy of an alpha-blocker for the treatment of nonneurogenic voiding dysfunction in women: an 8-week, randomized, double-blind, placebo-controlled trial. Int Neurourol J. 2018;22(1):30–40.
21. Schilit S, Benzeroual KE. Silodosin: a selective α1A-adrenergic receptor antagonist for the treatment of benign prostatic hyperplasia. Clin Ther. 2009;31(11):2489–502.
22. Villa L, Capogrosso P, Capitanio U, et al. Silodosin: an update on efficacy, safety and clinical indications in urology. Adv Ther. 2019;36(1):1–18.
23. Jung JH, Kim J, Macdonald R, Reddy B, Kim MH, Dahm P. Silodosin for the treatment of lower urinary tract symptoms in men with benign prostatic hyperplasia. Cochrane Database Syst Rev. 2017;11(11):CD012615.
24. Matsubara Y, Kanazawa T, Kojima Y, et al. Pharmacokinetics and disposition of silodosin (KMD-3213). Yakugaku Zasshi. 2006;126(special issue):237–45.
25. McNicholas TA, Speakman MJ, Kirby RS. Evaluation and nonsurgical management of benign prostatic hyperplasia. In: Wein AJ, Kavoussi LR, Partin AW, Peters CA, editors. Campbell-Walsh urology. 11th ed. Philadelphia: Elsevier; 2016. p. 2463–503.
26. Rogalski MJ, Kellogg-Spadt S, Hoffmann AR, Fariello JY, Whitmore KE. Retrospective chart review of vaginal diazepam suppository use in high-tone pelvic floor dysfunction. Int Urogynecol J. 2010;21(7):895–9.
27. Crisp CC, Vaccaro CM, Estanol MV, et al. Intra-vaginal diazepam for high-tone pelvic floor dysfunction: a randomized placebo-controlled trial. Int Urogynecol J Pelvic Floor Dysfunct. 2013;24(11):1915–23.
28. Holland MA, Joyce JS, Brennaman LM, Drobnis EZ, Starr JA, Foster RT. Intravaginal diazepam for the treatment of pelvic floor hypertonic disorder. Female Pelvic Med Reconstr Surg. 2019;25(1):76–81.
29. Chen CH, Hsiao SM, Chang TC, Wu WY, Lin HH. Clinical and urodynamic effects of baclofen in women with functional bladder outlet obstruction: preliminary report. J Obstet Gynaecol Res. 2016;42(5):560–5.
30. Xu D, Qu C, Meng H, et al. Dysfunctional voiding confirmed by transdermal perineal electromyography, and its effective treatment with baclofen in women with lower urinary tract symptoms: a randomized

double-blind placebo-controlled crossover trial. BJU Int. 2007;100(3):588–92.
31. He Y, Brunstrom-Hernandez JE, Thio LL, et al. Population pharmacokinetics of oral baclofen in pediatric patients with cerebral palsy. J Pediatr. 2014;164(5):1181.
32. Stetkarova I, Brabec K, Vasko P, Menel L. Intrathecal baclofen in spinal spasticity: frequency and severity of withdrawal syndrome. Pain Physician. 2015;18(4):E633–41.
33. Malanga G, Reiter RD, Garay E. Update on tizanidine for muscle spasticity and emerging indications. Expert Opin Pharmacother. 2008;9(12): 2209–15.
34. Hoogstraten MC, van der Ploeg RJO, vd Burg W, Vreeling A, van Marle S, Minderhoud JM. Tizanidine versus baclofen in the treatment of spasticity in multiple sclerosis patients. Acta Neurol Scand. 1988;77(3):224–30.
35. Bass B, Weinshenker B, Rice GPA, et al. Tizanidine versus baclofen in the treatment of spasticity in patients with multiple sclerosis. Can J Neurol Sci. 1988;15(1):15–9.
36. Groves L, Shellenberger MK, Davis CS. Tizanidine treatment of spasticity: a meta-analysis of controlled, double-blind, comparative studies with baclofen and diazepam. Adv Ther. 1998;15(4):241–51.
37. El-Hefnawy AS, Helmy T, El-Assmy MM, Sarhan O, Hafez AT, Dawaba M. Doxazosin versus tizanidine for treatment of dysfunctional voiding in children: a prospective randomized open-labeled trial. Urology. 2012;79(2):428–33.
38. Henney HR, Chez M. Pediatric safety of tizanidine: clinical adverse event database and retrospective chart assessment. Pediatr Drugs. 2009;11(6):397–406.
39. Kuo HC. Botulinun A toxin urethral sphincter injection for neurogenic or nonneurogenic voiding dysfunction. Tzu Chi Med J. 2016;28(3):89–93.
40. Kuo HC. Botulinum a toxin urethral injection for the treatment of lower urinary tract dysfunction. J Urol. 2003;170(5):1908–12.
41. Davids HR, Moberg-Wolff EA. What is the median lethal dose (LD50) of botulinum toxin? https://www.medscape.com/answers/325574-179844/what-is-the-median-lethal-dose-ld50-of-botulinum-toxin. Published 2019.

12 Urethral Dilatation and Minimally Invasive Surgical Options for Female Bladder Outlet Obstruction

T. Manasa

Learning Objectives

- Identify procedural consideration pertaining to the etiology of bladder outlet obstruction (BOO) in a female.
- Application of clinical concepts of female BOO in surgical practice.
- Techniques and outcomes of minimally invasive techniques in female BOO.

12.1 Introduction

Conventional teaching often overlooks urethral pathology as a frequent etiology of lower urinary tract symptoms (LUTS) in women. Anatomical obstruction of the bladder outlet is estimated to affect 2.7–8% of women presenting with voiding LUTS [1]; however, this may be significantly underdiagnosed or underreported. There is a lack of understanding of the pathophysiology of bladder outlet obstruction (BOO) in females with no clear consensus on the diagnostic criteria perhaps due to substantial variation in normal female voiding function. Obstruction can be broadly classified into anatomical and functional, despite the list of etiologies being diverse. Symptoms are myriad and have a low predictive value with 13–57% sensitivity and 18–38% specificity for elevated post-void residue (PVR) [2, 3]. Accurate clinical evaluation comprising of a detailed history, physical examination adequately supported by ancillary studies such as ultrasound, voiding cysto-urethrogram, and urodynamic studies aids in appropriate diagnosis.

Treating a female BOO appears to be as complex, with a multitude of options being available at present. The choice, however, should be based primarily according to the underlying pathophysiology with due consideration to disease characteristics and the needs of an individual. In contrast to men, in whom pharmacotherapy has been used extensively to treat outlet obstruction, its use in women is still limited. Alpha-adrenoreceptor blockers, including tamsulosin, alfuzosin and terazosin [4–6], have demonstrated their usefulness in women with voiding dysfunction(VD). Reduction in urethral resistance seems to be an efficacious treatment in women with functional bladder outlet obstruction as supported by evidence. Costantini et al. [7] reported a 71.4% improvement in voiding symptoms, 66.7% improvement in both voiding and storage symptoms, with a 62.5% decrease in PVR in women on tamsulosin for functional BOO. However, there is lack of clarity as to why alpha-blockers are beneficial in one woman but not in the other and as to why the symptomatic improvement seem to be better as compared to uroflowmetry results. Associated presence or absence of pelvic

T. Manasa (✉)
Ramaiah Medical College, Bengaluru, India

N. Khattar et al. (eds.), *Female Bladder Outlet Obstruction and Urethral Reconstruction*,
https://doi.org/10.1007/978-981-15-8521-0_12

floor dysfunction, or a missed underlying clinical pathology either mechanical or neurological, could be the reason.

12.2 Minimally Invasive Surgical Options in BOO

12.2.1 Urethral Dilatation (UD)

Urethral dilatation for female LUTS continues to be used despite lack of adequate evidence backing its use. It has been noted that 50% of the clinicians used UD overall 6 or fewer times per year, with the number of dilatations reaching as high as 30 times/year in 23.7% as revealed by a questionnaire-based survey carried out among 194 urologists of Texas in 1999 [8]. UD for BOO was first described by Lyon and associates in 1923, who, having postulated the presence of a distal urethral ring, recommended dilatation and rupture of this ring for relieving obstruction [9, 10]. Dilatation has since then found widespread use for the treatment of female LUTS, although lacking evidence from long-term, well-controlled outcome studies.

To this day, UD forms the cornerstone of treatment in female urethral stricture (FUS). In a large series on urethral dilation for FUS in 91 patients, Romman et al. have shown only a 51% success rate for initial dilation to 41 Fr. Prior UD was a statistically significant predictor of failure in this cohort [11]. A 57% success rate was reported by Smith et al. in seven women after dilatation to 30 Fr at a mean follow-up of 21 months [12]. Although most urologists dilate the urethra to 32 Fr [10, 13], there is no clear consensus about the exact size to which urethral dilatation needs to be performed. This lack of uniformity could be attributed to a surprisingly wide range of urethral caliber seen in normal women. As a result of absence of a set criteria and a definite urethral caliber cutoff to diagnose urethral stricture in women, the caliber at which a female urethra may require dilatation remains unanswered. However, the procedure itself can be carried out either as an office procedure with serial urethral dilators under local anesthesia or in the operation theatre under spinal anesthesia aided by cystoscopy. No difference in the outcomes have been noted. But post-dilatation, there is a higher rate of recurrence noted due to fibrosis and scarring [14, 15]. Extreme stretching of urethra may actually be counter-productive, especially the stretching that causes trauma where healing occurs by fibrosis. This can undo the benefits of stretching the stricture scar leading to recurrence. Hence **more and more urologists are opting for reconstructive procedures such as urethroplasty using vaginal or buccal graft owing to higher mean success rate (80–100%) when compared to UD (<50%) at any given time of follow-up** [16, 17].

In the algorithm for management of FUS, UD should therefore be reserved as an initial treatment or preferred method of treatment in patients unwilling or unsuitable for complex urethral procedures. It is prudent to avoid a repeat dilatation if prior dilatation has failed as increased scarring and peri-urethral fibrosis due to bleeding and extravasation are higher with repeat procedures leading to lower success rates [18]. Nevertheless, **periodic dilatation is advised if patients are unfit for or un-interested in surgery. It may also be an appropriate option for previous failed reconstructions.** On-demand UD seems to be as effective as periodic/intermittent dilatations with similar improvements in flow measurement while avoiding overtreatment [19].

SELF-CALIBRATION: **Urethral dilatation followed by chronic intermittent self-calibration is considered safe and effective for managing FUS** [12]. Though the ideal catheter size and the appropriate regimen of self-calibration are yet to be determined, calibration once daily to once or twice weekly is a common practice in patients requiring repeated urethral dilatations to prevent recurrence [12]. Though a routine practice among most urologists, literature is scarce in providing the statistical benefit of this procedure and no study to this date has evaluated the risk/cost benefit ratio. Conversely, Santucci et al. [13] are opposed to self-dilatation as they find the procedure uncomfortable, inconvenient, and disliked by most of their patients. The belief that long-term self-dilation regimens lead to urethral false passages and the unavailability of data proving its role in delaying the onset of urinary retention have also been enumerated [13]. However, in a prospective, randomized trial of 49 patients, those on self-calibration had higher urinary flow rates and better subjective quality-of-life scores when compared to patients on urethral dilatation with sounds for recurrent urethral strictures [20]. The rates of urinary tract infections were also lesser among the ones performing self-calibration.

UD still remains an accepted method of treatment among most urologists in conditions other than FUS [18]. However there is a paucity of literature suggesting the empirical use of UD in women who have significant LUTS without clear etiology will improve outcomes. UD is routinely practiced as it seems to be an easier option due to inadequate understanding of the disease processes causing voiding dysfunction along with no accepted cut off on urethral caliber. The rationale for the use of UD despite inadequate evidence is based on the transient symptomatic relief experienced by women following UD [21]. This could be due to the mechanical stretching of the urethral sphincter complex coupled with an increase in the urethral caliber [21]. It has been suggested that mechanical stretching causes local tissue proliferation, remodeling, and reorganization of neural reflexes. This may help promote a more sustained guarding reflex. As proposed by Shafik et al. [22], mild urethral distention occurring during voiding stimulates urethral stretch receptors and helps reflex bladder contraction.

Furthermore, such women request repeated dilatations despite its questionable efficacy in female LUTS. In a retrospective review by Yee et al. [23], 20 patients with LUTS diagnosed as primary (functional) BOO showed no significant change in Q_{max} (9.6 ± 2.8 vs. 9.7 ± 4.0 mL/s, $p = 0.869$) and postvoid residual urine (246 ± 196 vs. 263 ± 198 mL, $p = 0.753$) after urethral calibration. On the contrary, on urodynamics, PdetQ_{max} showed significant improvement (72.2 ± 39 vs. 50.2 ± 30.5 cmH_2O, $p = 0.013$). Thirteen (65%) underwent a repeat calibration for persistent symptoms. However, further studies with patient reported outcomes and long follow-up are required to identify the exact role of UD in functional BOO. Until then, the presumed favorable efficacy of UD is simply anecdotal.

12.2.2 Clean Intermittent Catheterization (CIC)

Intermittent catheterization is recommended for patients with functional BOO. CIC should be considered only if the biofeedback or bladder retraining therapy fails in dyscoordinated functional voiding. The exception to the rule being severe cases defined by PVR of >50% of the functional bladder capacity where CIC may be offered as an initial form of management [24]. In a setting of primary bladder neck obstruction (PBNO) a failed response to alpha-blocker therapy or patients unfit or unwilling for surgery should be offered CIC. For DSD, CIC still remains the standard therapy [25]. In the post-surgical setting, CIC is recommended in obstruction following anti-incontinence surgery, especially in patients with severe incontinence preoperatively, who do not want to risk recurrent incontinence [26].

12.2.3 Internal Urethrotomy

Internal urethrotomy involves incision of the stricture with an endoscopic knife, Otis urethrotome or laser. Urethrotomy in females owes its inception to Kerr and associates, who postulated the use of Otis urethrotome for cutting the distal contraction ring rather than dilating it with sounds [10]. However the evidence supporting its use for anatomical obstruction in females is scarce. Most urologists propose urethrotomy as an empirical treatment in women with voiding LUTS of unclear etiology. The rationale behind its routine use is based on the assumption that it may cause temporary partial paralysis of the external sphincter in patients with detrusor–sphincter dyssynergia [27] akin to anal dilatation/sphincterotomy in patients with high anal tone due to anal fissure while opening the urethral channel in cases of bladder neck or urethral stricture [28] and perhaps also causing urethral denervation due to dilatation [29]. **The classical technique involves incision at the 12 o'clock position through the fibrotic scar bundle to healthy tissue with the Otis urethrotome/cold knife urethrotome.** Nonetheless, the caliber to which Otis urethrotomy needs to be performed is yet to be defined. Laser urethrotomy requires a high-energy, high-frequency setting for making a deep sharp cut. Laser incisions are generally made at the 3 and 9 o'clock positions. An additional 12 o'clock incision is made if deemed necessary. Length of the incisions may differ based on the urethral site, however not more than 2 cm. A 16 Fr or larger urethral catheter is left in place postoperatively for several days. Self-calibration has been recommended by some after surgery to reduce the risk for recurrence; however, the ideal regimen and duration remain elusive [30, 31]. Serial dilatations until 40 Fr up to 6 times following urethrotomy has been shown to be more effective as compared to urethrotomy alone in women [32].

12.2.4 Endoscopic Core Through (Cut to the Light)

In traumatic obliterated strictures not amenable to urethrotomy, a "cut to the light" procedure can be performed. The procedure is preferred in more proximal or mid distal stricture. Antegrade identification of the true bladder neck with a flexible/rigid cystoscope is important for such a procedure [33]. For a complete distal urethral stricture, Dogra and Nabi [34] described a special technique where a puncture needle was passed from the presumed urethral meatus to the bladder neck transgressing the obliterated urethral segment under antegrade endoscopic guidance. A 0.038 inch guidewire was then passed and serial dilatation done till 18 Fr. A 16 Fr catheter was kept in situ for 6 weeks. At 6 weeks, urethroscopy was performed which showed an epithelialized urethra. Patient was placed on self-calibration for 3 months and was found to be continent and voiding well at 18 months. A prolonged postoperative catheterization is recommended to ensure complete healing and re-epithelialization in such cases [31]. A ventral urethrotomy to create a hypospadiac urethra has also been described for posttraumatic complete distal urethral stricture [33]. Such reports, however, are isolated and the success rates of such procedures are generally considered as dismal, and, wherever possible, a formal reconstruction gives the best outcome, although a standard treatment algorithm has not been established.

12.2.5 Sphincterotomy

The role of endoscopic urethral sphincterotomy in detrusor sphincter dyssynergia (DSD) is to reduce the outflow resistance by impairing the external sphincter. The current indications are limited only to neurogenic DSD associated with hydronephrosis, vesicoureteric reflux (VUR), recurrent UTIs, or autonomic dysreflexia [35]. Though it has not been attempted in neurologically intact women for dysfunctional voiding (DV) but has been tried in males for such indications with promising outcomes [36], it can be attempted as a last resort for refractory non-neurogenic DV in women.

The procedure involves resection/incision of the external sphincter with electrocautery or a cold knife. It is done at the 12 o'clock position to limit hemorrhage. It is, however, difficult to assess the depth of the incision. As recommended, the depth of incision should reach the plane of the periurethral venous sinuses [37]. Complications include bleeding, urinary extravasation, and prominence of bladder neck obstruction [38]. Failures can occur due to an inadequate sphincterotomy, underlying detrusor hypocontractility, or formation of urethral stricture [39].

12.2.6 Transurethral Incision/Resection of the Bladder Neck

Primary bladder neck obstruction (PBNO) accounts for 9–16% of women with BOO. The characteristic features of BOO include low flow rates with high voiding pressures on urodynamic studies, non-funneling of the bladder neck on fluoroscopy, and absence of significant electromyographic (EMG) activity [39, 40]. Alpha-blocker therapy should be initiated, failing which CIC or definitive treatment in the form of transurethral resection or incision of the bladder neck can be offered [41].

The concept of bladder neck incision was first described in 1973 by Turner-Warwick et al. [42]. Current consensus is that bladder neck incisions be placed at 5'o clock and 7'o clock positions with a Collings knife electrode [43]. The incisions extend from just inside the vesical neck through the proximal third of the urethra. A single incision at 6'O clock would sometimes suffice [43]. However, the ideal incision site remains debatable. Earlier an anterior or 12-o'clock position was also preferred in order to prevent vaginal wall perforation. Delaere et al. [44] performed anterior incisions in 32 women who had either detrusor failure (20 patients) or mechanical iatrogenic bladder neck obstruction (12 patients). Overall 18 (56%) women benefitted, 6 required a repeat incision, and 2 developed severe stress incontinence [44]. **With the standard procedure of 5- and 7-o'clock incisions overall reported satisfactory rate ranges from 76% to 100%** [41, 43, 45].

Use of potassium-titanyl-phosphate (KTP, green) laser for bladder neck incision has been recently reported. KTP laser bladder neck incision was performed by Fu et al. [46], who reported an improvement in IPSS (21.4 ± 4.7 vs. 11.7 ± 3.2, $p < 0.01$) and quality of life (4.5 ± 1.8 vs. 3.2 ± 0.9, $p < 0.05$) after surgery with 32/40 patients spontaneously voiding at a mean follow-up of 9.7 ± 2.7 months. Significant improvement in the maximal flow rate (13.4 ± 4.6 mL/s, $p < 0.01$) and voiding pressure (58.8 ± 24.6 cmH_2O, $p < 0.05$) was also noted.

Some authors have proposed more than two standard incisions. Jonas et al. [47] reported that 14% of women with 5-, 7- and 12-o'clock incisions on the bladder neck were reoperated [47]. Jin et al. have suggested bladder neck incision at 4 different sites, i.e., 3-, 6-, 9- and 12-o'clock positions [48]. The reoperation rate reportedly ranges from 18% with a single incision to 0% with four incisions [45, 47, 48]. Though multiple incisions are known to confer better results than the standard 5 and 7 o'clock incision with minimal complications, they are usually reserved for a second procedure when the standard technique fails. No study has directly compared the results of these incisions with respect to success rate or complications.

Though most urologists just incise the neck, **some prefer to resect the intervening tissue in between using a resectoscope** [49]. Blaivas et al. performed resection instead of incision in seven patients diagnosed with PBNO aged between 39 and 81 years. At a median follow-up of 3 years, 6 showed complete relief and 1 showed improvement [49]. In 2016, Shen et al. [50] described a novel technique of controlled transurethral resection and incision of the bladder neck in women. They measured the actual urethral length by inserting a single lumen urethral catheter after instilling 300 mL of physiological saline. The position of the resection was then marked, and a controlled resection of the bladder neck tissue was performed between 5 o'clock and 7 o'clock position from the bladder neck opening to the marked site. A catheter was placed for 4 days postoperatively. This technique is thought to shorten the urethra and release obstruction while maintaining continence. Fifty-nine patients reported significant improvement in flow rates from 7.2 ± 3.9 to 26.1 ± 5.2 mL/s [50].

Complications include urinary incontinence due to striated sphincter injury (6.2%) and vesicovaginal fistula due to perforation of the vaginal wall [44, 45, 49]. Limiting the incision to the proximal third of the urethra and use of a pediatric resectoscope could potentially avoid these complications [50].

12.2.7 Botulinum Toxin Injection

Botulinum neurotoxin (BoNT) is a neurotoxin secreted by *Clostridium botulinum* [51], which is a gram-positive, anaerobic, spore-forming, rod-shaped bacterium. BoNT causes paralysis of the affected neuromuscular junctions by disrupting neurotransmission of various neurotransmitters and neuropeptides [52]. Seven immunologically distinct serotypes of BoNTs from type A to type G [53] have been identified. BoNT-A and Type B are the most commonly used subtypes for medical purposes. BoNT-B appears to cause an incomplete and short-lasting effect of muscle paralysis compared to BoNT-A [54].The commercial forms containing BoNT-A used in clinical practice are onabotulinumtoxin A (Botox; Allergan, Dublin, Ireland), abobotulinumtoxin A (Dysport; Ipsen-Biotech, Paris, France), and incobotulinum toxin A (Xeomin; Merz Pharmaceuticals, Frankfurt, Germany). BoNT-A formulations also differ from each other due to underlying structural and formulation differences. One unit of Botox is reportedly equivalent to 2.5 or 3 U of Dysport [55].

After initial FDA approval of botulinum toxin for the treatment of blepharospasm and strabismus in 1989, it has been used extensively for various indications. Botulinum has demonstrated considerable effectiveness in urology to treat refractory overactive bladder, detrusor sphincter dyssynergia, recurrent urethral strictures, and more recently in Fowlers syndrome [56]. Chancellor's group [57] used botulinum toxin in 68 patients with BOO. Most had DSD and/or were physically unable to perform intermittent catheterization. A marked improvement in daytime and nocturnal voiding symptoms was noted. Dykstra et al. [58] explained that reversible chemical sphincterotomy could be performed with BoNT injections to reduce DSD in spinal cord injury patients for the first time. 8/11 showed improvement in urethral pressure profile and PVR. Urethral pressures decreased by an average of 27 cm H_2O, and PVR decreased by an average of 146 mL. No immediate or delayed side effects were observed, while the effect lasted for about 50 days. Jiang et al. [59] have studied treatment outcomes of patients with non-neurogenic ($n = 53$) and neurogenic ($n = 42$) urethral sphincter hyperactivity after the injection of botulinum toxin A to the external sphincter. They found a significant improvement in PVR and Q_{max} with a satisfactory outcome in 58% of non-neurogenic and 64% of neurogenic patients. Therapeutic duration was significantly longer in non-neurogenics vs. neurogenics (9.55 vs. 7.44 months) and development of de novo incontinence was higher in neurogenics.

A dose of 100–200 U of BoNT-A in 4 mL saline is used. A rigid cystoscope and a standard cystoscopic collagen injection needle are used to inject BoNT-A deep into the external sphincter at 3-, 6-, 9-, and 12-o'clock positions in approximate equal proportion. A fine-gauge spinal needle can also be used to inject BoNT-A periurethrally. Either way a deeper injection (compared to a standard collagen injection) is important to target the nerve terminals innervating the skeletal muscle [57, 58]. The procedure is well tolerated under local anesthesia and generally performed as an office-based procedure. A transperineal fine-gauge spinal needle can also be used instead of a trans-cystoscopic needle to inject BoNT-A periurethrally. The high cost of the toxin and its reversibility, requiring re-injections every 4–6 months, coupled with complications of the procedure such as stress incontinence and retention of urine, demand its judicious use.

12.2.8 Sacral Neuromodulation

Tanagho and Schmidt, in 1982, performed the first sacral neuromodulation (SNM) at the University of California in San Francisco [60]. However the US FDA approval came only in 1997 for the InterStim device (Medtronic, Minneapolis, MN, USA) to treat urge urinary incontinence (UUI) and later extended to urinary urgency frequency syndrome and non-obstructive urinary retention. Over the years, the InterStim device has seen considerable improvements in its technical design, leading to better lead placement and patient comfort [61].

SNM acts by electrical stimulation of the S3 nerve root that may activate or inhibit the neural reflexes associated with lower urinary tract function. The more detailed and exact mechanism of action of SNM is still not well understood. Several theories for mechanisms of action have been postulated. It may moderate both the overactivity and underactivity of reflex arc either by direct action on the disturbed reflex arc, or by stimulation of the afferent pathway to the brain area that controls bladder and sphincter function [62, 63].

SNM is still an emerging mode of therapy in functional female BOO. It may be an effective therapeutic alternative to CIC or indwelling catheterization. **Currently its use in female BOO is limited only to intractable Fowler's syndrome and pseudodyssynergia in women.** Following SNM, 72% of women are found to void spontaneously, with a mean PVR of <100 mL. Around half of them no longer require CIC [64]. **In women with the Fowler's syndrome, a form of DV, a higher success rate of 78% has been noted in women who continue to void spontaneously even at 10 years' follow-up** [64]. Nevertheless, neuromodulation is not bereft of complications. Failure occurs in 25% of patients and 30–50% require revision [65].

12.2.9 Indwelling Catheterization

Some women with BOO presenting with retention, incontinence, and recurrent UTI prefer an indwelling catheter instead of repeated dilatations. This is particularly true following failed definitive management. Although indwelling catheterization is often used as an immediate short-term measure, intermittent catheterization is preferable for longer-term care. This is particularly true for those who are able to learn and physically perform catheterization themselves or at least have a caregiver to do so. Long-term indwelling catheter, be it intraurethral or suprapubic, has an increased risk of morbidity [66–68].

12.3 Conclusion

The long-term efficacy of UD for anatomical urethral narrowing is poor, and it may not be justified as an effective treatment. Urethroplasty can be offered early on as an option in this setting. For functional disorders intermittent self-catheterization remains an option as the cause seems to be multifactorial. Most women would find long-term indwelling catheterization to be an unacceptable treatment method. Such patients can be evaluated and treatment tailored individually with minimally invasive options wherever feasible.

12.4 Case-Based Discussion

A 39-year-old female factory worker, with no associated co-morbidities, presented with voiding LUTS of 18 months duration. She voided four times by day with poor stream and ineffective emptying. Nocturia without urgency led to disturbed sleep. She had consulted a local urologist and was evaluated with ultrasonography which showed a post void residue of 166 cc with minimal bladder wall thickening. Her peak flow on uroflowmetry was 11 mL/s. She underwent multiple UDs with diagnosis of functional BOO and usually had transient relief in symptoms for up to 6 weeks upon dilatation. Periodic UDs were suggested to her. However, she demonstrated an unwillingness to undergo frequent dilatations and desired a definitive treatment.

On examination, she had an abdominal infraumbilical scar due to lower segment caesarean section 10 years back. Her local examination and per vaginal examination were normal. A voiding cystourethrogram gram demonstrated bladder

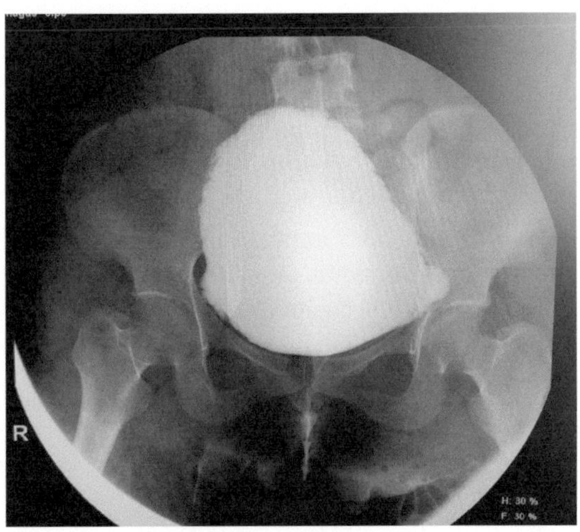

Fig. 12.1 VCUG showing non-funneling of bladder neck, irregular bladder wall with bladder diverticulae

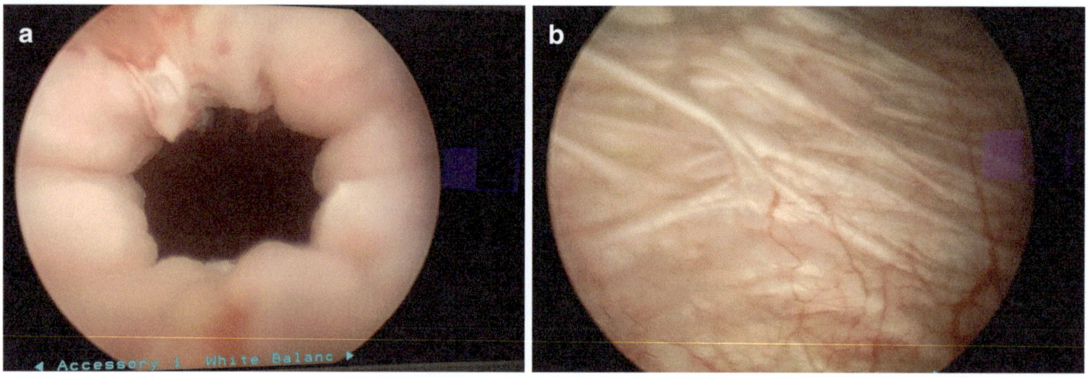

Fig. 12.2 Cystoscopy with 17 Fr rigid cystoscope demonstrating narrow bladder neck (**a**) with trabeculated bladder wall (**b**)

diverticulae, increased residual, and non-funneling of bladder neck (Fig. 12.1). Both filling and storage phases were normal on multi-channel urodynamics with electromyography, with synchronized sphincter activity during voiding. A diagnostic cystoscopy was done using a 17 Fr scope and revealed normal urethra, narrow bladder neck, and trabeculations in the urinary bladder (Fig. 12.2).

The diagnosis of PBNO was established based on corroborating the symptoms, with the findings on uroflowmetry, VCUG, and multichannel urodynamics. Alpha-blocker therapy(tamsulosin 0.4 mg) for 4 weeks did not improve symptoms or peak flow rates. Transurethral incision of the bladder neck (TUIBN) using Colling's knife with monopolar electrocautery in glycine was planned after thorough consideration. Incisions were made at 5 o'clock and 7 o'clock positions, and a catheter was left in situ postoperatively for 48 h. Follow-up, both immediate and long term, showed significant improvement in the flow rates, postvoid residue, and AUA scores. Patient complains of an occasional dribble on straining and coughing. At 3 years following TUIBN, patient remained symptom free with no nocturia and normal postvoid residual urine.

Key Learning Points

- Urethral dilatation is likely best reserved as an initial treatment for female urethral stricture. It may be preferred in patients unwilling or unsuitable for more complex urethral reconstruction. Its utility as a management option for functional BOO is unclear.
- Internal urethrotomy or core through procedure, although reported in select cases, may not have sustainable long-term results.
- Results with the use of botulinum toxin injection for functional BOO are poorer than neurogenic causes.
- SNM offers an effective alternative for Fowler's syndrome and pseudodyssynergia in women.

References

1. Carr LK, Webster GD. Bladder outlet obstruction in women. Urol Clin North Am. 1996;23:385–91.
2. Lowenstein L, Anderson C, Kenton K, Dooley Y, Brubaker L. Obstructive voiding symptoms are not predictive of elevated post void residual urine volumes. Int Urogynaecol J. 2008;19:801–4.
3. Al-Sharani M, Lovatis D. Do subjective symptoms of obstructive voiding correlate with the post void residual urine in women? Int Urogynaecol J. 2005;16:12–4.
4. Athanasopoulos A, Gyftopoulos K, Giannitsas K, Permenis P. Effect of alfuzosin on female primary bladder neck obstruction. Int Urogynecol J Pelvic Floor Dysfunct. 2009;20:217–22.
5. Kessler T, Studer U, Burkhard F. The effect of terazosin on functional bladder outlet obstruction in women: a pilot study. J Urol. 2006;176:1487–92.
6. Pischedda A, Pirozzi Farina F, Madenia M, et al. Use of alpha 1-blockers in female functional bladder outlet obstruction. Urol Int. 2005;74:256–61.
7. Costantini E, Lazzeri M, Bini V, Zucchi A, Fioretti F, Frumenzio E. Open-label, longitudinal study of tam-

sulosin for functional bladder outlet obstruction in women. Uro Int. 2009;83:311–5.
8. Lemack G, Foster B, Zimmern P. Urethral dilatation in women: a questionnaire based analysis of practice patterns. Urology. 1999;54:37–43.
9. Lyon RP, Smith DR. Distal urethral stenosis. J Urol. 1963;89:414–21.
10. Masarani M, Willis RG. Urethral dilatation in women: urologists' practice patterns in the UK. Ann R Coll Surg Engl. 2006;88:496–8.
11. Romman AN, Alhalabi F, Zimmern PE. Distal intramural urethral pathology in women. J Urol. 2012;188:1218–23.
12. Smith AL, Ferlise VJ, Rovner ES. Female urethral strictures: successful management with long-term clean intermittent catheterization after urethral dilatation. BJU Int. 2006;98:96–9.
13. Santucci R, Chen M. Evaluation and treatment of female urethral stricture disease. Curr Bladder Dysfunct Rep. 2013;8:123–7.
14. Migliari R, Leone P, Berdondini E, De Angelis M, Barbagli G, Palminteri E. Dorsal buccal mucosa graft urethroplasty for female urethral strictures. J Urol. 2006;176:1473–6.
15. Schwender CE, Ng L, McGuire E, Gormley EA. Technique and results of urethroplasty for female stricture disease. J Urol. 2006;175:976–80.
16. Blaivas JG, Santos JA, Tsui JF, Deibert CM, Rutman MP, Purohit RS, et al. Management of urethral stricture in women. J Urol. 2012;188:1778–82.
17. Osman NI, Mangera A, Chapple CR. A systematic review of surgical techniques used in the treatment of female urethral stricture. Eur Urol. 2013;64:965–73.
18. Santucci R, Payne C, Saigal C, et al. Office dilation of the female urethra: a quality of care problem in the field of urology. J Urol. 2008;180:2068–75.
19. Heidari F. Results and complications in women with urethral stricture. Nephrol Urol Mon. 2014;6(2):e15212.
20. Ngugi PM, Kassim A. Clean intermitent catheterisation in the management of urethral strictures. East Afr Med J. 2007;84(11):522–4.
21. Basu M, Jonathan R, A. Duckett. Effect of urethral dilatation on women with voiding dysfunction. Curr Bladder Dysfunct Rep. 2010;5:23–6.
22. Shafik A, El-Sibai O, Ahmed I. Effect of urethral dilation on vesical motor activity: identification of the urethrovesical reflex and its role in voiding. J Urol. 2003;69:1017–9.
23. Yee CH, Ho LY, Hung HH, Chan WH. The effect of urethral calibration on female primary bladder outlet obstruction. Int Urogynecol J. 2012;23(2):217–21.
24. Sinha S. Dysfunctional voiding: a review of the terminology, presentation, evaluation and management in children and adults. Indian J Urol. 2011;27(4):437–47.
25. Stoffel JT. Detrusor sphincter dyssynergia: a review of physiology, diagnosis, and treatment strategies. Transl Androl Urol. 2016;5(1):127–35.
26. Patel R, Nitti VW. Bladder outlet obstruction in women: prevalence, recognition, and management. Curr Urol Rep. 2001;2(5):379–87.
27. Seddon JM, Bruce AW. Cystourethritis. Urology. 1978;11:1–10.
28. Smith PJ. The management of the urethral syndrome. Br J Hosp Med. 1979;22:578–87.
29. Farrar DJ. An evaluation of otis urethrotomy in female patients with recurrent urinary tract infections. A review after 6 years. Br J Urol. 1980;52:68–74.
30. Rosenblum N, Nitti VW. Female urethral reconstruction. Urol Clin N Am. 2011;38(1):55–64.
31. Hartanto VH, Nitti VW. Recent advances in management of female lower urinary tract trauma. Curr Opin Urol. 2003;13:279–84.
32. Grivas N, Tsimaris I, Makatsori A, et al. The effectiveness of otis urethrotomy combined with six weeks urethral dilation until 40 Fr in the treatment of bladder outlet obstruction in women: a prospective study. Urol J. 2014;10:1063–6.
33. Hemal AK, Dorairajan LN, Gupta NP. Posttraumatic complete and partial loss of urethra with pelvic fracture in girls: an appraisal of management. J Urol. 2000;163:282–7.
34. Dogra PN, Nabi G. Endourologic reconstruction of post-traumatic obliterated urethral stricture in a young female: a point of technique. Urology. 2001;58:1053–5.
35. Reynard JM, Vass J, Sullivan ME, Mamas M. Sphincterotomy and the treatment of detrusor-sphincter dyssynergia: current status, future prospects. Spinal Cord. 2003;41(1):1–11.
36. Moreno-Palacios J, Maldonado-Alcaraz E, Montoya-Martínez G, Serrano-Brambila E. Outcomes and complications of sphincterotomy with bladder neck incision in neurologically healthy male patients with voiding dysfunction. Arch Esp Urol. 2012;65(2):244–50.
37. Mundy AR. Urodynamic and reconstructive surgery of the lower urinary tract, vol. 36. Edinburgh: Churchill Livingstone; 1996.
38. Hoag N, Chee J. Surgical management of female urethral strictures. Transl Androl Urol. 2017;6(Suppl 2):S76–80.
39. Kuo HC. Videourodynamic characteristics and lower urinary tract symptoms of female bladder outlet obstruction. Urology. 2005;66:1005–9.
40. Nitti VW, Tu LM, Gitlin J. Diagnosing bladder outlet obstruction in women. J Urol. 1999;161:1535–40.
41. Kumar A, Mandhani A, Gogoi S, Srivastava A. Management of functional bladder neck obstruction in women: use of alpha-blockers and pediatric resectoscope for bladder neck incision. J Urol. 1999;162:2061–5.
42. Turner-Warwick R, Whiteside CG, Worth PHL, et al. A urodynamic view of the clinical problems associated with bladder neck dysfunction and its treatment by endoscopic incision and transtrigonal posterior prostatectomy. Br J Urol. 1973;45:44–59.
43. Axelrod SL, Blaivas JG. Bladder neck obstruction in women. J Urol. 1987;137:497–9.
44. Delaere KP, Debruyne FM, Moonen WA. Bladder neck incision in the female: a hazardous procedure? Br J Urol. 1983;55:283–6.

45. Peng CH, Kuo HC. Transurethral incision of bladder neck in treatment of bladder neck obstruction in women. Urology. 2005;65:275–8.
46. Fu Q, Xu YM. Transurethral incision of the bladder neck using KTP in the treatment of bladder neck obstruction in women. Urol Int. 2009;82(1):61–4.
47. Jonas U, Petri E, Hohenfellner R. Indication and value of bladder neck incision. Urol Int. 1979;34:260–5.
48. Jin X, Qu H, Liu H, Li B, Wang J, Zhang Y. Modified trans-urethral incision for primary bladder neck obstruction in women: a method to improve voiding function without urinary incontinence. Urology. 2012;79(2):310–3.
49. Blaivas JG, Flisser AJ, Tash JA. Treatment of primary bladder neck obstruction in women with transurethral resection of the bladder neck. J Urol. 2004;171:1172–5.
50. Shen W. Controlled transurethral resection and incision of the bladder neck to treat female primary bladder neck obstruction: description of a novel surgical procedure. Int J Urol. 2016;23(6):491–5.
51. Leippold T, Reitz A, Schurch B. Botulinum toxin as a new therapy option for voiding disorders: current state of the art. Eur Urol. 2003;44:165–74.
52. Dong M, Yeh F, Tepp WH, Dean C, Johnson EA, Janz R, Chapman ER. SV2 is the protein receptor for botulinum neurotoxin A. Science. 2006;312:592–6.
53. Nigam PK, Nigam A. Botulinum toxin. Indian J Dermatol. 2010;55:8–14.
54. Aoki KR. Pharmacology and immunology of botulinum toxin serotypes. J Neurol. 2001;248(Suppl S1):3–10.
55. Mangera A, Andersson KE, Apostolidis A, Chapple C, Dasgupta P, Giannantoni A, Gravas S, Madersbacher S. Contemporary management of lower urinary tract disease with botulinum toxin A: a systematic review of botox (onabotulinumtoxinA) and dysport (abobotulinumtoxinA). Eur Urol. 2011;60:784–95.
56. Chapple C, Patel A. Botulinum toxin–new mechanisms, new therapeutic directions? Eur Urol. 2006;49:606–8.
57. Smith CP, Nishiguchi J, O'Leary M, Yoshimura N, Chancellor MB. Single-institution experience in 110 patients with botulinum toxin A injection into bladder or urethra. Urology. 2005;65:37–41.
58. Dykstra DD, Sidi AA, Scott AB, et al. Effects of botulinum A toxin on detrusor-sphincter dyssynergia in spinal cord injury patients. J Urol. 1988;139:919–22.
59. Jiang YH, Chen SF, Jhang JF, Kuo HC. Therapeutic effect of urethral sphincter onabotulinumtoxinA injection for urethral sphincter hyperactivity. Neurourol Urodyn. 2018;37(8):2651–7.
60. Juenemann KP, Lue TF, Schmidt RA, Tanagho EA. Clinical significance of sacral and pudendal nerve anatomy. J Urol. 1988;139(1):74–80.
61. Spinelli M, Giardiello G, Gerber M, Arduini A, Van Den Hombergh U, Malaguti S. New sacral neuromodulation lead for percutaneous implantation using local anesthesia: description and first experience. J Urol. 2003;170(5):1905–7.
62. Leng WW, Chancellor MB. How sacral nerve stimulation neuromodulation works. Urol Clin N Am. 2005;32(1):11–8.
63. Fowler CJ, Swinn MJ, Goodwin RJ, Oliver S, Craggs M. Studies of the latency of pelvic floor contraction during peripheral nerve evaluation show that the muscle response is reflexly mediated. J Urol. 2000;163(3):881–3.
64. Datta SN, Chaliha C, Singh A, Gonzales G, Mishra VC, Kavia RB. Sacral neurostimulation for urinary retention: 10-year experience from one UK centre. BJU Int. 2008;101:192–6.
65. Dasgupta, et al. Long-term results of sacral neuromodulation for women with urinary retention. BJU Int. 2004;94(3):335–7.
66. Turi MH, Hanif S, Fasih Q, Shaikh MA. Proportion of complications in patients practicing clean intermittent self-catheterization (CISC) vs indwelling catheter. J Pak Med Assoc. 2006;56:401.
67. Tang MW, Kwok TC, Hui E, Woo J. Intermittent versus indwelling urinary catheterization in older female patients. Maturitas. 2006;53:274.
68. Hunter KF, Bharmal A, Moore KN. Long-term bladder drainage: suprapubic catheter versus other methods: a scoping review. Neurourol Urodyn. 2013;32:944.

Applied Anatomy for Female Urethral Reconstruction

13

Nikhil Khattar and Rishi Nayyar

Learning Objectives

- To understand the female anatomy as conceptually unified to the male anatomy.
- Where exactly is the female external sphincter? What keeps continence preserved in dorsal (anterior) onlay approaches and what keeps it intact in ventral (posterior)-based onlay approaches. Can the urethrotomy be extended into the bladder neck without jeopardizing the continence?
- To understand the vascularity of female urethra. After complete obliteration or transection, what keeps the two ends of the urethra vascularized.
- What bed provides vascular support to the graft on dorsal and ventral side in onlay procedures?
- Which anatomical structures are responsible for female sexual function and how are they potentially affected during female urethral reconstructive procedures?

N. Khattar (✉)
Female Urology, Reconstructive Urology and Neurovesical Dysfunction, Medanta, The Medicity, Gurugram, India

R. Nayyar
Department of Urology, All India Institute of Medical Sciences, New Delhi, India

13.1 Concepts Suggesting Unification of Male and Female Genitourinary Anatomy

Female urethral reconstructions demand a clear understanding of female external genital and urethral anatomy. The anatomy textbooks have always maintained a clear compartmentalization between sections of male and female genital anatomy as if they were two separate boxes of information. However, it is known that embryologically till the 8th week of gestation [1], the anatomy is similar in both sexes before the male external genitalia evolve (Fig. 13.1). All female genital structures, therefore, have a corresponding homologue from the male and have defined urinary and sexual functions. The main difference in anatomy is the undeveloped anterior urethra and scrotum because of non-fusion of inner genital and labioscrotal folds (Fig. 13.1). **The structures that form the external urethra in males are all present in females in the form of vestibule of the vagina, the corpus spongiosum of the clitoris and vestibular bulbs, the inner surfaces of labia minora and the clitoral body.** If they get adequate androgenic stimulation as in women with congenital adrenal hyperplasia (CAH), they get virilized to various degrees (Fig. 13.2) [2] and some completely virilized XX females have even been reared as males with

N. Khattar et al. (eds.), *Female Bladder Outlet Obstruction and Urethral Reconstruction*,
https://doi.org/10.1007/978-981-15-8521-0_13

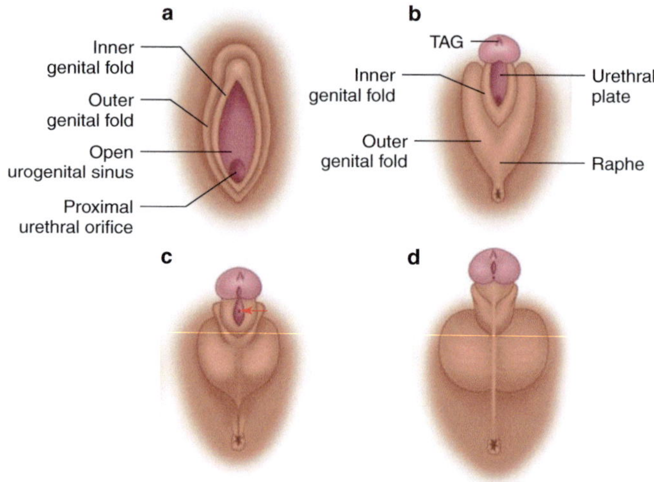

Fig. 13.1 Development of male genitalia: Appearance of external genitalia in both the sexes is similar till early gestation (8th week) as in (**a**). In males, under the effect of androgens over the next few weeks (**b**–**d**), the inner genital fold tubularizes from posterior to anterior to form the urethra and the outer genital fold fuses over it to form the scrotal sac. The genital tubercle elongates to form the phallus

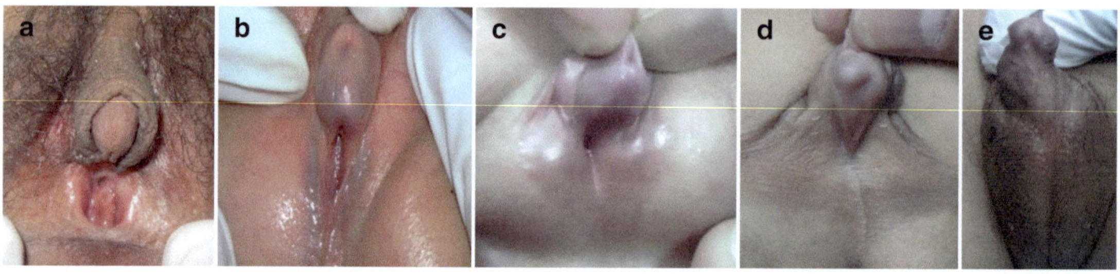

Fig. 13.2 Spectrum of virilization in females with Congenital Adrenal Hyperplasia (CAH): from only clitoromegaly in (**a**) to progressive fusion of labia minora (inner genital fold) in (**b**, **c**), fusion of labia majora (outer genital fold) to form scrotum like sac and finally completely developed phallus in extreme virilization (**e**). [*Reproduced with permission from AbouZeid AA, Mohammad SA. Transformation of the female genitalia in congenital adrenal hyperplasia: MRI study. J Pediatr Surg. 2020;55(5):977–984*] [2]

ability to perform satisfactory sexual intercourse [3].

On the contrary, in severe perineal hypospadias where the male genitals appear feminized, there is also a higher frequency of the persistent prostatic utricle [4]—the "male vagina" is a homologue of female vagina derived from urogenital sinus (and not Mullerian duct remnant as previously thought) [5, 6]. Interestingly, metaidoioplasty techniques for creating a neophallus during female to male gender reassignment surgeries treat the female external genitalia as a form of severe degree of hypospadias and require release of chordee after androgen stimulation before using vestibular mucosa for tubularization [7].

The embryology provides a different perspective to the female urethral and genital anatomy. The *genital tubercle*, which forms the glans, corpora cavernosa, dorsal penile skin, and dorsal prepuce in males, in turn forms the glans clitoris, corpora cavernosa of the glans, and prepuce of the clitoris in females. The *inner genital fold (urethral fold)* forms vestibular skin, corpus spongiosum, and labia minora in females, whereas in males it forms the penile urethra and corpus spongiousum. The *labioscotal swellings* form the labia majora in females, whereas in males they form the ventral aspect of the penile skin and scrotum (Fig. 13.3). **Actual female urethra corresponds only to the prostatic urethra in male from bladder neck till the veru montanum (colliculus seminalis). The opening of the seminal colliculus in males itself corresponds to the hymen in the female** [1].

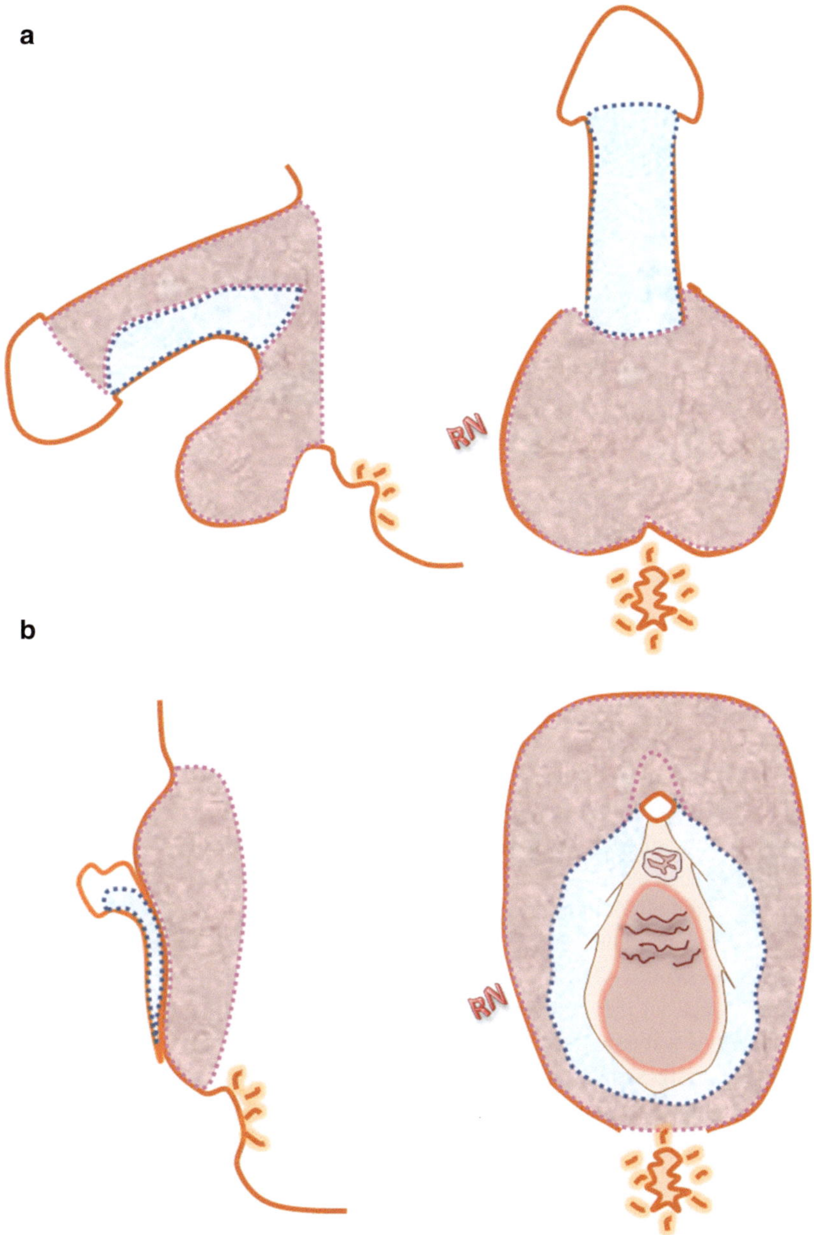

Fig. 13.3 Corresponding portions of male (**a**) and female (**b**) external genitalia derived from inner genital fold (shaded blue) and labioscrotal swellings (shaded brown). [*Adapted with permission from Puppo V. Embryology and anatomy of the vulva: the female orgasm and women's sexual health. Eur J Obstet Gynecol Reprod Biol. 2011 Jan;154(1):3–8*]

In effect, the adult female urethra is reminiscent of the primitive urethra which is separated as the cranial part of the primitive urogenital sinus once the fused paramesonephric ducts join it at the Mullerian tubercle. The caudal portion is the urogenital sinus (Fig. 13.4). The entire primitive urethra is surrounded by a mesenchymal tissue which later forms the striated sphincter. **Unlike in males, where the development of prostate later rearranges and displaces the sphincter to the membranous area, the adult female urethra remains surrounded by the striated rhabdosphincter throughout its length (thickest in mid-urethra)** as we shall see in detail in further subsection [8, 9].

The Skene's glands in the female urethra have been identified as homologous to the male prostate. Periurethral glands with cells staining for prostatic

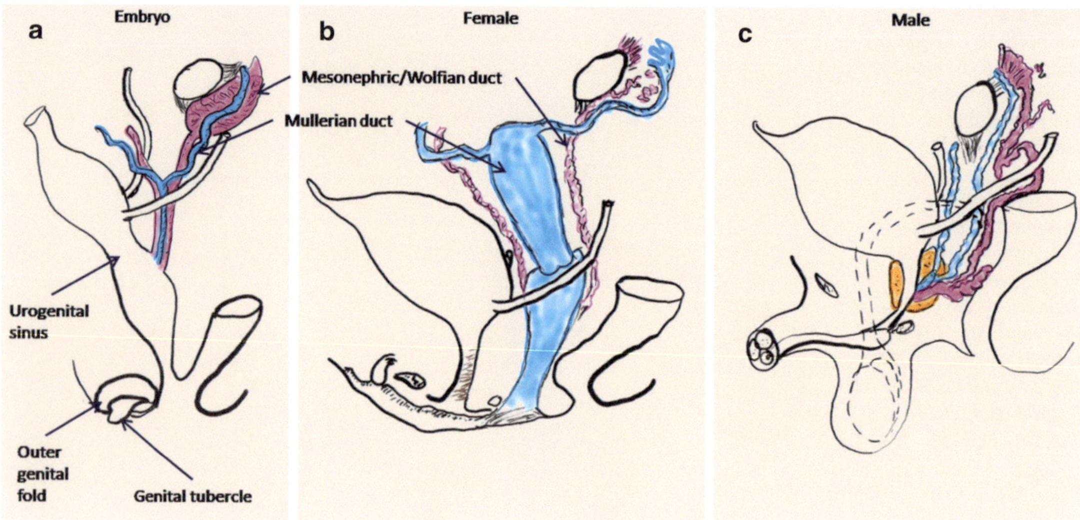

Fig. 13.4 Development of urethra from primitive urogenital sinus. The point of joining of fused Mullerian ducts (Mullerian tubercle) divides the primitive urogenital sinus to primitive urethra cranially and urogenital sinus caudally (**a**). Female urethra is reminiscent of the primitive urethra (**b**), while in males (**c**) the corresponding portion is till the verumontanum and rest of the urethra is derived from tubularization of urogenital sinus

acid phosphatase (PAP) or prostate specific antigen (PSA) can be identified in 66–80% of females at autopsy from all age range (fetal to octogenarian). They, however, do not mature with age and retain their rudimentary appearance throughout life unlike in males where they organize to form a prostate under the effect of androgens [10]. Very rarely a developed prostate can be identified in 46 XX individuals with CAH [11]. These glands serve no known function; they, however, may be important as source of some urethral and periurethral pathologies like urethral diverticulum, urethritis, and possibly female urethral stricture.

The presence of corpus spongiosum in female has been a debated topic. Some researchers have been affirmative about a layer of cavernous tissue rich in veins at the submucosal level of urethra with claims that it has a role in continence [12] and even engorges during sexual arousal [1], whereas others refute the claim. **Histological studies on fresh human female cadavers confirm the spongiosum to be arising from vestibular bulbs (which is a homologue of the urethral bulb in male) on each side of the urethra and then extending anteriorly underneath the vestibular mucosa to the undersurface of glans** (Figs. 13.5 and 13.17). The same tissue hypertrophies in androgenized females as pars intermedia [13]. **Corpus spongiousum, thus, does not form a layer around the urethra unlike in men.**

13.2 Layers of Female Urethra: Histological and MR Perspectives

Urethral, peri-urethral, and paraurethral anatomical descriptions have continuously evolved over time. Figure 13.6 shows the urethra with its layers with rhabdosphincter and immediate relations to the vagina, the erectile structures of clitoris along with the dual nerve supply. DeLancey had described in his cadaveric studies the four portions of urethra as intramural urethra (0–20%, part that traverses the bladder wall), mid-proximal urethra (20–60%, part related to rhabdosphincter, pubourethral ligaments, and vagino-levator muscle), mid-distal urethra (60–80%, part related to urogenital diaphragm and compressor urethrae), and distal urethra (80–100%, part related to vestibular bulbs and bulbocavernosus muscles) [14]. The availability of ultrasonography and magnetic resonance imaging (MRI) with their refinements has paved the way for further understanding of female urethra, correlating the anatomical to physiological and clinical aspects [15].

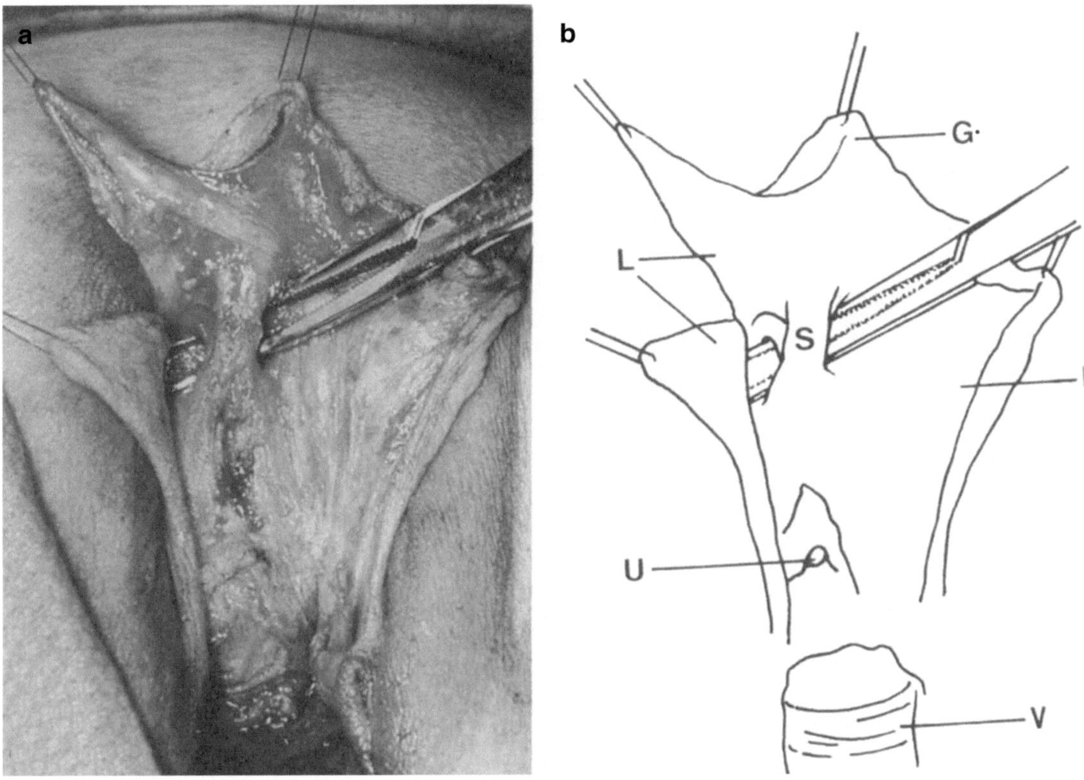

Fig. 13.5 Dissection under the vestibular mucosa during metaidoioplasty reveals tethering cords which represent corpus spongiosal tissue. *S* spongiosa, *U* urethral orifice, *V* vaginal wall, *L*+ labium minus and *G* glans clitoris. [Reproduced with permission from *van Turnhout AA, Hage JJ, van Diest PJ. The female corpus spongiosum revisited. Acta ObstetGynecol Scand. 1995 Nov;74(10):767–71*] [13]

Microdissection and microanatomic studies of human female urethra on cadavers have shown that the female urethra has two layers comprising of inner longitudinal and outer circular smooth muscle fibers at the proximal levels of the urethra. These layers are direct continuation of detrusor muscles. Smooth muscle bundles were seen throughout all levels of urethra and did not change from one level to another. Below the mid-urethra level, smooth muscle fibers end by gaining insertion into dense collagenous tissue and distal fourth of urethra is mainly composed of elastic and collagenous tissues [16]. Other researchers opine that the smooth muscles in continuation with the detrusor are condensed posteriorly and extend to a variable extent in the adult female urethra [17]. On imaging with a 1.5 T MRI, urethral layers can be delineated with precision on T2 weighted images. Such images from human female cadavers have been correlated with histology and also with nulliparous continent women. The urethral mucosa is seen as a T2 "bright" layer and in contrast the submucosa as T2 "dark." The longitudinal and circular layers of smooth muscle are collectively seen as a T2 "bright" layer and is in continuation with the detrusor. Another T2 "dark" layer of varying thickness is seen outside this layer and collectively represents the connective tissue matrix and the striated muscle layer (rhabdosphincter) (Fig. 13.7). *All these layers together give the urethra a "target" like appearance. Toward the distal urethra the target-like appearance disappeared and the bright smooth muscle layer did not extend to the distal urethra. Also, the striated muscle layer fanned out laterally and merged with the compressor urethrae muscle.* The density of striated muscle decreases with age [18]. In a study by Macura et al. using intraurethral MRI on adult nulliparous women, the researchers were able to demonstrate the urethral

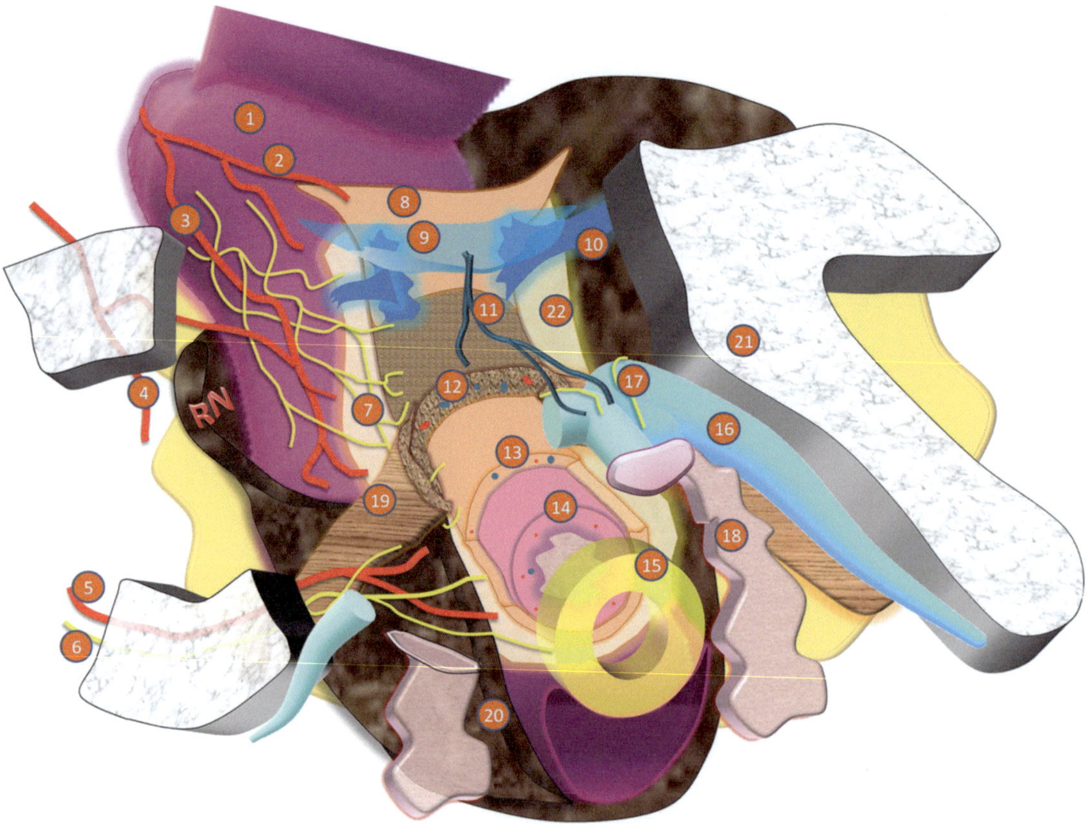

Fig. 13.6 View of female urethra seen after removing right pubic bone. *1*. Vagina. *2*. Inferior vesical artery. *3*. Vaginal artery. *4*. Obturator artery. *5*. Internal pudendal artery. It runs in the Alcock's canal along with pudendal nerve. *6*. Pudendal nerve. *7*. Nerves from the pelvic plexus entering into urethra at 4 or 8 o'clock position. *8*. Urethra. The detrusor fibers merge with the inner longitudinal and outer circular smooth muscle layer of urethra. *9*. Endopelvic fascia. *10*. Pubourethral ligaments. *11*. Deep vein of clitoris. *12*. Rhabdosphincter. It is thicker in its anterior aspect. *13*. Outer circular smooth muscle layer of urethra. *14*. Inner longitudinal smooth muscle layer of urethra. *15*. Outermost collagenous portion of urethra (Lyon's ring). *16*. Left crus of the Clitoris. *17*. Dorsal nerve of clitoris (Terminal branch of pudendal nerve). *18*. Vestibular bulb. *19*. Compressor urethrae. *20*. Pubovaginalis portion of Levator ani. *21*. Pubic bone. *22*. Pubovaginal fascia

anatomy in a detailed manner and confirm that the **striated muscle layer is thickest anteriorly** [19] (Fig. 13.7c, d). Fascia outside of these muscular elements are discussed in a further section.

The urethral mucosal lining is stratified squamous near the external meatus and transitional epithelium near the bladder neck. The line of this transition moves up with age and so in elderly, almost entire urethra may be lined with stratified squamous epithelium. The urethral submucosa is rich in elastic fibers and has smooth muscle cells in it. **This layer is extensively vascular and when fully engorged there is a noticeable increase in the volume of this layer along with a decrease in the urethral lumen. This vascularity may contribute up to 30% of closure forces of the urethra and is hormone-sensitive** and hence age-dependent decrease is noticed [20].

13.3 Female Sphincters and Continence Mechanisms

A thorough understanding and due regard for the continence mechanisms is expected before undertaking female urethral reconstructive or other endoscopic procedures to relieve bladder outlet obstruction (BOO) in women. Female urethroplasties have been described from all possible approaches (anterior/dorsal, posterior/ventral,

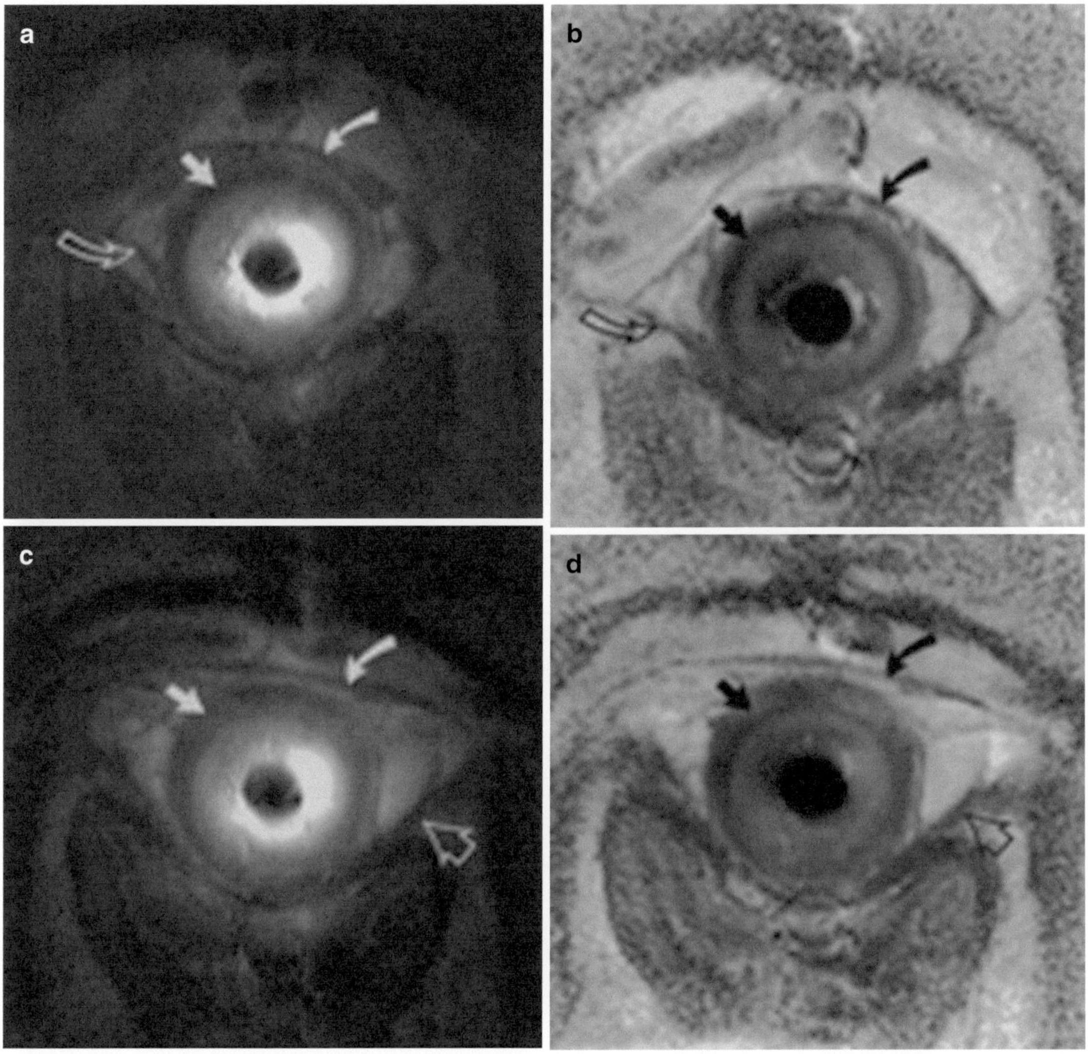

Fig. 13.7 Intraurethral MRI (T2 weighted images) of an adult nulliparous continent woman showing the target-like appearance of the urethra. The left-sided images (**a**, **c**, **e**) are T2W images, and the right-sided images (**b**, **d**, **f**) are intensity-corrected versions of the same image on left. On the intensity-corrected images, the mucosa can be identified as T2 bright layer around the coil, submucosa as hypointense layer followed by a hyperintense smooth muscle and again a hypointense striated muscle. (**a**, **b**) Cross-sections of proximal urethra. Here the circularly oriented striated muscle layer is equally distributed around the urethra. (**c**, **d**) Cross-sections of mid-urethra. The rhabdosphincter is anteriorly thickened (black arrow). (**e**, **f**) Images of the distal urethra. Urethra assumes an ovoid shape and the rhabdosphincter fans out and fibers start merging with the compressor urethrae. Urethral support ligaments can be identified anterior to the urethra (curved arrow). Fascial tissue posterior and lateral to the urethra (open arrow) forms the hammock for urethal support. [Reproduced with permission from *Macura KJ, Genadry R, Borman TL, Mostwin JL, Lardo AC, Bluemke DA. Evaluation of the female urethra with intraurethral magnetic resonance imaging. J MagnReson Imaging JMRI. 2004 Jul;20(1):153–9*] [19]

onlay, inlay, end to end) without jeopardizing the continence, although all the described procedures potentially disrupt the striated sphincter or its innervation. Similarly, radical cystectomy with orthotopic neobladder, bladder neck incisions, and bladder neck resections have been carried out without causing de novo incontinence in women if principles are adhered to. *Functionally these areas can be demonstrated as separate continence zones on video-urodynamics and urethral pressure profilometry respectively, but the anatomical aspects of these two continence zones*

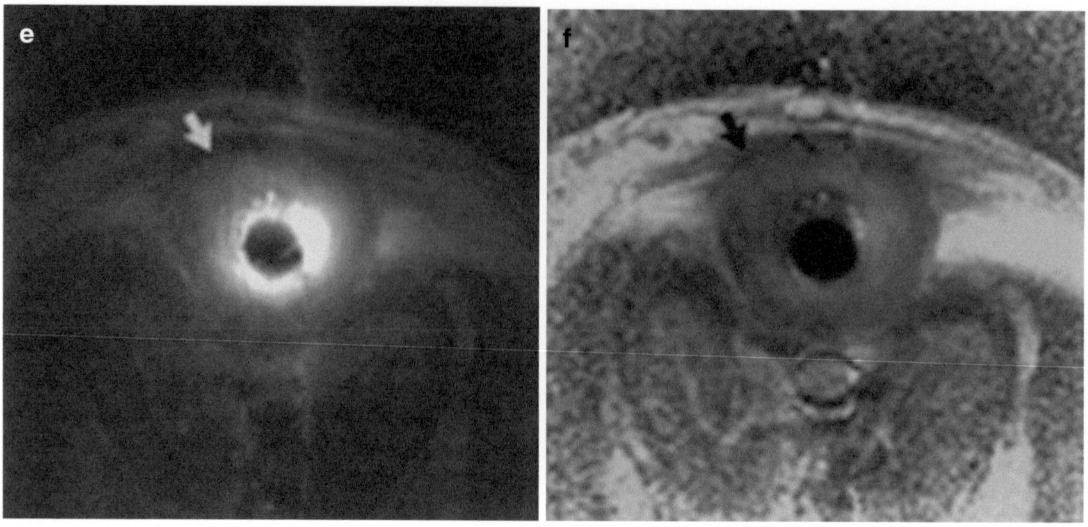

Fig. 13.7 (continued)

are poorly understood. The following section discusses the anatomical context of the female sphincters and continence mechanisms.

The continence in women is provided by *permanent closure forces* (which provide the resting tone), the *adjunctive closure forces* (which come into play at the time of any increase in pressure during various activities), and the *sealing effect* provided by the mucus because of rich submucosal vascular plexus as described above.

13.3.1 Bladder Neck

Anatomy of the bladder neck has been under debate. Some researchers believe that the multilayered detrusor fibers rearrange in a circular fashion toward the neck, but they do not encircle completely and hence there is no structural entity as sphincter at the bladder neck and the continence at this level is by passive forces [21]. Others, however, believe that the smooth muscle fibers of the bladder not only rearrange toward the neck to completely encircle it but also have dense mixture of cholinergic and noradrenergic innervation which is unlike most of the bladder which has only cholinergic nerve fibers [22]. Embryological studies, however, confirm that there is indeed a circular orientation of smooth muscles at the neck, but they are of trigonal origin extending up to the proximal urethra [23]. The autonomic innervation of the bladder is richest in the bladder neck and proximal urethra in both males and females as shown by 3D reconstruction models of nervous tissue using cadaver histology further confirming that the smooth muscle of internal sphincter is different from that of bladder and has active continence mechanism [24].

Like in males, in females too the bladder is anteriorly tilted over the proximal urethra making a vesicourethral angle which is being realized as one of the continence mechanisms and when lost can cause stress incontinence. Yucel and Baskin [25], using 3D reconstruction of immunohistology from males and female fetuses, observed that this angulation is held in place by the outer longitudinal coat of detrusor muscles in both the sexes. These fibers are prominent on anterior surfaces of bladder which descend up to the proximal urethra. In males they merge with the prostate while in females they surround the anterior and lateral surfaces of the neck and proximal urethra outside the external sphincteric muscles. They are said to have a prominent role in the dynamic changes at the bladder neck region during bladder filling and voiding. Tanagho and Smith, in their cadaveric studies, had observed that these longitudinal fibers descend and throw loops around the proximal urethra which were incomplete rings and open on one side (Fig. 13.8a). Many such loops from various

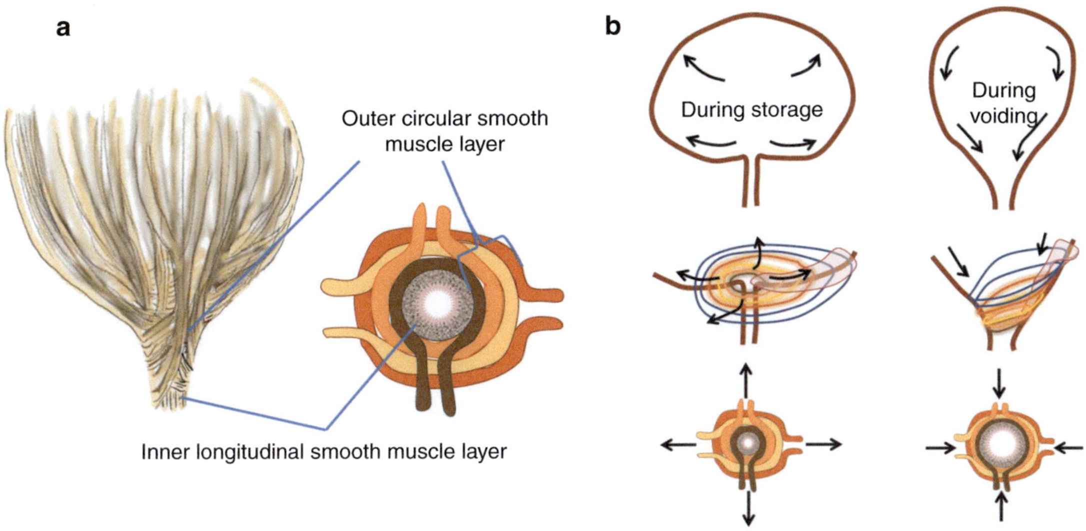

Fig. 13.8 Plausible explanation of a passive functional bladder neck in addition to an autonomic control. The outer longitudinal layer of detrusor throws interlacing loops around the bladder neck from all sides (**a**) predominantly anterior and lateral. During storage phase the distention of the bladder further pulls these loops squeezing the neck. During voiding, when the neck funnels, these loops slide over each other and loosen the grip over the neck (**b**). [*Redrawn with permission from Tanagho EA, Smith DR. The anatomy and function of the bladder neck. Br J Urol. 1966 Feb;38(1):54–71*] [21]

sides were seen to intermingle with each other and with bladder filling would tighten further, thus maintaining the bladder neck integrity. During initiation of voiding as the bladder neck is turned to a funnel, these loops slide over each other and lose their grip on the neck (Fig. 13.8b) [21]. The funneling as such is believed to be a function of the longitudinal smooth muscles which on contraction bring about shortening of the urethra and funneling at the neck [20].

Hence, **the bladder neck is structurally and functionally different from the rest of the bladder and may have both an active and passive sphincter mechanism, but the resting closure pressures at the neck are significantly less than the mid-urethra** [26].

13.3.2 External Urethral Sphincter (Rhabdosphincter)

The smooth muscles of the urethra contribute very little to the resting tone and overall continence and are known only to provide some compensatory increase in tone when the striated sphincter mechanisms are damaged as in child birth injuries [27]. It is the striated muscle of the urethra, *the rhabdosphincter* which is responsible for maximum closure pressures along the entire urethra [28]. The rhabdosphincter muscle has two components namely *pars urethralis (or sphincter urethralis)* and the *pars urethrovaginalis*. Both the parts are in continuity with each other as they surround the *anteriorly concave urethra* (Fig. 13.9).

The *pars urethralis* or the "striated sphincter proper" begins at the base of the bladder and has fibers in circular orientation which completely surround the urethra in embryo and female child but are deficient posteriorly in adults where most of the bulk is anteriorly (Fig. 13.10). Note the similarity of cross-sectional anatomy on cadaveric histology and adult MRI as in Fig. 13.7. In the posterior midline, the fibers attach to a thin linear tendinous raphe which provides a fixed structure for the sphincteric muscles to contract. The maximum thickness of this sphincter is at the mid-urethra level and corresponds with the site of maximum urethral closure pressure in the urethra. Some superficial fibers merge with the

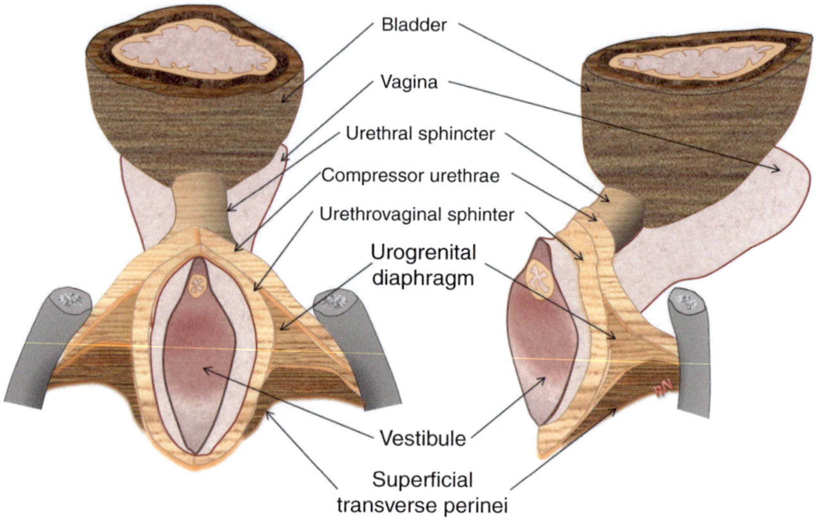

Fig. 13.9 The rhabdosphincter in a female with its components of urethral sphincter proper, compressor urethrae, and urethrovaginal sphincter. [*Redrawn with permission from Oelrich TM. The striated urogenital sphincter muscle in the female. Anat Rec. 1983 Feb;205(2):223–32*] [8]

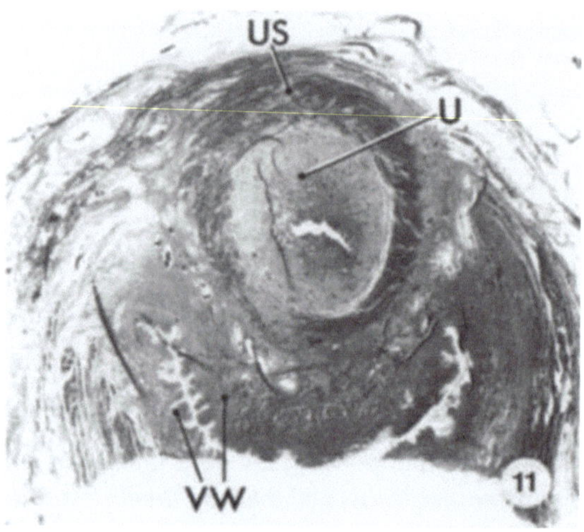

Fig. 13.10 1.8 times magnified cross-sectional view of urethra and anterior vaginal wall (VW) of an adult female cadaver, age 33 years. Urethral smooth muscle wall (U) is surrounded by striated muscle urethral sphincter (US). Notice the anteriorly bulky urethral sphincter muscle and an apparent septum posteriorly. [*Reproduced with permission from Oelrich TM. The striated urogenital sphincter muscle in the female. Anat Rec. 1983 Feb; 205(2):223–32*] [8]

anterior vaginal wall. The caudal fibers are continuous with the pars urethrovaginalis. *The human female striated sphincter consists of a mixture of slow and fast twitch type fibers where slow twitch fibers are predominant (up to 87%). The slow twitch fibers are useful for maintaining the consistent resting tone as they are resistant to fatigue* [29].

The *pars urethrovaginalis* consists of two important thin striated muscles, both of which wrap the urethra only anteriorly. The bundles of *compressor urethrae* are in direct continuity with the rhabdosphincter and instead to encircling the urethra they are directed inferolaterally toward the ischiopubic rami on either side (Fig. 13.9). Just caudal to the bundles of compressor urethrae are the fibers of *urethrovaginal sphincter muscle* which go posteriorly and encircle the vagina as well (Fig. 13.9). Both these muscles help to retract and elongate the urethra and complement the pelvic floor which keeps the bladder neck lifted. The urethral length achieved thereby is independently crucial in maintaining the continence [8].

Three-dimensional reconstruction models of the sphincteric mechanisms also confirm the above arrangement of striated sphincter as interpreted from cadaveric studies (Fig. 13.11). In males the development of the prostate does not allow the cranial portions of the sphincteric complex to develop well; it is the compressor urethrae (in fact is the most powerful but a thin portion in females) and the urethrovaginal sphincter regions which develop well and are the homologue of the membranous urethral sphincter [9, 25].

While all the striated sphincteric muscles are related to the pelvic portion of the urethra, the most distal one fourth of the urethra lies

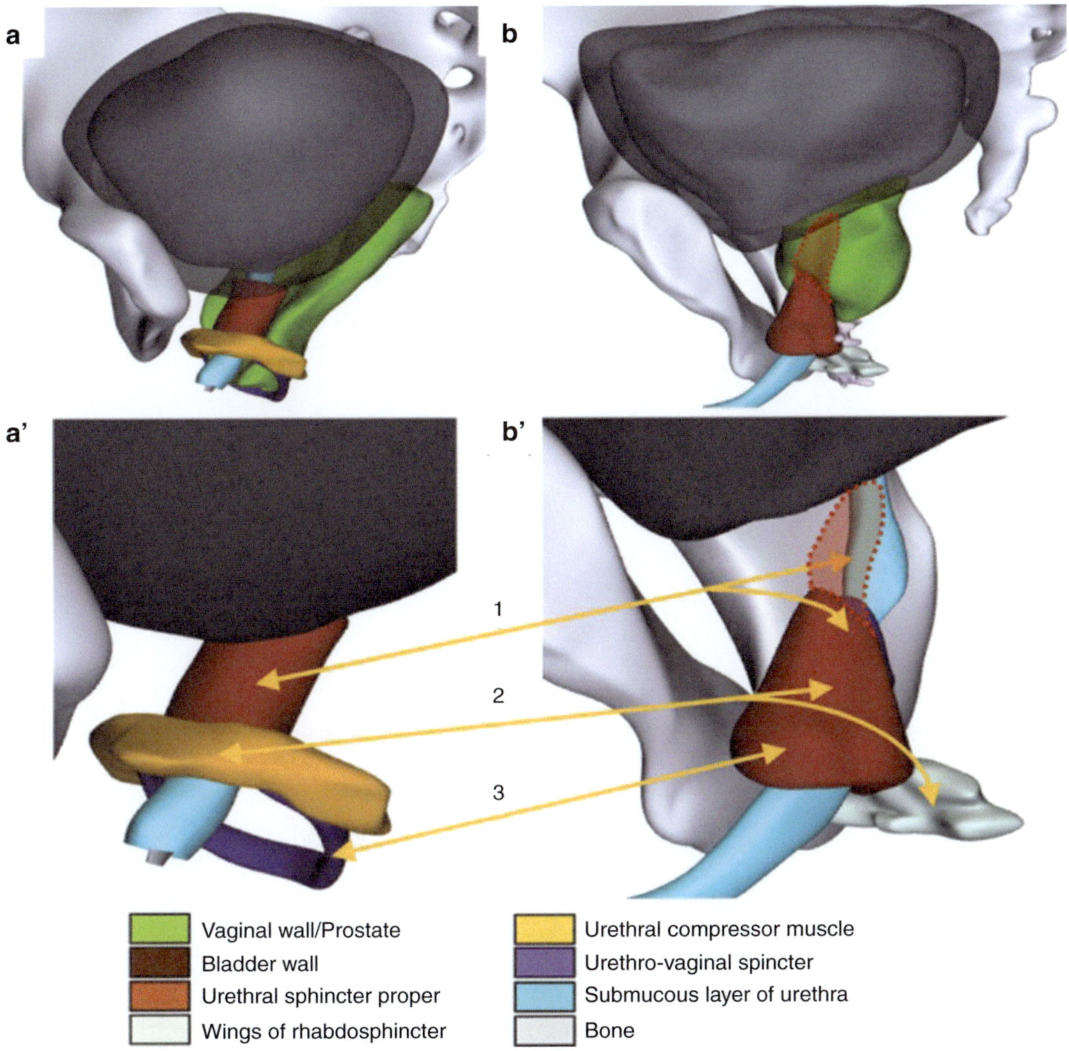

Fig. 13.11 The striated sphincter in females (**a**, **a′**) and males (**b**, **b′**) showing homologous components of male and female urethra marked with arrows in **a′** and **b′**. In both the sexes, the striated sphincter muscle extends from bladder neck to cover the entire pelvic portion of the urethra. Whereas in females the middle part is more well developed as rhabdosphincter, in males the inferior part is most well developed. [*Reproduced from Wu Y* et al. *Interactive three-dimensional teaching models of the female and male pelvic floor. Clin Anat N Y N. 2020 Mar;33(2):275–85*] [9] (Creative commons license)

below the perineal membrane, i.e., in the perineum and does not have the extension of either the smooth muscle layers or the striated sphincter cover. This portion is related to the bulbs of the vestibule (see Fig. 13.14 below) which are the erectile bodies and are covered with the bulbospongiosus muscle on either side.

13.3.3 Innervation of the Sphincters

Immunohistochemical staining of thin sections of the urethra in female fetuses followed by 3D reconstruction has shown that the urethra is supplied by both autonomic and somatic nerves. The autonomic nerves are derived from the pelvic plexus and travel through the lateral vaginal

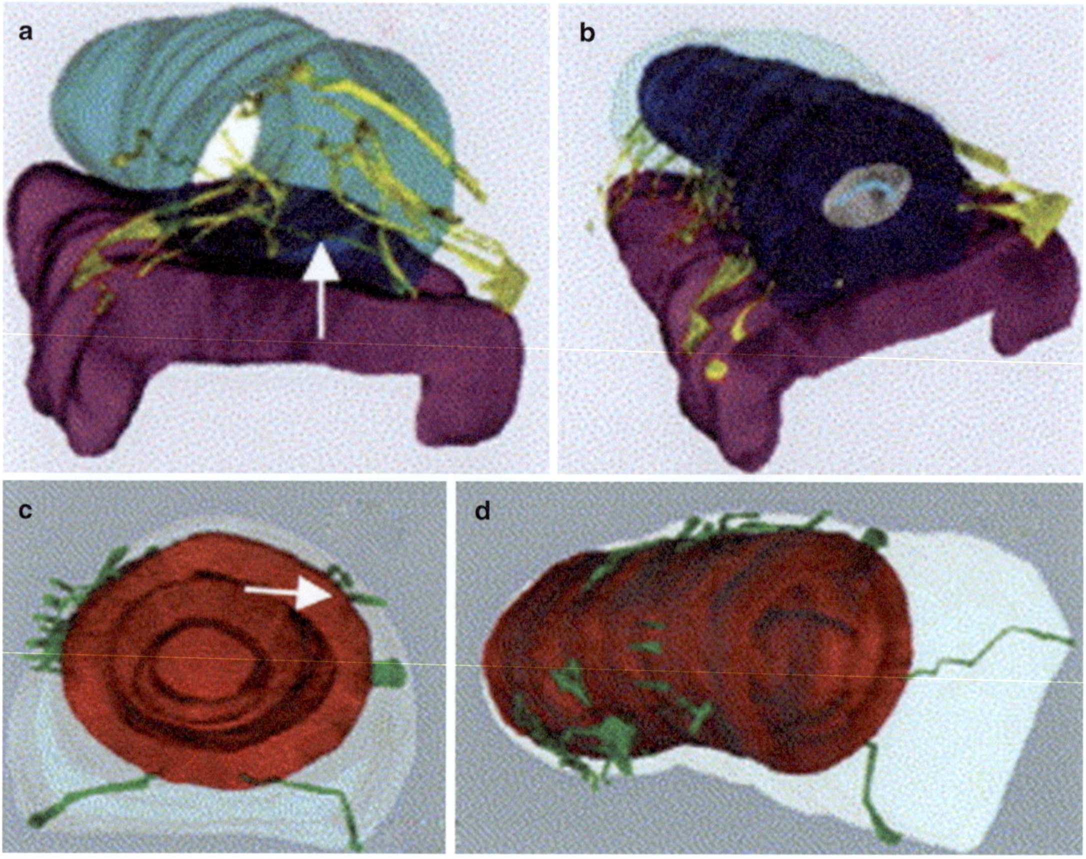

Fig. 13.12 3D reconstruction after immunohistochemical staining of serial sections of female fetus. (**a**, **b**) Unmyelinated autonomic fibers (yellow) traveling from the lateral vaginal wall enter the periurethral connective tissue (light blue) predominantly at 4 and 8 o'clock to supply the smooth musculature of the urethra (in dark blue). (**c**, **d**) Myelinated somatic nerve fibers (green) enter the periurethral connective tissue at 3 and 9 o'clock and supply the striated sphincter (in red). [*Reproduced with permission form Karam* et al. *Innervation of the Female Human Urethral Sphincter: 3D Reconstruction of Immunohistochemical Studies in the Fetus. Eur Urol. 2005 May;47(5):627–34*] [30]

walls to a space between the posterior surface of urethra and the anterior vaginal wall. They enter the urethra throughout the urethral length predominantly at the 4 and 8 o'clock positions and supply the urethral smooth muscle (Fig. 13.12 a, b). The somatic nerves reach the striated sphincter urethra through the periurethral connective tissue and penetrate the striated sphincter predominantly at the 3 and 9 o'clock positions (Fig. 13.12 c, d). These somatic nerves are derived from the pudendal nerve and reach the urethra either through intrapelvic (supralevator) pathway or through the extrapelvic (infralevator) pathway (Fig. 13.13) [30]. Out of the two, the Infralevator extrapelvic pathway has a more predominant contribution to the innervation of striated sphincter [31].

13.3.4 Role of Pelvic Floor Muscles

The contemporary understanding is that the *pelvic floor muscles do not encircle the urethra completely (there being significant dense connective tissue and vascular network between the pubis and anterior urethra) and consequently they do not play an active role as a permanent closure force of the urethra* [32]. At the level of distal striated sphincter (urethrovaginalis sphincter level), the lower edges of the sheet like levator

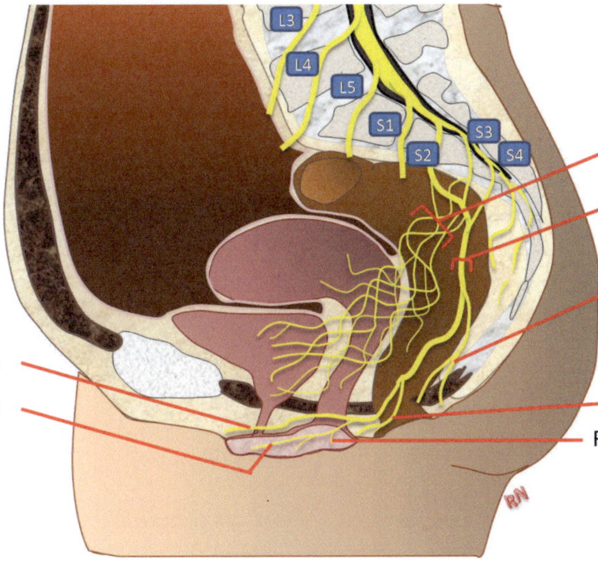

Fig. 13.13 Nerves to the urethra arise from sacral segments S2–4 and course either through pelvic plexus to run over lateral vaginal wall (supralevator pathway) or through the pudendal nerve (infralevator pathway)

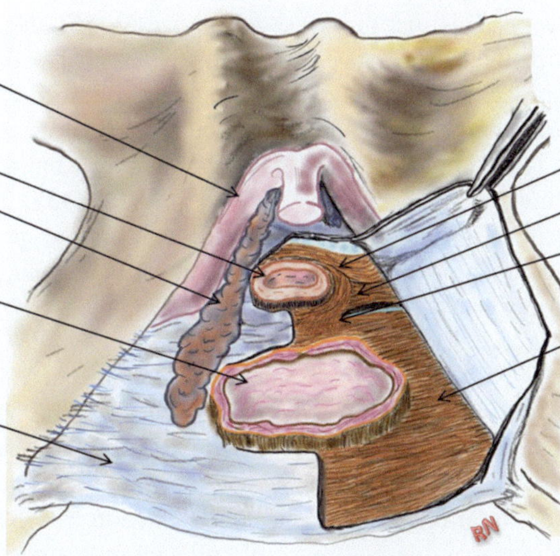

Fig. 13.14 The inferior-most portion of urethra below the perineal membrane is the perineal part of urethra. It is not surrounded by any sphincteric muscle but is flanked on either side by vestibular bulbs

ani muscles condense to form a sling like structure (the urogenital hiatus), which plays only an adjunctive role to the striated sphincter [25]. The anatomical existence of a urogenital diaphragm has also been refuted time and again [8, 25]; a perineal membrane is, however, identified. In both the sexes an elastic fiber-rich connective tissue sheath extends over the entire rhabdosphincter to encage it in a thin sheath. Inferiorly, it condenses to form a broad sheet-like membrane *(perineal membrane)* on which the lowermost fibers of the striated sphincter are enmeshed. Consequently, in females the lowermost fibers of the urethrovaginal sphincter muscle are enmeshed into this membrane which extends from one ischiopubic ramus to the other (Fig. 13.14). *The fibers of the levators are also attached to this membrane and not directly to the rhabdosphincter. It is through the perineal membrane that the forces of levator are transferred to the rhabdosphincter* [33]. *Below this membrane, the perineal part of the urethra begins.*

13.3.5 Surgical Implications of sphincteric anatomy

As most of the bulk of the striated sphincter is anterior, the anterior (dorsal) onlay approach for urethroplasty poses more theoretical risk to the rhabdosphincter mechanism. Whether a plane can be developed between the smooth and striated sphincteric muscles to avoid damage to rhabdosphincter is uncertain and unlikely. Posterior (ventral) onlay approach poses less potential of damage to rhabdosphincter. However, because the development of de novo sphincteric incontinence after urethroplasties is very rare, it is possible that the bladder neck mechanisms provide the backup. As both anterior and posterior approaches are confined to the midline, any extensive nerve damage to the sphincters is avoided. It is also prudent to avoid tempering with both the mechanisms at the same time as may appear justified in strictures extending up to the bladder neck. The depth of incision for inlay approaches may not be consistent, and it is not sure whether it reaches up to the external sphincter level.

Additionally, in proximal urethra, sphincter lies in a circular orientation and distally it changes the configuration to form the urethrovaginal sphincter or extends along the inferior pubic ramus above the perineal membrane (urogenital diaphragm) as the compressor urethra. So, while it is easy to separate urethra in its upper posterior third from the adjacent vagina its lower portion is fused with the wall of the vagina. Therefore, a ventral onlay approach for a distal stricture is surgically more demanding and the flaps often get thinned out. On the dorsal aspect, however, the distal urethra is only juxtaposed to the clitoral structures, which must be carefully preserved during dissection [34].

13.4 Fascial Supports of the Urethra

Anatomical studies correlating the MRI findings of alive female with cadaveric images and histology have made the understanding of concepts of fascial supports of the urethra and their possible role in continence easy [35, 36].

13.4.1 On The Dorsal (anterior Side)

The urethra is supported by three sets of ligaments.

(a) *Pubourethral/Pubovesical ligaments:* these extend as fascial condensations on either side of midline in the space of Retzius from posterior surface of the pubis to the vesicourethral junction. This condensation has been described as superior pubourethral ligament in one study [35] and pubovesical ligament in the other [36] . Two more components supporting the mid- and distal urethra with the pubis have been described in cadaveric dissections but cannot be identified on normal female MRI [35]. Free downward movement between the pubis and the anterior urethral wall on dynamic MRI in nulliparous female volunteers also confirms the absence of stiff ligamentous attachment between these structures at mid- or distal urethral level. Pubourethral/pubovesical ligaments can be identified by naked eye in the space of Retzius (Fig. 13.15) are best identified on a sagittal section of MRI. They are composed of collagen with smooth muscle fibers interspersed in them.
(b) *Periurethral ligaments:* they are transversely oriented structure connecting with the puborectalis muscle on either side and coursing as a ventral (anterior) sling in front of the urethra (Fig. 13.7). On histology it is composed of only connective tissue. In histological and anatomical studies of the fetus this is identified as ventral urethral fascia [36].

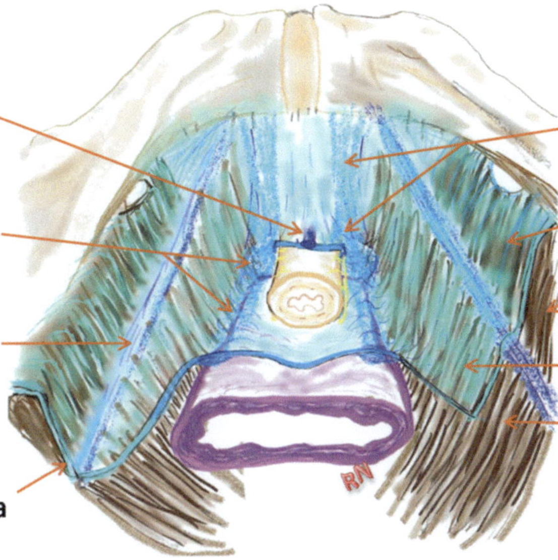

Fig. 13.15 Pubourethral ligaments as identified from space of Retzius

(c) *Paraurethral ligaments:* they are relatively poorly defined structures connecting the lateral wall of urethra to the periurethral ligaments.

The space in front of the ventral urethral fasciae and the pubis is filled with extracellular matrix rich loose areolar tissue.

13.4.2 On the Ventral (Posterior) Side

The *suburethral ligament* is like a hammock underneath the urethra most prominent in mid- and distal urethral level. This shelf-like structure is anterior to vagina and extends laterally to the pelvic side wall to the same site as the origin of levator ani. A plane of cleavage is visible on MRI between this ligamentous structure and the anterior vaginal wall (Fig. 13.7). It contains striated muscle fibers interspersed in collagen [35]. The existence of such structure, however, is not consistent in other studies [37] However, we know from our suburethral dissections during incontinence and urethral diverticular surgeries that there is a prominent fascial layer between the urethra and the anterior vaginal wall.

The role of the pubourethral/pubovesical ligaments is to maintain the position of the bladder neck and provide support to the anterior wall of urethra. They may provide the anchor point for the urethral continence mechanisms to act. The periurethral ligaments being laterally attached to the muscles provide support to the entire urethra and the suburethral ligament may be providing the backboard over which the urethral compression can be achieved during straining.

13.4.3 Surgical Implications

The periurethral or the lateral urethropelvic ligaments mark a division between the dorsal (Anterior) and Ventral (posterior) approaches. The semicircular perimeatal incision during the anterior approach should not cross this limit to reach the posterior compartment and vice versa. During dorsal (anterior) approaches, one should avoid severing the endopelvic fascia and superior pubourethral ligament to drop the bladder neck and thereby help preserving the normal suspension of urethra.

The dorsally (anteriorly) placed grafts over proximal two-third of urethra in onlay approaches get no support from any defined structure but may be fixed only over a loose areolar tissue in their proximal part (Fig. 13.16). More distally, however, the clitoral structures would be providing the bed.

13.5 Urethral Blood Supply

The urethra has a dual blood supply. *The proximal three-fourth of the urethra (the intrapelvic portion) derives its supply trough the inferior vesical and vaginal arteries. The distal fourth of urethra (perineal portion) is supplied by branches*

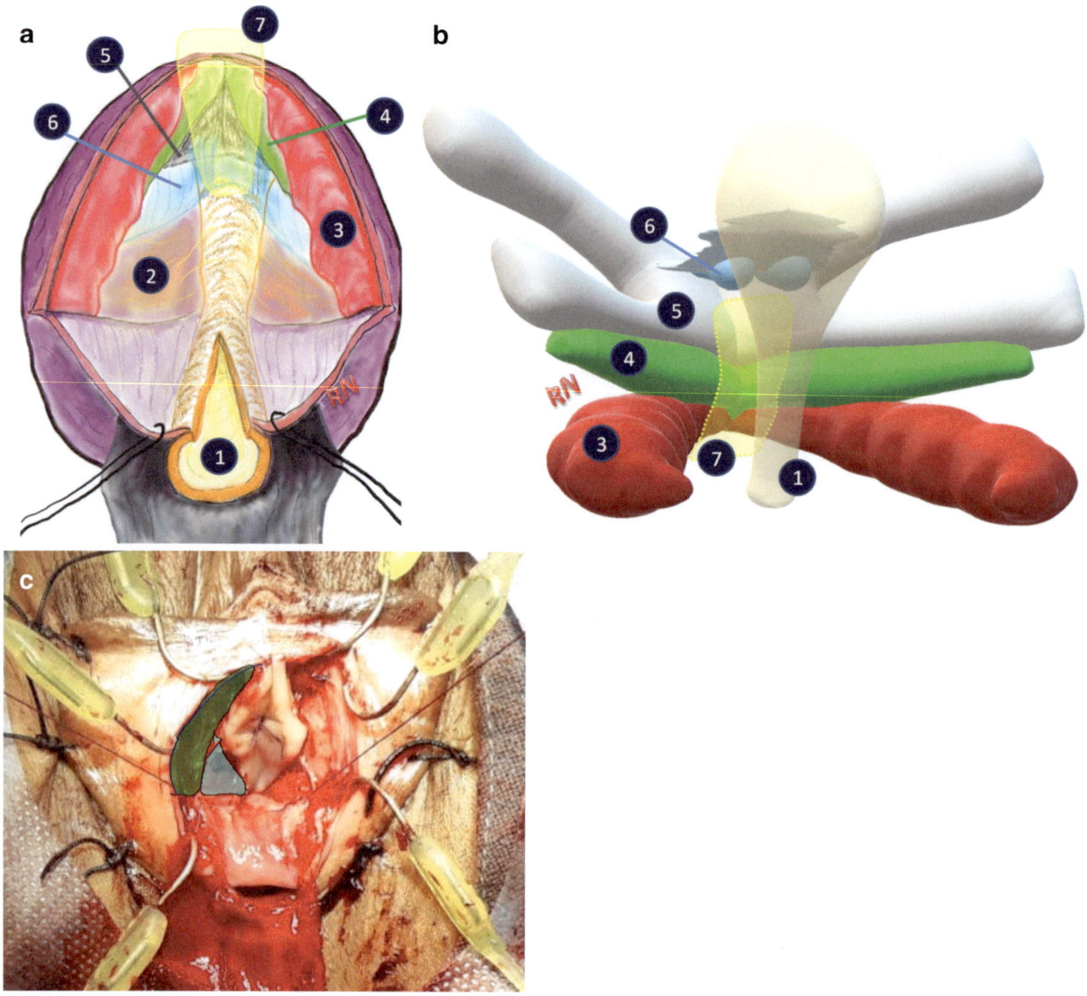

Fig. 13.16 (**a**) Dorsally dissected and dropped down urethra (*1*) during a dorsal (anterior) onlay urethroplasty showing the periurethral ligaments (*2*) laterally which hold the urethra to pelvic wall in entire course, The clitoral structures, viz. vestibular bulb (*3*) and clitoral crus (*4*) form the distal bed for the graft. More proximally, the bed is formed by retropubic fibrofatty tissue over the pubis (*5*). The endopelvic fascia with underlying pubourethral ligaments (*6*) lies deep near the bladder neck. The extent of base for dorsal placement of graft is depicted as a yellow rectangle (*7*). (**b**) Posterolateral view of dorsal graft bed for female urethroplasty. (**c**) Intraoperative photograph of dorsal onlay graft urethroplasty. The clitoral structures are marked with green patch on the patient's right and can be identified in corresponding location on the left. The area marked with triangular patch is the retropubic fibrofatty tissue. Buccal graft is seen sutured in anterior midline

of the pudendal artery. Both the segments therefore are supplied by the internal iliac artery. As the arterial twigs from these vessels approach urethra, they arborize to supply the urethra in three tunics: Fascial, muscular, and mucous.

The urethral microvascularity [38] in the *fascial tunic* consists of longitudinal vessels descending and ascending from pelvic and perineal portion respectively and anastomosing at various levels longitudinally as well as transversely. They are most prominent in the anterior and lateral urethral walls. The fascial networks are absent in the lower fourth. The *muscular tunic* has transverse running microvessels in the circular coats and longitudinal running vessels in the longitudinal muscle layer and anastomose freely. The vessels in this tunic are also most abundant in anterior and lateral walls. The *mucous tunic* is the richest in terms of microvascularity. It has a mucosal and a submucosal component. The vessels in the submucosa run longitudinally along the mucosal folds with little cross-column anastomoses. The veins are of larger caliber and fill the longitudinal folds and are thereby involved in the modulation of the urethral lumen. *Throughout the urethra, the vessels first enter the fascial tunic and then pierce through the muscular tunic to supply the mucosal tunic. This rich vasculature is least developed in the lower urethra where posterior urethral and vaginal walls are merged.* The vessels of the lower urethra freely communicate with those of the erectile bodies and the vaginal wall. The overall vascularity of the urethra decreases with age and is significantly less in post-menopausal as compared to premenopausal women as demonstrated by translabial contrast-enhanced ultrasonography of the urethra [39]. The mucosal seal is responsible for one third of permanent closure forces of the urethra and the effect decreases with age making women more prone for stress incontinence.

13.5.1 Surgical Implications

As urethra is rich in both ascending and descending blood supply with microvaculature freely anastomosing at all levels except the lowermost urethra; urethral transaction at any level understandably leaves a viable portion on either end. As the vessels first enter the outer tunic and then pierce to the inner tunics, stripping the urethra off its outer layers during mobilization may jeopardize the entire vascularity of the urethra.

13.6 Sexual Anatomy in the Female

O'Çonnell [40] described clitoral anatomy in healthy, nulliparous volunteers using MRI imaging with fat saturation techniques to enhance cavernous techniques. Clitoral structures were seen as a bright erectile tissue which lie ventrolateral to urethrovaginal complex and provide strong dorsal support to distal urethra. The clitoris is a multiplanar structure with: *two corporal bodies* which arise from ischiopubic rami and join together as they approach midline. *Bulbs of clitoris (vestibular bulbs)* flank the anterolateral surface of the distal vaginal wall and lowermost urethra to join ventral to urethra and extend as a sheet of corpus spongiousum underneath the vestibular mucosa till the undersurface of glans, where it enlarges to cover the terminal portion of corporal bodies as the glans clitoris. A succinct graphical description of female urethra in relation to the clitoral structures is given in Fig. 13.17.

13.6.1 Surgical implications

Of particular concern to a surgeon regarding dorsal approach to urethra is possible injury to neurovascular bundle. These large bundles ascend along the ischiopubic ramus on either side to the under surface of the pubic symphysis in the midline, from which they run along the cephalad surface of the clitoral body toward the glans. So, these neurovascular bundles are located at safe distance away from dissection area and a dorsal approach does not jeopardize the sexual function [41]. A ventral (posterior) approach also may affect these structures and rather a far lateral mobilization of vaginal flaps and paravaginal tissues during a ventral/posterior approach may put neurovascular bundles at more risk.

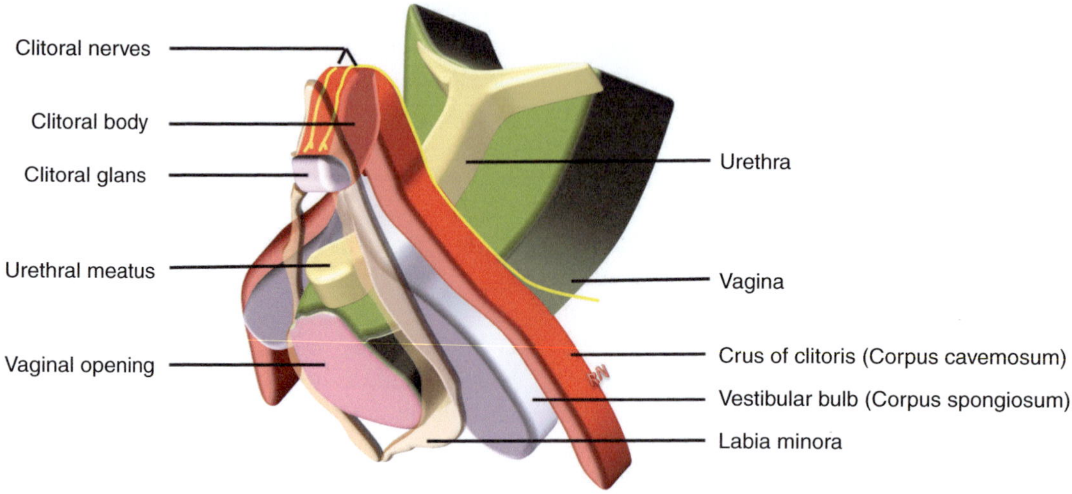

Fig. 13.17 Graphical illustration showing female urethra in relation to the clitoral anatomy

The dorsal curvilinear incision to approach the anterior surface of the urethra should be close to the meatus so that the space is entered below the confluence of vestibular bulbs. The graft thus placed will find its bed distally under the confluence of vestibular bulbs. Incision lines further away from the anterior edge of the meatus will help develop flaps based on vestibular mucosa and may also have underlying corpus spongiosum.

Key Learning Points

- The female urethra developmentally corresponds to the prostatic and membranous urethra in males.
- External female genitalia are developmentally similar to severe perineal hypospadias in male.
- The bladder neck and external urethral sphincter (rhabdosphincter) are the two main continence zones.
- Bladder neck possibly has both an active and a passive mechanism of continence.
- The rhabdosphincter is distinct from the pelvic floor muscles and extends from proximal urethra to cover the entire pelvic portion of urethra with maximum bulk in mid-urethra.
- The pelvic floor muscles play an adjunctive role for both sphincter contraction and relaxation.
- Female urethra has dual blood supply from inferior vesical and vaginal arteries from above and pudendal arteries from below. There is a rich vascular network in the tunics of the urethra.
- The mucosal seal effect which helps in continence is produced by large-caliber veins running longitudinally in the submucosa and becomes less prominent with age.
- Anterior fascial attachments of urethra provide an anchor point which may play an important role in continence mechanisms.

The clitoris is a multiplanar structure with the clitoral corpora, vestibular bulbs, and the glans as its components, and the clitoral neurovascular bundle appears anatomically safe from harm's way during most of the female urethral reconstructive procedures.

References

1. Puppo V. Embryology and anatomy of the vulva: the female orgasm and women's sexual health. Eur J Obstet Gynecol Reprod Biol. 2011;154(1):3–8.
2. AbouZeid AA, Mohammad SA. Transformation of the female genitalia in congenital adrenal hyperplasia: MRI study. J Pediatr Surg. 2020;55(5):977–84.
3. Apóstolos RAC, Canguçu-Campinho AK, Lago R, Costa ACS, Oliveira LMB, Toralles MB, et al. Gender

identity and sexual function in 46,XX patients with congenital adrenal hyperplasia raised as males. Arch Sex Behav. 2018;47(8):2491–6.
4. Shima H, Yabumoto H, Okamoto E, Orestano L, Ikoma F. Testicular function in patients with hypospadias associated with enlarged prostatic utricle. Br J Urol. 1992;69(2):192–5.
5. Shapiro E, Huang H, McFadden DE, Masch RJ, Ng E, Lepor H, et al. The prostatic utricle is not a Müllerian duct remnant: immunohistochemical evidence for a distinct urogenital sinus origin. J Urol. 2004;172(4 Pt 2):1753–6; discussion 1756.
6. Puppo V, Puppo G. Male vagina is a more accurate term than prostatic utricle. Int J Urol. 2016;23(1):108.
7. Hage JJ. Metaidoioplasty: an alternative phalloplasty technique in transsexuals. Plast Reconstr Surg. 1996;97(1):161–7.
8. Oelrich TM. The striated urogenital sphincter muscle in the female. Anat Rec. 1983;205(2):223–32.
9. Wu Y, Hikspoors JPJM, Mommen G, Dabhoiwala NF, Hu X, Tan L-W, et al. Interactive three-dimensional teaching models of the female and male pelvic floor. Clin Anat. 2020;33(2):275–85.
10. Wernert N, Albrech M, Sesterhenn I, Goebbels R, Bonkhoff H, Seitz G, et al. The "female prostate": location, morphology, immunohistochemical characteristics and significance. Eur Urol. 1992;22(1):64–9.
11. Fang BXH, Cho FKY, Lam WWM. Prostate gland development and adrenal tumor in a female with congenital adrenal hyperplasia: a case report and review from radiology perspective. J Radiol Case Rep. 2013;7(12):26–34.
12. Berkow SG. The corpus spongeosum of the urethra: its possible role in urinary control and stress incontinence in women. Am J Obstet Gynecol. 1953;65(2):346–51.
13. van Turnhout AA, Hage JJ, van Diest PJ. The female corpus spongiosum revisited. Acta Obstet Gynecol Scand. 1995;74(10):767–71.
14. DeLancey JO. Correlative study of paraurethral anatomy. Obstet Gynecol. 1986;68(1):91–7.
15. el-Sayed RF, Morsy MM, el-Mashed SM, Abdel-Azim MS. Anatomy of the urethral supporting ligaments defined by dissection, histology, and MRI of female cadavers and MRI of healthy nulliparous women. AJR Am J Roentgenol. 2007;189(5):1145–57.
16. Baggish MS, Steele AC, Karram M. The relationships of the vestibular bulb and corpora cavernosa to the female urethra: a microanatomic study part 2. J Gynecol Surg. 1999;15(4):171–8.
17. Hinata N, Murakami G, Abe S, Honda M, Isoyama T, Sejima T, et al. Detailed histological investigation of the female urethra: application to radical cystectomy. J Urol. 2012;187(2):451–6.
18. Strohbehn K, Quint LE, Prince MR, Wojno KJ, Delancey JO. Magnetic resonance imaging anatomy of the female urethra: a direct histologic comparison. Obstet Gynecol. 1996;88(5):750–6.
19. Macura KJ, Genadry R, Borman TL, Mostwin JL, Lardo AC, Bluemke DA. Evaluation of the female urethra with intraurethral magnetic resonance imaging. J Magn Reson Imaging JMRI. 2004;20(1):153–9.
20. Haderer JM, Pannu HK, Genadry R, Hutchins GM. Controversies in female urethral anatomy and their significance for understanding urinary continence: observations and literature review. Int Urogynecol J Pelvic Floor Dysfunct. 2002;13(4):236–52.
21. Tanagho EA, Smith DR. The anatomy and function of the bladder neck. Br J Urol. 1966;38(1):54–71.
22. Gosling JA, Dixon JS. The structure and innervation of smooth muscle in the wall of the bladder neck and proximal urethra. Br J Urol. 1975;47(5):549–58.
23. Dröes JT. Observations on the musculature of the urinary bladder and the urethra in the human foetus. Br J Urol. 1974;46(2):179–85.
24. Spradling K, Khoyilar C, Abedi G, Okhunov Z, Wikenheiser J, Yoon R, et al. Redefining the autonomic nerve distribution of the bladder using 3-dimensional image reconstruction. J Urol. 2015;194(6):1661–7.
25. Yucel S, Baskin LS. An anatomical description of the male and female urethral sphincter complex. J Urol. 2004;171(5):1890–7.
26. Gosling JA. The structure of the bladder neck, urethra and pelvic floor in relation to female urinary continence. Int Urogynecol J Pelvic Floor Dysfunct. 1996;7(4):177–8.
27. Furuta A, Suzuki Y, Asano K, de Groat WC, Egawa S, Yoshimura N. Urethral compensatory mechanisms to maintain urinary continence after pudendal nerve injury in female rats. Int Urogynecology J. 2011;22(8):963–70.
28. Thind P. The significance of smooth and striated muscles in the sphincter function of the urethra in healthy women. Neurourol Urodyn. 1995;14(6):585–618.
29. Partin AW, Dmochowski RR, Kavoussi LR, Peters CA, editors. Campbell-Walsh-Wein urology. 12th ed. Philadelphia: Elsevier; 2020.
30. Karam I, Droupy S, Abd-Alsamad I, Uhl J-F, Benoît G, Delmas V. Innervation of the female human urethral sphincter: 3D reconstruction of immunohistochemical studies in the fetus. Eur Urol. 2005;47(5):627–34.
31. Colleselli K, Stenzl A, Eder R, Strasser H, Poisel S, Bartsch G. The female urethral sphincter: a morphological and topographical study. J Urol. 1998;160(1):49–54.
32. Gosling JA, Dixon JS, Critchley HOD, Thompson S-A. A comparative study of the human external sphincter and periurethral levator ani muscles. Br J Urol. 1981;53(1):35–41.
33. Hinata N, Murakami G. The urethral rhabdosphincter, levator ani muscle, and perineal membrane: a review. Biomed Res Int. 2014;2014:1–18.
34. Migliari R, Leone P, Berdondini E, De Angelis M, Barbagli G, Palminteri E. Dorsal buccal mucosa graft urethroplasty for female urethral strictures. J Urol. 2006;176(4):1473–6.
35. El Sayed RF, Morsy MM, El Mashed SM, Abdel-Azim MS. Anatomy of the urethral supporting liga-

ments defined by dissection, histology, and MRI of female cadavers and MRI of healthy nulliparous women. Am J Roentgenol. 2007;189(5):1145–57.
36. Fritsch H, Pinggera GM, Lienemann A, Mitterberger M, Bartsch G, Strasser H. What are the supportive structures of the female urethra? Neurourol Urodyn. 2006;25(2):128–34.
37. Mazloomdoost D, Westermann LB, Mutema G, Crisp CC, Kleeman SD, Pauls RN. Histologic anatomy of the anterior vagina and urethra. Female Pelvic Med Reconstr Surg. 2017;23(5):329–35.
38. Sery FG, Wolfram-Gabel R, Sick H. Microvascularization of the female urethra in fetuses, neonates and infants. Surg Radiol Anat. 2002;24(5):271–6.
39. Siracusano S, Bertolotto M, Cucchi A, Lampropoulou N, Tiberio A, Gasparini C, et al. Application of ultrasound contrast agents for the characterization of female urethral vascularization in healthy pre- and postmenopausal volunteers: preliminary report. Eur Urol. 2006;50(6):1316–22.
40. O'Connell HE, Delancey J. Clitoral anatomy in nulliparous, healthy, premenopausal volunteers using unenhanced magnetic resonance imaging. J Urol. 2005;173(6):2060–3.
41. Manasa T, Khattar N, Tripathi M, Varshney A, Goel H, Sood R. Dorsal onlay graft urethroplasty for female urethral stricture improves sexual function: short-term results of a prospective study using vaginal graft. Indian J Urol. 2019;35(4):267–72.

Dorsal (Anterior) Onlay Urethroplasty for Female Urethral Stricture

14

Rishi Nayyar, Prashant Kumar, and Bharti Uppal Nayyar

Learning Objectives

- To understand the key steps and surgical approach for dorsal onlay repair of female urethral stricture.
- To understand the possible advantages of using a dorsal approach for female urethral reconstruction.
- To understand the current status of dorsal graft placement approach for female urethral stricture disease.

Dorsal buccal mucosal free graft urethroplasty was first described in males by Barbagli et al. in 1996 [1]. He used it in patients with long penile (>1 cm) or bulbar strictures (>2 cm) where primary end-to-end anastomosis will lead to chordee. Dorsal placement of the graft maintained urethral patency and, since the graft was supported on the corpora cavernosa, it avoided diverticula formation. On a similar principle, dorsal approach in female urethral stricture offers mechanical support and vascular bed to the graft and thus minimizes formation of diverticula or urethrovaginal fistula. Dorsal approach to female urethra and use of free graft to augment the urethra were first described in 2006 by two separate groups [2, 3]. It is also a more physiological approach as it directs urinary stream away from vagina and spares ventral urethra for any anti-incontinence procedure in future [3]. Additionally, the blood supply to urethra comes from posterior and posterolateral aspect; therefore, not mobilizing the plane between urethra and vagina may also preserve some blood supply besides avoiding risk to posterolateral neurovascular bundles. Furthermore, the dorsal plane of dissection of urethra is easy to develop. On the contrary, ventral dissection may be difficult particularly in the distal urethra, where the urethral and vaginal walls are more densely fused together and may be difficult to separate [4]. Possible advantages of a dorsal urethroplasty are given in Table 14.1. We shall discuss the salient anatomical considerations and surgical steps of a typical dorsal onlay urethroplasty in this chapter.

R. Nayyar (✉) · P. Kumar
Department of Urology, All India Institute of Medical Sciences, New Delhi, India

B. U. Nayyar
Department of Obstetrics and Gynecology, All India Institute of Medical Sciences, New Delhi, India

14.1 Surgical Technique

Pre-op preparation: Establishing the diagnosis may sometimes be difficult, particularly in soft mid-urethral strictures in females. Once confirmed by a combination of history/examination, imaging, urodynamics, and endoscopy, dorsal free graft augmentation urethroplasty technique is appropriate for distal urethral strictures. However, there is now increasing trend to utilize this approach even for strictures requiring mobi-

N. Khattar et al. (eds.), *Female Bladder Outlet Obstruction and Urethral Reconstruction*,
https://doi.org/10.1007/978-981-15-8521-0_14

Table 14.1 Proposed benefits of dorsal approach to female urethroplasty

• Sturdy, vascular and immobile tissue bed, avoiding any diverticulum
• No hypospadiac meatus, urine flow remains directed anteriorly, avoids vaginal pooling and post-void dribbling
• Posterior urethral plane remains untouched for any subsequent surgery, if required
• Double-faced graft can also be placed easily, by combining with ventral inlay procedure
• Doesn't require steep Trendelenburg positioning
• Urethral vascular supply is least affected
• Easier dissection for distal strictures
• No vaginal breach (may be important in children)

lization of urethra till bladder neck [3, 5]. We practice perineal hair clipping 1 day prior and also give vaginal douche. Urine culture is ensured to be sterile.

Anesthesia and patient position: Regional anesthesia is preferred in most cases at our center, except where buccal graft is to be harvested. Patient is placed in dorsal lithotomy position as for any perineal surgery taking care for appropriate padding at all pressure points. Trendelenburg positioning is generally not required because the plane of dissection is dorsal and looked down from above.

Planning the surgery: Urethroscopy may be repeated with a ureteroscope, even if already done earlier. If stricture is passable, length and proximal extent of stricture should be established. However, it may not always be passable till the stricture is incised. If the stricture caliber is too low (less than 7 Fr), it may be better to use either a double-faced graft (combined dorsal onlay and ventral inlay grafts) [6] or a tubularized graft/flap approach [7, 8]. Assessment of available urethral caliber also helps to find out the width of graft necessary to achieve a final caliber of about 30 Fr. A graft contraction rate of approximately 20% should also be borne in mind. Shrinkage is expectedly more in skin graft than buccal, vaginal, bladder, or bowel graft [9, 10].

Surgical steps: An illustration of surgical steps is given in Fig. 14.1. Stay sutures are taken at external urethral meatus to help provide longitudinal traction on the urethra during initial dissection. An integument deep hemi-circle incision is given surrounding the upper half of meatus (Fig. 14.1a, b). Incision may be extended in an inverted "Y" manner depending upon the depth of urethra to which exposure is required. Catheter may or may not be placed depending upon the available caliber of the urethra and surgeon's preference. Urethral tube is dissected with Metzenbaum scissors held longitudinally along the urethra with the curved tip pointing away from urethra (Fig. 14.1c). Dissection is done by separating the jaws of scissors. Cutting is required only occasionally. Far lateral urethral mobilization should be avoided. Some surgeons prefer to instill this plane with 10–20 mL of adrenaline saline (1:200,000) before dissection. However, we prefer not to use saline hydro-dissection as it makes tissue planes soggy and difficult to follow. Precise coagulation also becomes difficult because of edematous tissues. While the plane of dissection may initially appear to be bloodless, the vessels would be prone to bleed once the effect of adrenaline wears off.

The distal half of urethra is easily separable and is surrounded on its lateral and anterior aspects by the vestibular bulbs (equivalent of bulb of penis and corpus spongiosum in males) inferiorly and cavernosal bodies superiorly (Fig. 14.2). They all join together to form the clitoral body and also provide a good vascular bed for the graft to take up. Proximally the urethra is hinged on the pubis bone through the periurethral and paraurethral ligaments [11]. One should not cut extensively through these ligaments which may have an important bearing on continence mechanisms. Rather, these should be moved laterally starting from midline, using the "opening of jaws" movement of Metzenbaum scissors or dissecting forceps. The neurovascular bundle of clitoris runs on the dorsolateral aspect of cavernosal bodies and is therefore not in direct relation to the correct dissection plane. Followed proximally, the plane of dissection enters the subsphincteric plane, thereby preserving the external sphincter as well. There have been no reports of sexual dysfunction or de novo stress incontinence after a dorsal graft procedure, though this area remains understudied in literature. Manasa et al have reported an improvement of sexual function after dorsal urethroplasty [12].

Incision is given at the 12 o'clock position to open the urethra to include the entire longitudinal length of stricture and 5 mm beyond it (Fig. 14.1d). It helps to progressively take stay sutures on proximal urethra on either flap. Unlike strictures in males, most female strictures lack deep spongiofibrosis and mucosal texture may also not be visibly different between healthy and unhealthy stricture zone. Thus, the surgeon often has to resort to apparent caliber of urethra to ensure that incision reaches the normal urethra beyond the stricture area. The urethra may be recalibrated with 30 Fr Hegar dilator to check for adequacy of incision (Fig. 14.1e). The dilator should tend to fall into the bladder with its own weight. Suture is then taken at the apex on either

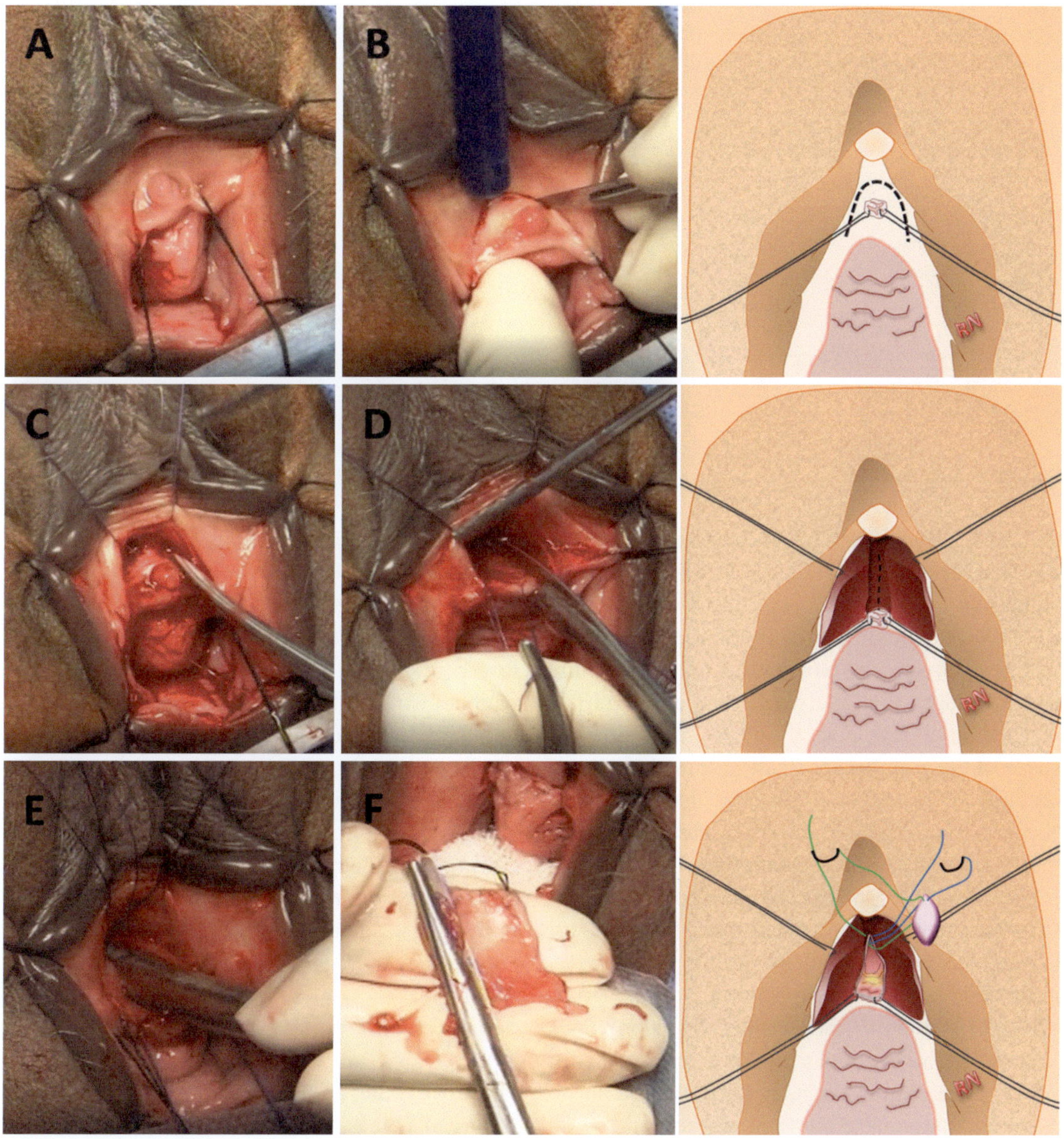

Fig. 14.1 Pictorial and graphical description of surgical steps of dorsal onlay graft urethroplasty for female urethral strictures. (**A**, **B**) Semi-circular incision on dorsal aspect of urethral meatus. (**C**, **D**) Dissection of urethra in its dorsal plane and longitudinal incision across stricture. (**E**, **F**) Adequate spatulation of urethra is and appropriate sized defatted graft is parachuted on sutures. (**G**, **H**) The graft is fixed to urethral edges and quilted to its bed. (**I**, **J**) Incision edges are closed and dressing done over a catheter

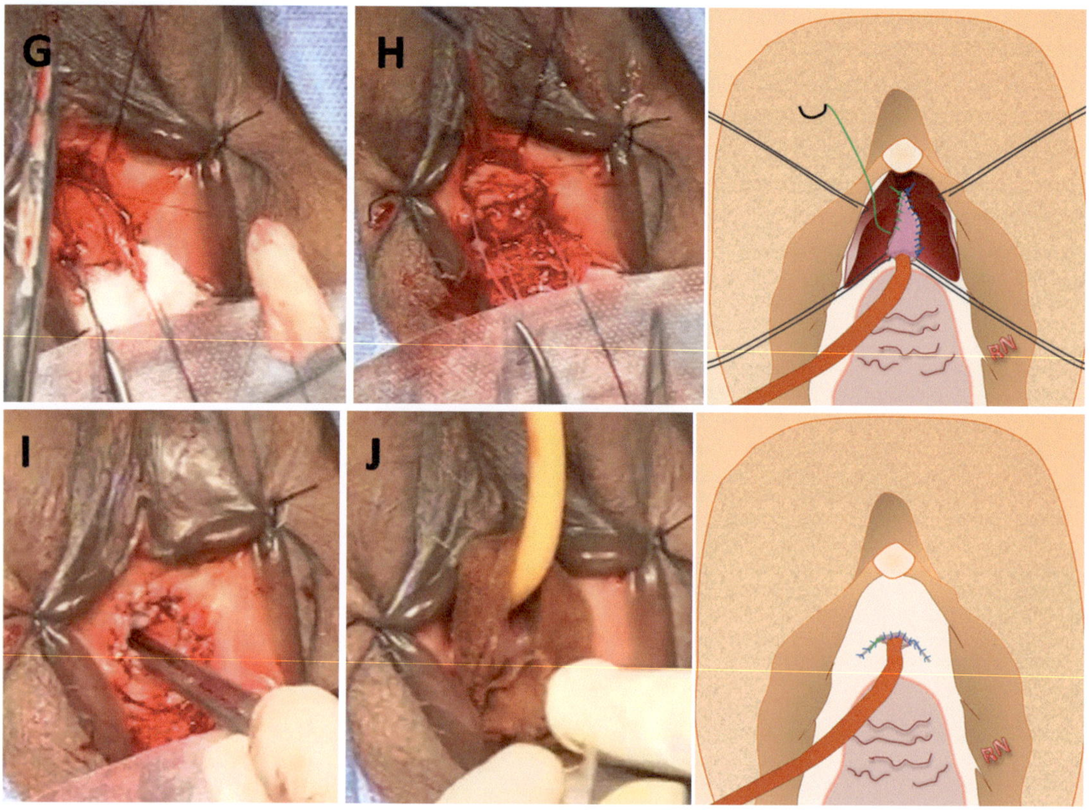

Fig. 14.1 (continued)

flap with 4-O absorbable monofilament suture. The harvested graft (Fig. 14.1f) is then parachuted on these sutures to fix the apex on either side. The ipsilateral suture is continued on respective sides to sew the entire graft length with the urethral flaps (Fig. 14.1g). If large, the graft is meshed at a few places before suturing. The shape of the graft is kept/made elliptical (for mid-urethral strictures) and the size is reduced to accommodate easily in the space created for urethral cavity without any crumpling.

A few quilting sutures are taken to fix the graft to its base and avoid any dead space (Fig. 14.1h). It helps to pre-place these quilting sutures on graft bed before starting suturing of the graft. Meatus is then closed along incision lines (Fig. 14.1i). Vagina and introitus are cleaned with saline once again. We generally keep a loose povidone-iodine-soaked vaginal pack and wrap its end around the catheter as antiseptic dressing for 1 day (Fig. 14.1j).

Peri-operative care: An 18 Fr catheter is placed and the tube is snugly anchored on the lower abdomen. We generally discharge the patient next morning. Oral antibiotics are continued for 5 days and catheter is usually kept for 2–3 weeks. We advise catheter and meatal care to all patients as a routine.

Follow-up: Follow-up is done at 3 months with uroflowmetry and post-void residue assessment. Subsequent follow-up may be decided on individual case basis.

14.2 Graft Harvest

For most young adult females, a vaginal mucosal graft can be easily harvested. It is wet, is easily available at donor site, and entails minimal donor

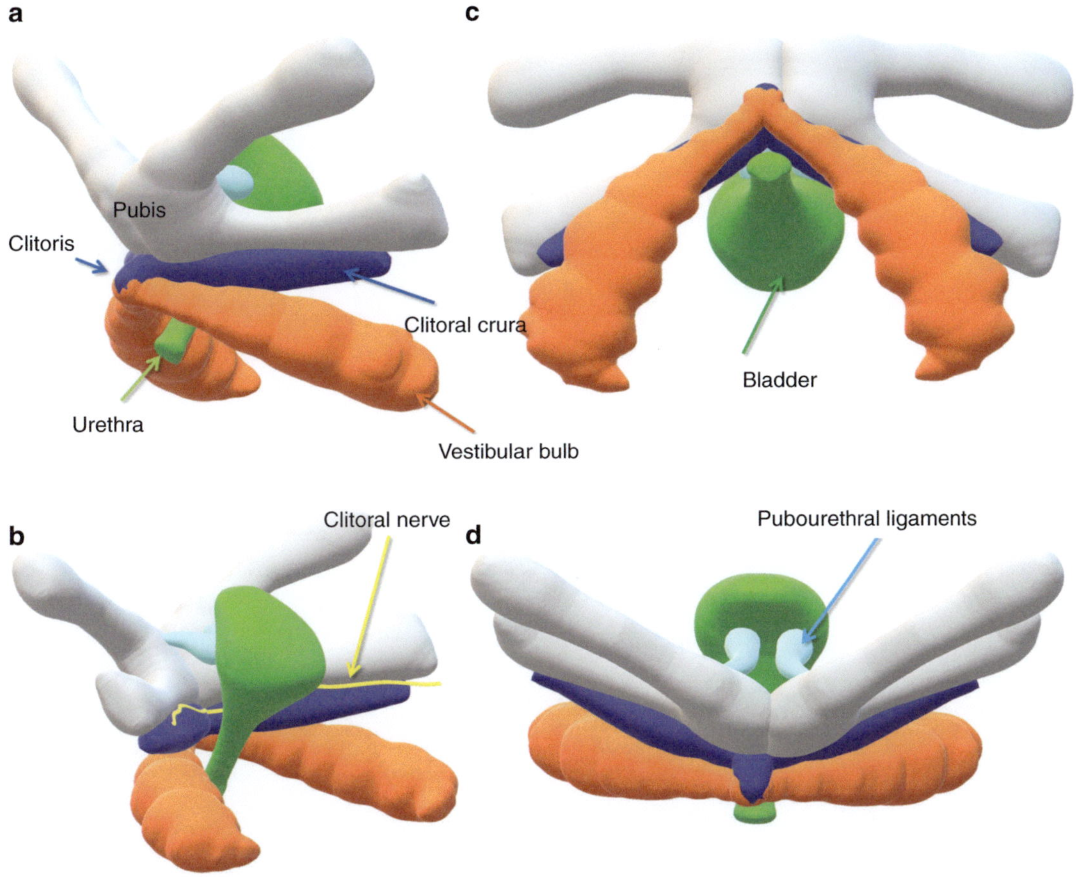

Fig. 14.2 Graphical illustration showing female urethra in relation to the clitoral anatomy. (**a**) Antero-lateral oblique view (**b**) Poster-lateral oblique view (**c**) Inferior/surgical view (**d**) Anterior view

site morbidity. The take properties of the graft are also as good as an oral mucosal graft with dense pan-laminar plexus of capillaries, though head-to-head comparison studies in this regard are lacking. Anterior distal one-third vagina is not very suitable as a donor site because mucosa here is thick and rugose. Besides, one would not like to alter the tissue planes here for any future requirement of incontinence surgeries. We prefer either middle anterior or posterior vagina to harvest the graft (Fig. 14.3). The donor site can easily be closed primarily. Skin graft from the inner aspect of labia minora is also a suitable donor site, but preferably avoided in cases of senile vaginitis or lichen sclerosus. Oral (buccal, labial, or lingual) graft is another very suitable donor site, especially in children or young females who may not accept vaginal breach or elderly with senile vaginitis.

14.3 Current Status of Dorsal Graft Urethroplasty

The use of dorsal graft approach to female urethral stricture has gradually increased over the last decade, and currently it is the most studied technique in literature. Nonetheless, the experience is limited to short case series only given the rarity of disease itself. A concise review of some

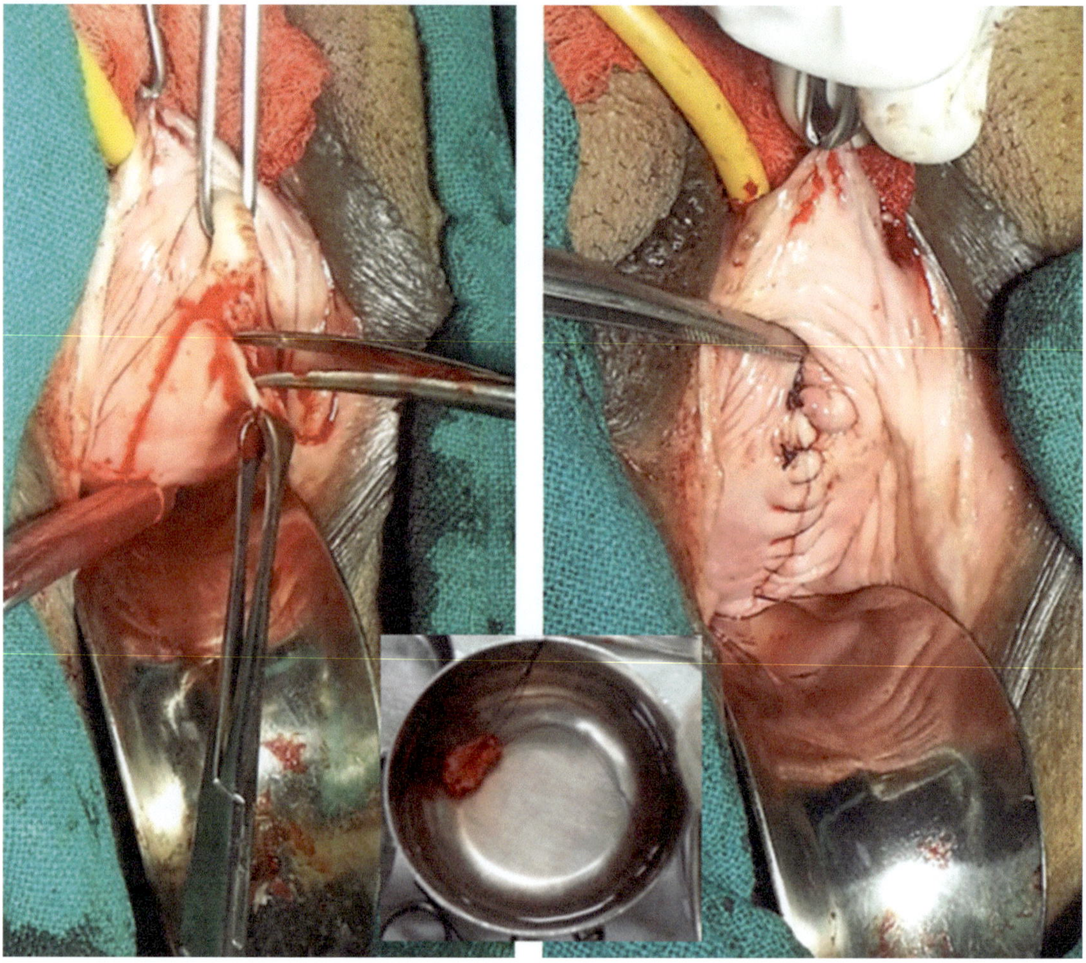

Fig. 14.3 Vaginal graft provides an easily accessible donor site for female urethral reconstruction. Distal vagina, particularly the anterior aspect related to urethra, should be avoided. We decide the graft length and width as per the stricture calibration at the time of surgery itself. A 30 Fr caliber should be obtained combining native urethral caliber with graft width. At least 5 mm additional length of graft should be taken beyond the stricture length at either end. The ends of the graft may be trimmed into an oval shape, particularly for grafts placed in mid-urethra. Meshing of graft may be done for larger grafts.

reported outcomes is given in Table 14.2. Graft lengths of 1.5–5 cm have been used for strictures of all kinds of etiologies with consistent success rates of 80% and above. No graft site morbidities have been reported. The reported follow-up remains relatively short- or intermediate-term. Post-radiotherapy strictures have typically shown poor results with graft technique.

In conclusion, dorsal onlay urethroplasty is a versatile technique which has been shown in literature to provide acceptable results for passable female urethral stricture, irrespective of length of stricture. The choice of donor site (vagina, labia, or oral mucosa) for substitution depends on the health of local tissue and hygiene. Harvesting graft from any of these local sites does not lead to functional or cosmetic problems, and all are easily available for urethral reconstruction. However, a longer follow-up should be gathered given the very limited follow-up duration in literature.

Table 14.2 Reported results from various studies of dorsal graft urethroplasty for female urethral stricture

Authors	Year	Study type	Number of cases	Urethral stricture site	Graft donor site	Follow-up (months)	Complications
Tsivian et al. [2]	2006	Retrospective	3	Distal	Vaginal/ buccal	12 (1–27)	None
Migliari et al. [3]	2006	Retrospective	3	Not specified	Buccal	6	None
Sharma et al. [13]	2009	Retrospective	15	Not specified	Lingual	12	None
Petrou et al. [14]	2012	Retrospective	11	Not specified	Vaginal	22.7 (6–46)	New onset urgency—1 Single time dilation—2 Self-daily calibration—1
Singh et al. [15]	2013	Retrospective	16	Mid	Vaginal	24.5 (6–36)	Single time dilation—1
Goel et al. [16]	2013	Retrospective	8	Mid or distal	Buccal	14.8 (3–24)	Restricture—2 (25%) at 12 and 18 months (defined as inability to pass an 18 Fr catheter)
Hampson et al. [5]	2019	Multi-institutional, retrospective	39	Distal: 6, mid-distal: 7, mid: 15, mid-proximal: 5, pan-urethral: 5	Buccal	33 (7–106)	Restricture—9 (23%) at mean of 14 months (defined as inability to pass a 17 Fr cystoscope) Incontinence—none
Manasa et al. [12]	2019	Prospective	13	Distal: 2, mid: 11	Vaginal	8.5 (6–14)	Restricture—3 (23%) by 6 months
Gomez et al. [17]	2019	Retrospective	17	Not specified (full length urethral grafting)	Buccal	15 (2–149)	Restricture—4 (23%) [2 post-radiotherapy cases] Blood transfusion—1 case (post-radiotherapy)

References

1. Barbagli G, Selli C, Tosto A, Palminteri E. Dorsal free graft urethroplasty. J Urol. 1996;155(1):123–6.
2. Tsivian A, Sidi AA. Dorsal graft urethroplasty for female urethral stricture. J Urol. 2006;176(2):611–3.
3. Migliari R, Leone P, Berdondini E, De Angelis M, Barbagli G, Palminteri E. Dorsal buccal mucosa graft urethroplasty for female urethral strictures. J Urol. 2006;176(4):1473–6.
4. Baggish MS, Steele AC, Karram M. The relationships of the vestibular bulb and corpora cavernosa to the female urethra: a microanatomic study part 2. J Gynecol Surg. 1999;15(4):171–8.
5. Hampson LA, Myers JB, Vanni AJ, Virasoro R, Smith TG 3rd, Capiel L, Chandrapal J, Voelzke BB. Dorsal buccal graft urethroplasty in female urethral stricture

disease: a multi-center experience. Transl Androl Urol. 2019;8(Suppl 1):S6–S12.
6. Joshi PM, Kulkarni SB. A new technique of double-face buccal graft urethroplasty for female urethral strictures. Turk J Urol. 2019;46(2):165–8.
7. Singh RK, Kaushal D, Khattar N, Nayyar R, Manasa T, Sood R. Pediatric pelvic fracture urethral distraction defect causing complete urethrovaginal avulsion. Indian J Urol. 2018;34(1):76–8.
8. Sawant A, Kasat GV, Kumar V, Pawar P, Tamhankar A, Bansal S, Kapadnis L, Savalia A. Reconstruction of female urethra with tubularized anterior vaginal flap. J Clin Diagn Res. 2016;10(7):PC01–3.
9. Filipas D, Fisch M, Fichtner J, Fitzpatrick J, Berg K, Störkel S, Hohenfellner R, Thüroff JW. The histology and immunohistochemistry of free buccal mucosa and full-skin grafts after exposure to urine. BJU Int. 1999;84(1):108–11.
10. Gardikis S, Giatromanolaki A, Ypsilantis P, Botaitis S, Perente S, Kambouri A, Efstathiou E, Antypas S, Polychronidis A, Touloupidis S, Sivridis E, Simopoulos C. Comparison of angiogenic activities after urethral reconstruction using free grafts in rabbits. Eur Urol. 2005;47(3):417–21.
11. El-Sayed RF, Morsy MM, el-Mashed SM, Abdel-Azim MS. Anatomy of the urethral supporting ligaments defined by dissection, histology, and MRI of female cadavers and MRI of healthy nulliparous women. AJR Am J Roentgenol. 2007;189(5):1145–57.
12. Manasa T, Khattar N, Tripathi M, Varshney A, Goel H, Sood R. Dorsal onlay graft urethroplasty for female urethral stricture improves sexual function: short-term results of a prospective study using vaginal graft. Indian J Urol. 2019;35(4):267–72.
13. Sharma GK, Pandey A, Bansal H, Swain S, Das SK, Trivedi S, Dwivedi US, Singh PB. Dorsal onlay lingual mucosal graft urethroplasty for urethral strictures in women. BJU Int. 2010;105(9):1309–12.
14. Petrou SP, Rogers AE, Parker AS, Green KM, McRoberts JW. Dorsal vaginal graft urethroplasty for female urethral stricture disease. BJU Int. 2012;110(11c):E1090–5.
15. Singh M, Kapoor R, Kapoor D, Kapoor R, Srivastav A, Chipde S. Dorsal onlay vaginal graft urethroplasty for female urethral stricture. Indian J Urol. 2013;29(2):124–8.
16. Goel A, Paul S, Dalela D, Sankhwar P, Sankhwar SN, Singh V. Dorsal onlay buccal mucosal graft urethroplasty in female urethral stricture disease: a single-center experience. Int Urogynecol J. 2014;25(4):525–30.
17. Gomez RG, Segura FJ, Saavedra A, Campos RA. Female urethral reconstruction: dorsal buccal mucosa graft onlay. World J Urol. 2019. [Epub ahead of print].

Ventral (Posterior) Onlay Augmentation Urethroplasty for Female Urethral Stricture

15

Hemant Kumar Goel, Varun Katiyar, and Varun Gunavanthe

Learning Objectives

- How to perform ventral onlay augmentation urethroplasty.
- How to choose between vaginal and buccal mucosal graft.
- How to preserve urethral meatus in this technique.
- Surgical anatomy of the approach.
- Follow-up after surgery.

Urethral stricture is an uncommon cause of voiding lower urinary tract symptoms (LUTS) in females. However, urethroplasty procedures still remain largely underutilized as unfamiliarity with female urethral anatomy, surgical procedures, lack of standardized protocols for the evaluation and management of this disease, and concerns for incontinence lead most surgeons to avoid these procedures [1–12].

Ventral onlay graft urethroplasty in female urethral stricture (FUS) is principally same as that in male and easily reproduces all principles of augmentation urethroplasty. Potential advantages are avoidance of dissection around the dorsal neurovascular bundle and predominantly dorsal sphincter complex, possibility of meatus preservation, relatively avascular field and familiarity with urogynaecologists. Potential disadvantages are theoretical possibility of urethrovaginal fistulae, creation of hypospadiac meatus (when meatus is not preserved).

Here we describe the steps of ventral onlay mucosal graft urethroplasty in female urethral stricture.

15.1 Surgical Steps: Ventral Onlay Graft Urethroplasty

15.1.1 Pre Op Preparation

Evaluation includes a baseline AUA symptom score, uroflowmetry, micturating urethrogram and urodynamic study. After documenting obstruction on this workup, we always do a urethroscopy for visual demonstration of urethral stricture (should be less than 14 Fr) within 2 weeks of definitive management.

Mucosal graft site should be decided after examination of vaginal cavity, buccal mucosa, history of tobacco exposure and consultation with patient about her preference.

Vaginal douching by 5% povidone-iodine solution is done twice daily 2 days prior to surgery. Also, any vaginal infection needs to be ruled out.

H. K. Goel (✉) · V. Katiyar
Department of Urology, Dr Ram Manohar Lohia Hospital and ABVIMS, New Delhi, India

V. Gunavanthe
Department of Urology, Bombay Hospital, Mumbai, India

N. Khattar et al. (eds.), *Female Bladder Outlet Obstruction and Urethral Reconstruction*,
https://doi.org/10.1007/978-981-15-8521-0_15

Second-generation cephalosporins are used for preoperative prophylaxis.

15.1.2 Anaesthesia

Regional anaesthesia in the form of spinal or epidural is adequate in most of the cases. Even a small buccal mucosal graft can be taken under local anaesthesia.

15.1.3 Patient Positioning and Exposure

The patient is put in a standard lithotomy with 20-degree Trendelenburg position. The labia majora is sutured to skin with silk suture; Lone Star retractor and weighted Sims speculum are used to provide adequate exposure.

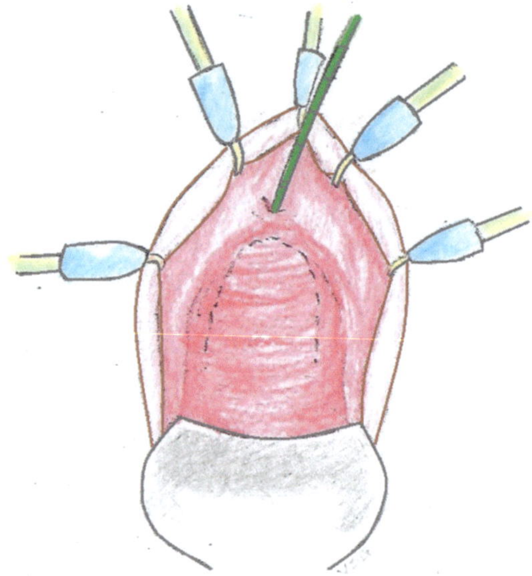

Fig. 15.1 Exposure of anterior vaginal wall with Sims speculum and Lone Star retractor. A ureteric access catheter is placed in the urethra and an inverted U-shaped incision is marked on the anterior vaginal wall

15.1.4 Stricture Re-evaluation

A pre-operative urethroscopy is performed with a 6 Fr ureteroscope taking care not to dilate the stricture site. After re-confirmation of the extent of stricture, a guidewire is passed under vision and a 5 Fr ureteric catheter is passed over it into the bladder (Fig. 15.1).

15.1.5 Incision and Raising Anterior Vaginal Wall Flap

An inverted U-shaped incision is made in the anterior vaginal wall with apex of 'U' near the urethral meatus and base till the bladder neck (Fig. 15.1). Anterior vaginal wall flap including only the vaginal mucosa is developed to access the ventral aspect of urethra.

15.1.6 Paraurethral Flap

A transverse incision is then made in paraurethral tissue and paraurethral tissue flaps are raised to expose the ventral urethra (Fig. 15.2).

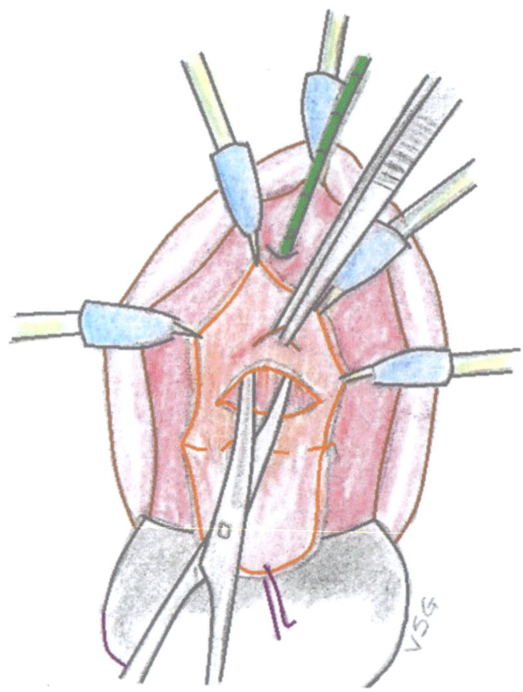

Fig. 15.2 A paraurethral tissue flap is raised after making a transverse incision. The underlying urethra is preserved

This layer is later used for quilting of graft and providing secure closure, avoiding an overlapping suture line.

The creation of paraurethral tissue flap may not be possible in all cases due to poor tissue quality in some or in distal urethral strictures where urethral and vaginal walls are more densely fused together. Alternatively, a longitudinal/linear incision on paraurethral tissue can be given. After exposure of the urethra we calibrate with a 16 Fr catheter to mark the distal extent of stricture for beginning our stricturotomy.

15.1.7 Stricturotomy

Ventral longitudinal stricturotomy is made at the 6 o'clock (on the ventral urethra, sparing the paraurethral flap) till a healthy mucosa is encountered on either end and a 30 Fr dilator is easily admissible.

Stricturotomy can be meatus-preserving or meatus-cutting depending on the location of stricture. For meatal strictures, meatotomy is necessary but the resultant meatus formed may result in a splayed urinary stream, as with any other repair. Thus, we practice the meatus-sparing approach wherever feasible (Fig. 15.3).

Three polyglactin 5–0 stay sutures are placed at the proximal healthy mucosa for easier subsequent placement of mucosal graft. A cystoscopy is now done to confirm the adequacy of stricturotomy.

15.1.8 Graft Harvest

A vaginal/buccal mucosa of sufficient length and width corresponding to the stricturotomy is harvested. For a vaginal graft, saline is injected submucosally in the posterolateral (author preference as this site is away from the operative field) wall of vagina after marking the mucosa as per the required graft size (we prefer buccal mucosa over vaginal mucosa wherever feasible and try to achieve a calibre of 26–28 Fr after augumentation) (Fig. 15.4). The underlying defect is sutured primarily with absorbable sutures after proper

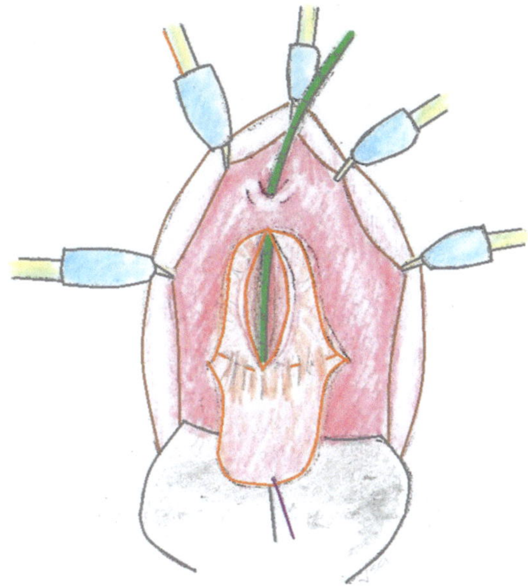

Fig. 15.3 Ventral longitudinal stricturotomy is made in the urethra keeping the overlying paraurethral flap intact (not shown in this picture)

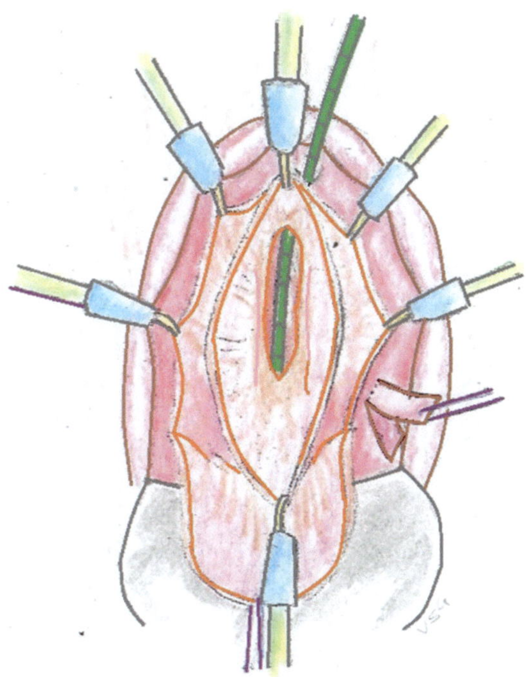

Fig. 15.4 A vaginal graft is harvested as per the dimensions of the stricturotomy. Graft is being harvested from the left posterolateral vaginal wall in this case

haemostasis. The buccal graft harvest site, when utilized, can be left open to heal secondarily. Graft is de-fattened prior to its application. Meshing of the graft is based on the surgeon's preference.

15.1.9 Graft Placement and Anastomosis

The mucosal graft is now placed and sutured to the opened urethral mucosa keeping the unmeshed graft mucosa towards the luminal side of urethra by first taking interrupted sutures from 3 preplaced sutures on the proximal urethra and then by interrupted or continuous polyglactin 5–0 suture to complete first layer of closure.

14/16 Fr Foley's catheter is then placed (Figs. 15.5 and 15.6).

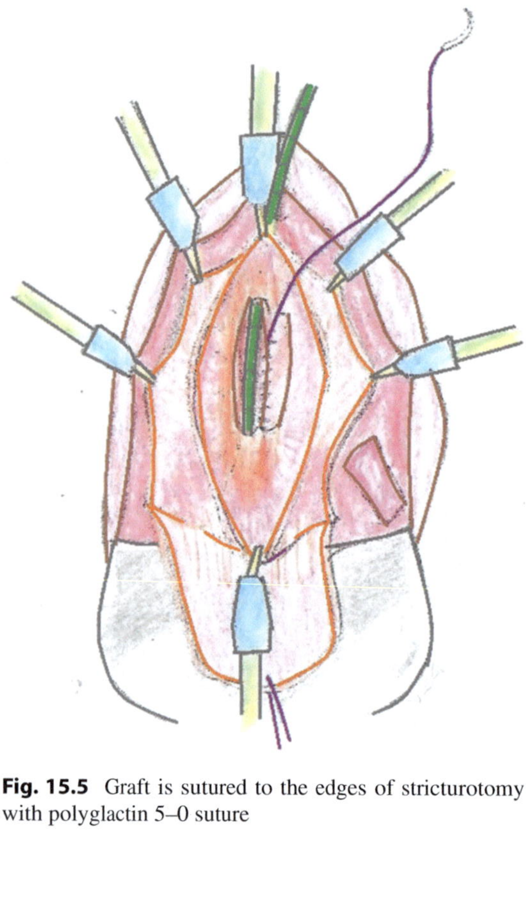

Fig. 15.5 Graft is sutured to the edges of stricturotomy with polyglactin 5–0 suture

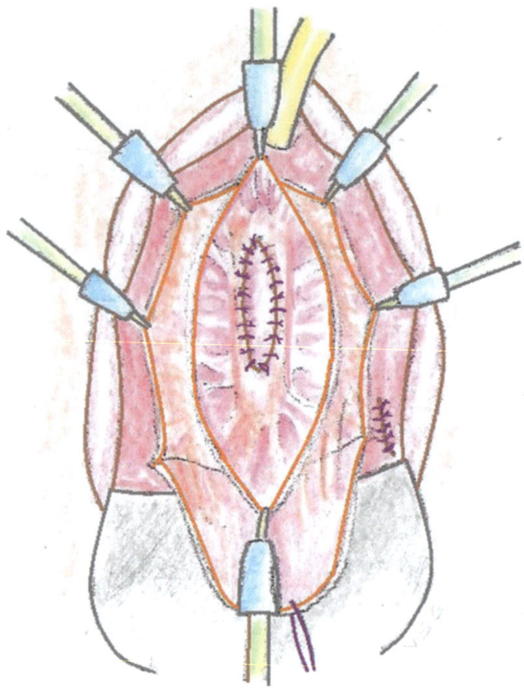

Fig. 15.6 The graft is completely sutured over a 16 Fr urethral catheter

15.1.10 Paraurethral Tissue Closure

Paraurethral tissue flap closure is done transversely over the urethra with continuous polyglactin 4–0 sutures (Fig. 15.7). This avoids overlapping of suture lines.

If paraurethral flap creation was not possible, then this layer is longitudinally closed by interrupted sutures.

Each suture takes the paraurethral tissue flap on either side and the graft tissue medially, thereby quilting the mucosal graft while closing this layer. So the paraurethral tissue will form a graft bed which is the most vascular layer.

15.1.11 Anterior Vaginal Wall Reconstruction

Anterior vaginal wall is closed with continuous polyglactin 3–0 sutures (Fig. 15.8). In the cases where the vaginal wall is atrophic, a Martius flap

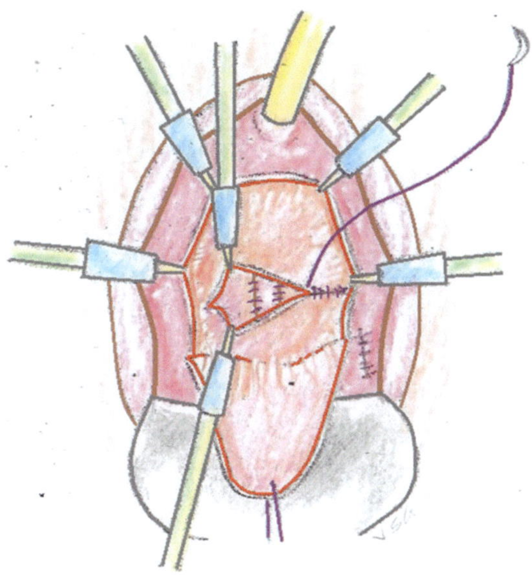

Fig. 15.7 Transverse closure of paraurethral tissue flap to cover longitudinal urethral suture lines

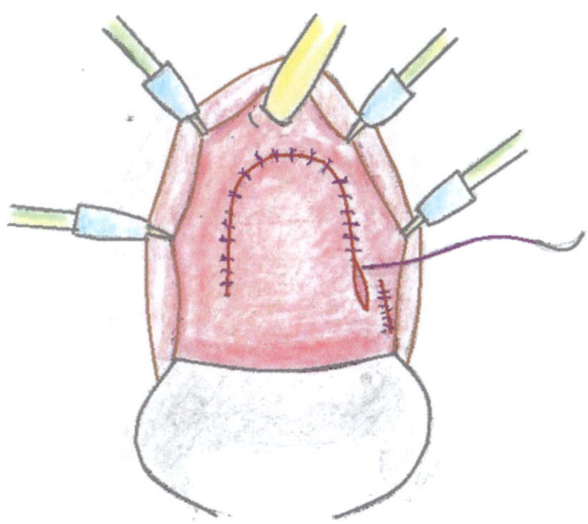

Fig. 15.8 Completed closure of anterior vaginal wall flap and posterolateral graft harvest site

is harvested and placed between the paraurethral tissues and the vaginal flap to ensure better soft tissue support, and to reduce chances of a urethrovaginal fistula.

A vaginal pack is placed, to be removed the next morning.

15.1.12 Post-operative Care and Follow-Up

The patient can be discharged on catheter on second post-operative day. Catheter is removed on post-operative day 21 after vaginal examination and ensuring healthy suture lines. She is asked to maintain perineal hygiene and avoid sexual intercourse for 3 months.

Patient is followed up by symptom assessment and uroflowmetry at 1 month, 3 months and 6 months post-surgery. Recurrence of symptoms is the most important factor for re-evaluation of these patients for stricture recurrence.

15.2 Current Status of Ventral Onlay Graft Urethroplasty

Among the largest existing descriptions of FUS management, Mukhtar et al. [13] have described their approach to ventral urethroplasty in female strictures using a similar technique. They utilized a midline incision over the anterior vaginal wall for exposure and to develop paravaginal planes. A ventral stricturotomy at the 6 o' clock, followed by the placement of buccal mucosal graft, was done. They interposed a modified Martius labial fat pad harvested over its posterior pedicle and tunnelled along the lateral vaginal wall in all cases to provide a more vascular graft bed for the graft. They reported a very good outcome in their series of 22 patients undergoing ventral onlay buccal graft urethroplasty with only 1 recurrence, thus reporting a success rate of over 95%.

In our experience, we have performed 12 cases of ventral onlay graft augmentation urethroplasty (unpublished data). The average stricture length in our series was 1.7 cm. The stricture distribution was distal in 4 patients (33%), mid-urethral in 3 (25%), involving both distal and mid-urethra in 4 (33%) and pan-urethral in 1 patient (8%). We achieved good results in majority of our patients with only one recurrence of stricture till date. There was significant improvement in post-operative uroflowmetry, symptomatology as well as preservation of sexual function post-surgery. Meatus preservation is an advantage in this approach. However, in cases the meatus is involved and needs to be incised, the ventral approach may result in a hypospadiac meatus with resultant splaying of urine. Meatus involvement is very rare in FUS and could be preserved in majority of our cases.

References

1. Malde S, Solomon E, Ockrim JL, Greenwell TJ. Female bladder outflow obstruction: an increasing but under-diagnosed phenomenon. Eur Urol Suppl. 2015;14:2.
2. Carr LK, Webster GD. Bladder outlet obstruction in women. Urol Clin North Am. 1996;23:385–91.
3. Spilotros M, Malde S, Solomon E, et al. Female urethral stricture: a contemporary series. World J Urol. 2017;35:991–5.
4. Groutz A, Blaivas JG, Chaikin DC. Bladder outlet obstruction in women: definition and characteristics. Neurourol Urodyn. 2000;19:213–20.
5. Kuo HC. Video-urodynamic characteristics and lower urinary tract symptoms of female bladder outlet obstruction. Urology. 2005;66:1005–9.
6. Waterloos M, Verla W. Female urethroplasty: a practical guide emphasizing diagnosis and surgical treatment of female urethral stricture disease. BioMed Res Int. 2019;2019:6715257.
7. Tanello M, Frego E, Simeone C, CoscianiCunico S. Use of pedicle flap from the labia minor for the repair of female urethral strictures. Urol Int. 2002;69:95–87.
8. Montorsi F, Salonia A, Centemero A, et al. Vestibluar flap urethroplasty for strictures of the female urethra. Impact on symptoms and flow patterns. Urol Int. 2002;69:12–6.
9. Blaivas JG. Vaginal flap urethral reconstruction: an alternative to the bladder flap neourethra. J Urol. 1989;141:542–5.
10. Kowalik C, Stoffel JT, Zinman L, et al. Intermediate outcomes after female urethral reconstruction: graft vs flap. Urology. 2014;83:1181–5.
11. Osman NI, Mangera A, Chapple CR. A systematic review of surgical techniques used in the treatment of female urethral stricture. Eur Urol. 2013;64:965.
12. Osman NI, Chapple CR. Contemporary surgical management of female urethral stricture disease. Curr Opin Urol. 2015;25:341–5.
13. Mukhtar MB, Spilotros M, Malde S, Greenwell TJ. Ventral-onlay buccal mucosa graft substitution urethroplasty for urethral stricture in women. BJU Int. 2017;120(5):710–6.

16 Dorsal (Anterior) Inlay Technique for Buccal Mucosal Graft for Female Urethroplasty

Arabind Panda

Learning Objectives

- To learn the surgical technique of dorsal inlay graft urethroplasty in female urethral strictures.

16.1 Introduction

The female urethra is of approximately 4 cm length, extending from the neck of the bladder to the external urethral meatus. It is elastic, with baseline diameter of about 6 mm, but should the need arise, can be easily dilated up to a diameter of 1 cm. Female urethral stricture is uncommon but causes significant morbidity in an affected individual.

16.2 Instruments Required

16.2.1 Perineal Surgery

1. Struycken nasal speculum or equivalent–blade length 90 mm [Fig. 16.1]. This speculum has thin long jaws, which are curved in the inside till the tip, increasing the working diameter, a bevelled distal segment, which improves access inside the urethra.
2. Two good needle holders (with tungsten-carbide inserts in the jaws)—7 and 8 inch. [Fig. 16.2].
3. Integrated cystoscope—14 or 17 Fr.
4. Lone Star retractor (Cooper Surgical®, 3304G) or equivalent with silicon stays.
5. Additional illumination—either a headlight or cold light using a sterile light cable.
6. Magnification—Using loupes (2.5×) is recommended.

16.2.2 For Harvesting the Buccal Mucosal Graft

1. Mouth retractor.
2. Fine scissors (5 or 6 in.).

16.2.3 Sutures Required

1. Polydioxanone (PDS-II®) 4–0 monofilament with 17 mm, taper point ½ circle needle—for fixation of the graft and quilting.
2. Silk 3–0/2–0 as stay sutures.

16.2.4 Miscellaneous

1. Inj. Lignocaine (2%) with adrenaline (1:100,000).
2. Marking pen.

A. Panda (✉)
Urology and Renal Transplantation, Krishna Institute of Medical Sciences, Secunderabad, Telangana, India

N. Khattar et al. (eds.), *Female Bladder Outlet Obstruction and Urethral Reconstruction*,
https://doi.org/10.1007/978-981-15-8521-0_16

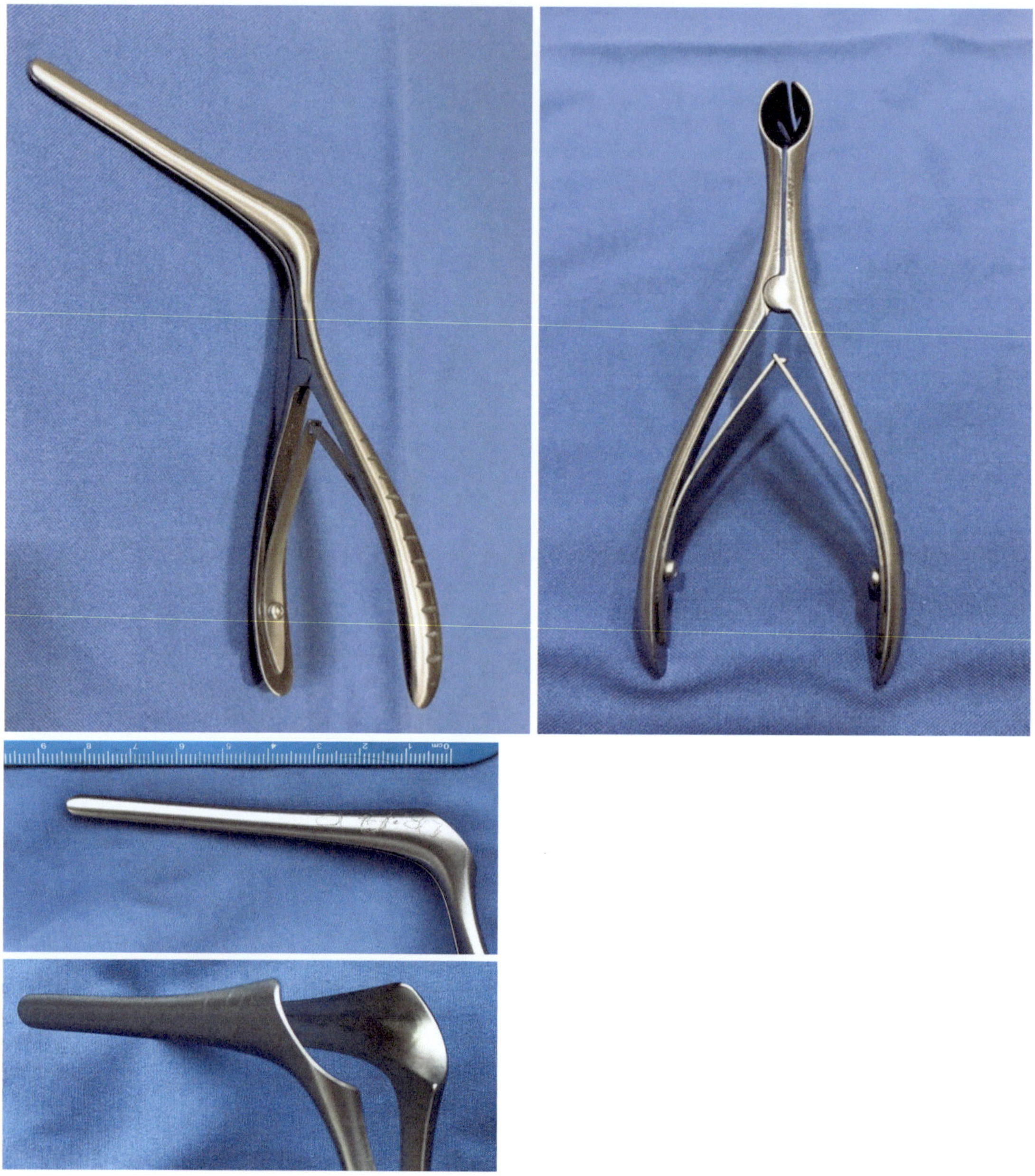

Fig. 16.1 Struycken nasal speculum—blade length 90 mm. (**a**) Struycken nasal speculum—thin long jaws, which are curved in the inside till the tip, increasing the working diameter, a bevelled distal segment, which improves access inside the urethra

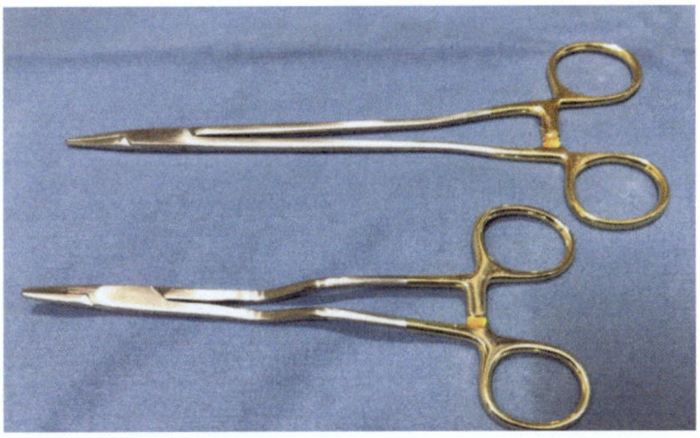

Fig. 16.2 Needle holders. One with a broad tip and other with a narrower tip

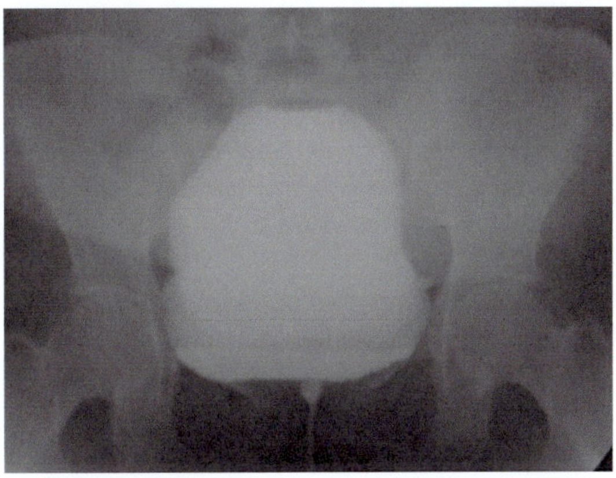

Fig. 16.3 Micturating cystourethrogram showing a long segment stricture

16.3 Pre-operative Evaluation

Preoperatively, it is important to document the stricture with a micturiting cystourethrogram (Fig. 16.3) and cystoscopy. A uroflowmetry with a post void residual urine provides a pre-operative baseline. While it is not essential to perform urodynamics before surgery and prove bladder outlet obstruction, the results of the surgery may be suboptimal in patients with an underactive detrusor. It helps in the pre-operative counselling and is not a reason to deny them the procedure.

If the patient is on regular urethral dilatation or intermittent self-calibration, she is advised to stop urethral dilatation 2 months before the surgery to enable more accurate delineation of the stricture segment [1].

Urine culture is essential and if there is a urinary tract infection, it must be treated before surgery. In the event of growth of Pseudomonas or beta haemolytic Streptococcus, it is best to defer surgery until the subsequent urine culture is documented to be sterile [2, 3].

In case of a sterile urine culture, prophylactic antibiotics are used for 48 h, starting on the day of surgery. Any systemic disease must be optimized, in particular Type 2 diabetes mellitus. Informed consent must be documented.

16.4 Surgical Technique

The patient is placed in the lithotomy position with the pressure points well padded. A silicone gel sheet is place under the gluteal and sacral area for more optimal distribution of pressure.

As an initial step, stay sutures are placed on the external meatus at 11 and 1 o' clock positions. A guidewire is placed through the stricture into the bladder.

With a sharp blade (surgical scalpel blade no. 11), the urethra is incised at the 12 o' clock from the inner mucosal surface [Fig. 16.4]. The nasal speculum is inserted after the initial incision and opened to visualize the inner dorsal/anterior surface of the urethral mucosa. The incision is made

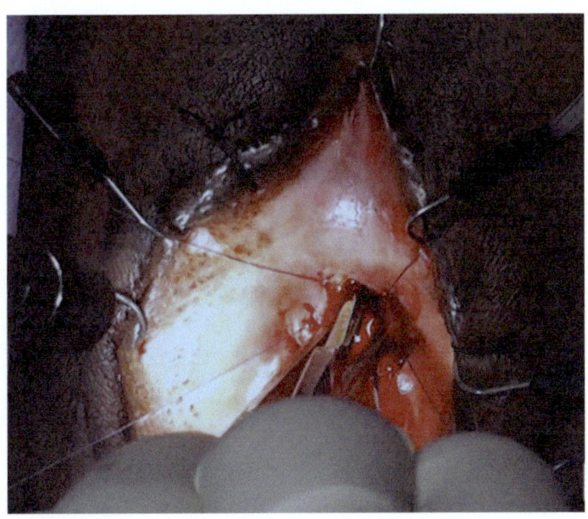

Fig. 16.4 The initial incision into the dorsal urethra from the inside. Note the stay sutures

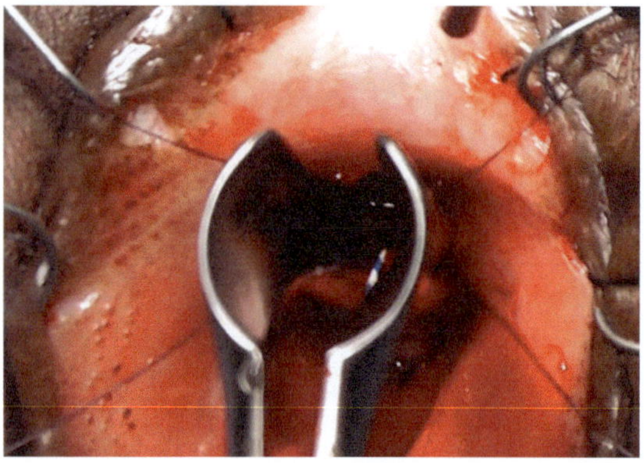

Fig. 16.5 The speculum is inserted into the incised urethra and opened

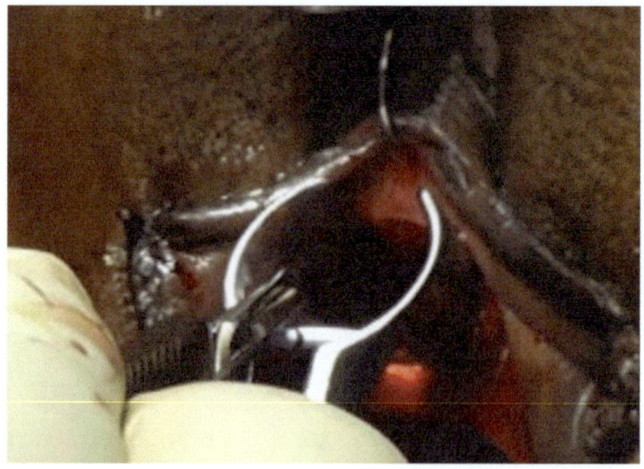

Fig. 16.6 The urethra is further incised in segments under vision to well beyond the stricture. Urethroscopy before extension of the incision with an integrated scope is mandatory to avoid injury to the bladder neck

in short segments. The female urethra is very vascular, and it is best to place stay sutures after each extension of the incision. The stay sutures keep the urethra open increasing exposure, reduce bleeding, and improve vision. The incision is then deepened full thickness. Opening the nasal speculum helps to incise the dorsal inner mucosal surface under vision. It gives an excellent view of the incised urethra and the proximal bladder neck (Fig. 16.5).

The female urethra lacks landmarks (unlike the male urethra with the verumontanum) and it is easy to inadvertently extend the incision to beyond the bladder neck. It is therefore vital to perform urethroscopy each time the dorsal incision is extended proximally. The incision is carefully extended to 0.5–1 cm beyond the stricture (depending on the location of the stricture) but just short of the bladder neck (Fig. 16.6). It is imperative to visualize the normal mucosa well beyond the incised segment. In general, it is better to err on the side of caution and extend the incision well beyond the stricture segment to prevent recurrence. As long as the bladder neck is intact, we have not observed any case of post operative urinary incontinence after urethroplasty.

The urethral edges are spread away from the midline by opening of the speculum and minimal additional sharp dissection from inside the urethra. No dissection is done around the urethra, the dorsal and lateral surfaces not being detached from the surrounding tissue. This preserves the vascular supply from the top and sides and avoids injury to the clitoral bodies and neurovascular bundles that traverse close to the dorsal urethral surface.

A needle with a ski configuration is required for placing the initial five sutures. A normal 17-mm ½-circle needle is straightened in the middle to produce the ski needle [Fig. 16.7]. We prefer to place five sutures (compared to the conventional three) at the proximal end of the incision and slide the defatted buccal graft inside. Placing five sutures ensures that the graft does not warp or fold at the apex as this can adversely affect graft take. A monofilament suture is essential to be able to parachute the graft into the apex of the incision.

Five 4–0 PDS-II sutures are placed using a ski needle in an outside-in fashion using the reverse Webster technique; one at the apex of the incision, 2 each on either side (Fig. 16.8). The reverse Webster's technique to place a suture at the depth of the incised urethra requires two needle holders. The modified needle (17mm, 1/2 circle) is held as shown in Fig. 16.9 with an extended wrist. The needle is inserted into the required area, flexing the wrist in the process. As the tip of the needle protrudes into the lumen, it is grabbed by the second needle holder, which is then pushed forward towards the bladder (while holding the needle) to bring the suture out of the

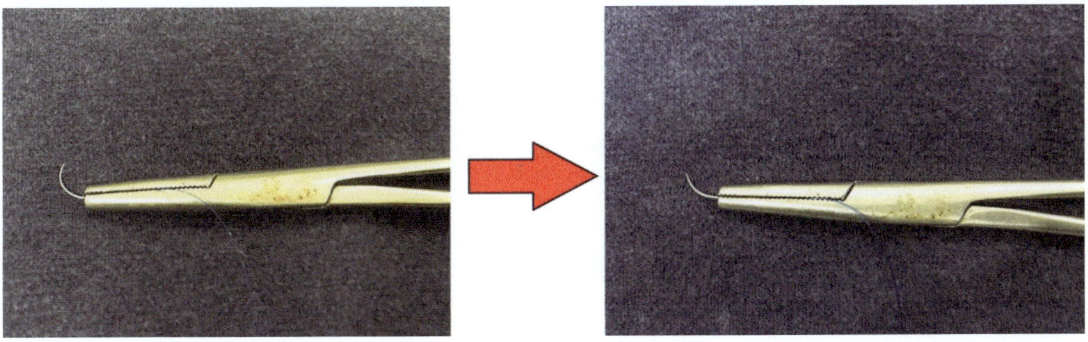

Fig. 16.7 Making a ski needle - the proximal curve of the needle is straightened, keeping the distal curve intact

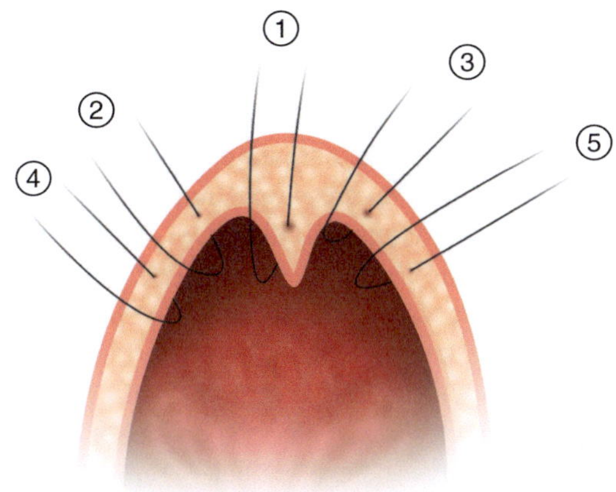

Fig. 16.8 Placement of the five apical sutures. The reverse Webster technique is used to place them proximal to the cut urethra

urethral wall and then it is withdrawn out of the urethra [Fig.16.9].

The buccal mucosal graft is then harvested from one of the cheeks. A mouth retractor is placed on the side opposite to site of graft harvest. Stay sutures are placed on the cheek and on the graft to provide traction and counter traction during the harvesting process. We take care to mark the Stenson duct and the area to be harvested before incising into the buccal mucosa. It is imperative to have sufficient width and length of the graft so that it is enough to augment the incised urethral segment. After the initial superficial marking incision, the area is infiltrated with 2% Lignocaine and adrenaline and the incision deepened till the Buccinator muscle. The graft is defatted and placed in saline. The team harvesting the graft must be isolated from the team performing the perineal surgery as the mouth is relatively unsterile. Exchange of instruments between the two teams is to be discouraged.

A defatted buccal mucosal graft of appropriate size is inserted in the pre-placed monofilament sutures (Fig. 16.10). It is then parachuted inside with its tip sutured with the apical stich and the other four sutures on either side. The edges are then sutured to the sides of the urethra and the graft quilted to fix the graft and also to achieve haemostasis. It is important to quilt extensively (Fig. 16.11) to prevent the graft moving and to prevent any haematoma in bed in the post-operative period. Fenestrating the graft is optional and we do not routinely do it.

The distal end of the graft is tailored and fixed to the vestibular mucosa with interrupted sutures and a18 Fr silicon catheter is placed in the bladder (Fig. 16.11) and fixed on the abdomen. We augment the entire incised segment, including the meatus with the graft. The meatus is therefore much wider than before. We believe that attempts to reduce the size of the meatus can result in a smaller breadth of graft with the inlay technique. A paraffin gauze dressing is applied on the graft and held in place with sutures. A pack soaked with povidine-iodine is placed in the vagina and removed after 24 h. A drain is not necessary.

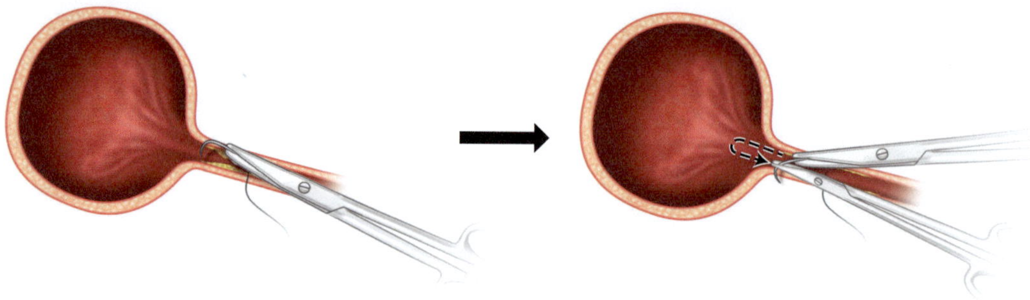

Fig. 16.9 The reverse Webster's technique to place a suture at the depth of the incised urethra. Note the path of the second needle holder (dotted line)

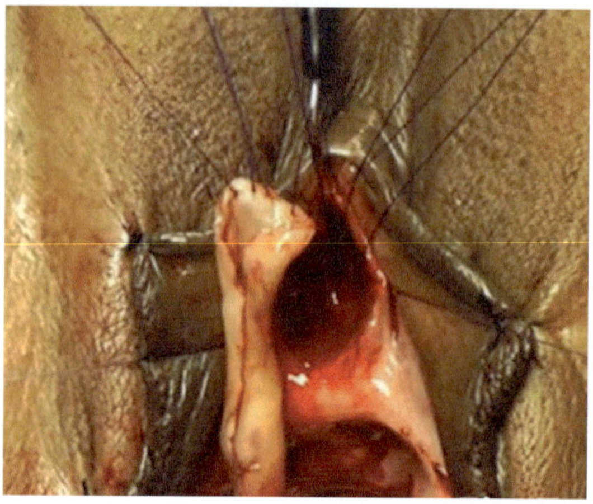

Fig. 16.10 The defatted graft is inserted in the pre-placed monofilament sutures and parachuted into the incised urethra

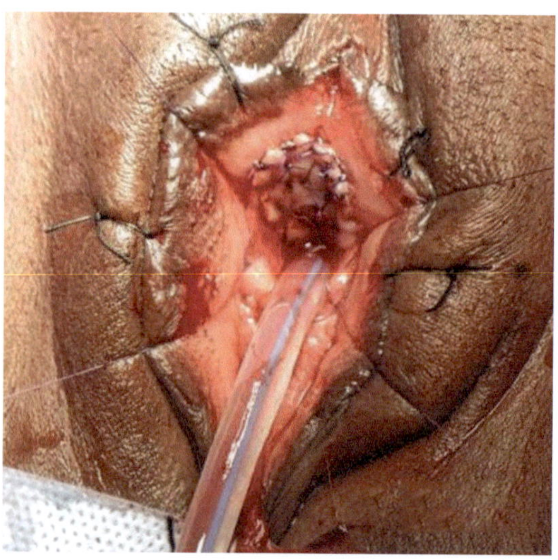

Fig. 16.11 The quilted graft with the catheter at the end of the procedure

16.5 Follow-Up

The patient is discharged after 48 h. All patients are followed up in the outpatient department after 2 days. The paraffin dressing is removed, and the catheter is refixed on the abdomen. The graft is inspected periodically (if needed cleaned regularly with a saline/flush) and the patient is instructed to keep the area clean. A urine culture (catheter sample) is done after 2 weeks and the patient is treated with culture specific antibiotics starting 3 days before catheter removal and 2 days after it. The catheter is removed at 3 weeks.

She is followed up with 6 monthly uroflowmetry and post void residual urine estimation. If the Q_{max} drops below 15 mL/s, a urethral calibration with an 18-Fr Foley catheter is done.

16.6 Advantages of the Dorsal Inlay Technique

A dorsal inlay technique has significant advantages. It avoids circumferential dissection and preserves the blood supply with resultant less ischemia. The extensive nerve supply around the urethra and clitoris is better preserved as the dissection is from inside the urethra. Careful complete incision of the strictured segment with cystoscopic confirmation prevents inadvertent injury to the bladder neck and incontinence. The incision of the urethra and subsequent lateral spreading ensures an adequate lumen. The highly vascular base ensures a good take of the buccal mucosal graft.

Compared to a ventral placement of graft; there is no chance of a urethrovaginal fistula. Furthermore, if needed in the future, subsequent incontinence procedures (a mid urethral sling) can be undertaken ventrally.

16.7 Our Experience

We have done 14 cases of dorsal inlay urethroplasty till date with a maximum follow-up of 6 years. Twelve of the 14 continue to void well with a Q_{max} above 15 mL/s without subjective voiding lower urinary tract symptoms. One patient with an underactive detrusor had recurrence of stricture. She was offered redo urethroplasty but preferred to be on periodic redilatation.

References

1. Terlecki RP, Steele MC, Valadez C, Morey AF. Urethral rest: role and rationale in preparation for anterior urethroplasty. Urology. 2011;77(6):1477–81.
2. Wilson GR, French GW, Sully L. Loss of split thickness skin grafts due to non-group a beta-haemolytic streptococci. Ann R Coll Surg Engl. 1988;70(4):217–9.
3. Høgsberg T, Bjarnsholt T, Thomsen JS, Kirketerp-Møller K. Success rate of split-thickness skin grafting of chronic venous leg ulcers depends on the presence of Pseudomonas aeruginosa: a retrospective study. PLoS One. 2011;6(5):e20492. Epub 2011.

Ventral (Posterior) Inlay Technique for Female Urethroplasty

17

Prasant Nayak and Swarnendu Mandal

Learning Objectives
- Surgical technique of Ventral Inlay Graft Urethroplasty in Female Urethral Strictures.
- Pros and cons of ventral inlay technique.

17.1 Introduction

Female Urethral Stricture has been a hitherto-ignored and largely undiscussed topic in urological literature. Many women with primary urethral strictures and some with lower urinary tract symptoms have been subjected to indiscriminate use of periodic urethral dilatation. These practices can result in urethras having reasonable calibers developing iatrogenic secondary strictures and ultimately the patient becomes dependent on regular periodic dilatation.

Of late, many urologists have taken a keener look into female patients with complaints of lower urinary tract symptoms with a focus on accurate diagnosis of genuine primary and iatrogenic strictures and have managed to develop ingenious surgical techniques to deal with this disease. The details of these diagnostic modalities and other surgical techniques are detailed elsewhere in this book. We limit ourselves to the description of Ventral Inlay Buccal Mucosal Graft Urethroplasty (VIBMGU), first described by Hoag et al. [1]. The technique aims to simplify the approach by avoiding periurethral dissection, thereby avoiding the putative risks of sphincteric injury and urethro-vaginal fistula formation.

17.2 Preoperative Evaluation

The most important diagnostic test in a case of suspected female urethral stricture is the inability to successfully calibrate the urethra with a 12 Fr Foley's catheter [2] and is confirmed on cystoscopy. It is also essential to rule out a neurogenic bladder and we largely rely on the assessment of symptoms of neurogenic dysfunction with a focused neurologic examination, reserving urodynamic testing if the initial assessment and examination flags these patients for the presence of neurogenic dysfunction. Patients who are deemed candidates for surgery are assessed for their oral hygiene as is routine prior to harvest of oral mucosa in any case of buccal mucosal graft (BMG) urethroplasty. A baseline uroflowmetry, renal function test and ultrasonogram (USG) for post-void residue and upper tract changes are done. Micturating cystourethrogram is a minimally invasive test, which gives images that corroborate with stricture disease. Though it is not

P. Nayak (✉) · S. Mandal
Department of Urology, All India Institute of Medical Sciences, Bhubaneswar, Odisha, India
e-mail: urol_prasant@aiimsbhubaneswar.edu.in; urol_swarnendu@aiimsbhubaneswar.edu.in

N. Khattar et al. (eds.), *Female Bladder Outlet Obstruction and Urethral Reconstruction*,
https://doi.org/10.1007/978-981-15-8521-0_17

confirmatory of stricture, still it gives an idea of the location of the stricture. Urodynamic study, though not mandatory before surgical management, if it is available, it could be performed to rule out a hypocontractile urinary bladder and give overall baseline bladder function.

A patient with symptoms of obstructive voiding, confirmed to have a genuine stricture on calibration and without features of neurogenic dysfunction, is further assessed for anesthetic fitness and consent is obtained for VIBMGU. A suitable antibiotic (second or third generation Cephalosporin) is started on the morning of surgery and continued for 3–5 days post-operatively.

17.3 Surgical Technique

Intraoperatively, cystoscopy is done with a pediatric cystoscope to confirm the diagnosis. The site and the length of the stricture is confirmed. The strictured/unhealthy mucosa is identified by its whitish color as compared to pink normal/healthy mucosa. Also, the caliber gives only an indirect evidence of unhealthy mucosa. A 20 Fr urethra is generally considered healthy and a caliber below 12 Fr is considered unhealthy. The goal of urethroplasty is to achieve a native urethral size of around 16–24 Fr.

A hydrophilic guide wire is passed through the urethra and coiled in the urinary bladder. The urethra is now progressively dilated to just allow insertion of a nontoothed forceps across the urethral length. The entire length of strictured urethral mucosa and periurethral tissue is then incised at 6 o' clock position with an 11-number blade (Fig. 17.1a) until the urethral caliber is widened enough to allow a nasal speculum (Fig. 17.1b) to be inserted. Free opening of the nasal speculum can even be considered an objective sign that fibrous tissue has been incised adequately. Cutting is restricted to the periurethral tissue as cutting any deeper would lead to cutting of the entire urethra and vaginal wall, leading to fistulation. However, we feel that a significant thickness of periurethral tissue exists ventrally and it would be a gross surgical misstep to land in a ventral urethra-vaginal fistula while performing VIBMGU.

Hemostasis is achieved with sparse use of bi-polar cautery. Now the incised urethral bed (Fig. 17.1a) is ready for placement of the buccal mucosal graft, which is generally harvested from a single cheek, never exceeding 4 cm in length (depending on the stricture length). A rectangular graft with an approximate length 2 cm larger than the stricture length and with a width of approximately 1.5 cm is chosen. The normal 5–0 PDS needle (Fig. 17.1c) is straightened as shown in Fig. 17.1d, akin to the Turner-Warwick needle used for placing deep proximal urethral stitches. This maneuver of straightening the needle helps in taking stitches at the proximal end of the incised urethra, to fix the buccal mucosa. The buccal mucosa is fixed to the urethra at four points, two at the proximal edge (Fig. 17.1e) of the incised urethra and two mirrored sutures at the external meatus (Fig. 17.1f). Additional stitches are taken laterally, if necessary (Fig. 17.1f). Quilting is generally not required, however can be taken distally. Bipolar cauterization to minimize ooze from the graft-bed eliminates the need for quilting.

Final appearance of the buccal mucosa attached to the bed is as shown in Fig. 17.1g. A 16 Fr silicon Foley's catheter is placed to drain the bladder and provide extrinsic compression for the buccal mucosa on to the urethral bed.

Ventral inlay can be performed even for pan-urethral strictures; however, the proximal stitches have to be taken from the bladder neck, which is a bit difficult. However, the J-shaped needle and the Turner-Warwick technique of needle holding, as is done for tackling the proximal end of the urethra in a pelvic fracture associated urethral distraction defect (PFUDD), makes this suturing feasible.

Post-operative oral rehabilitation is similar to any other case involving BMG harvest.

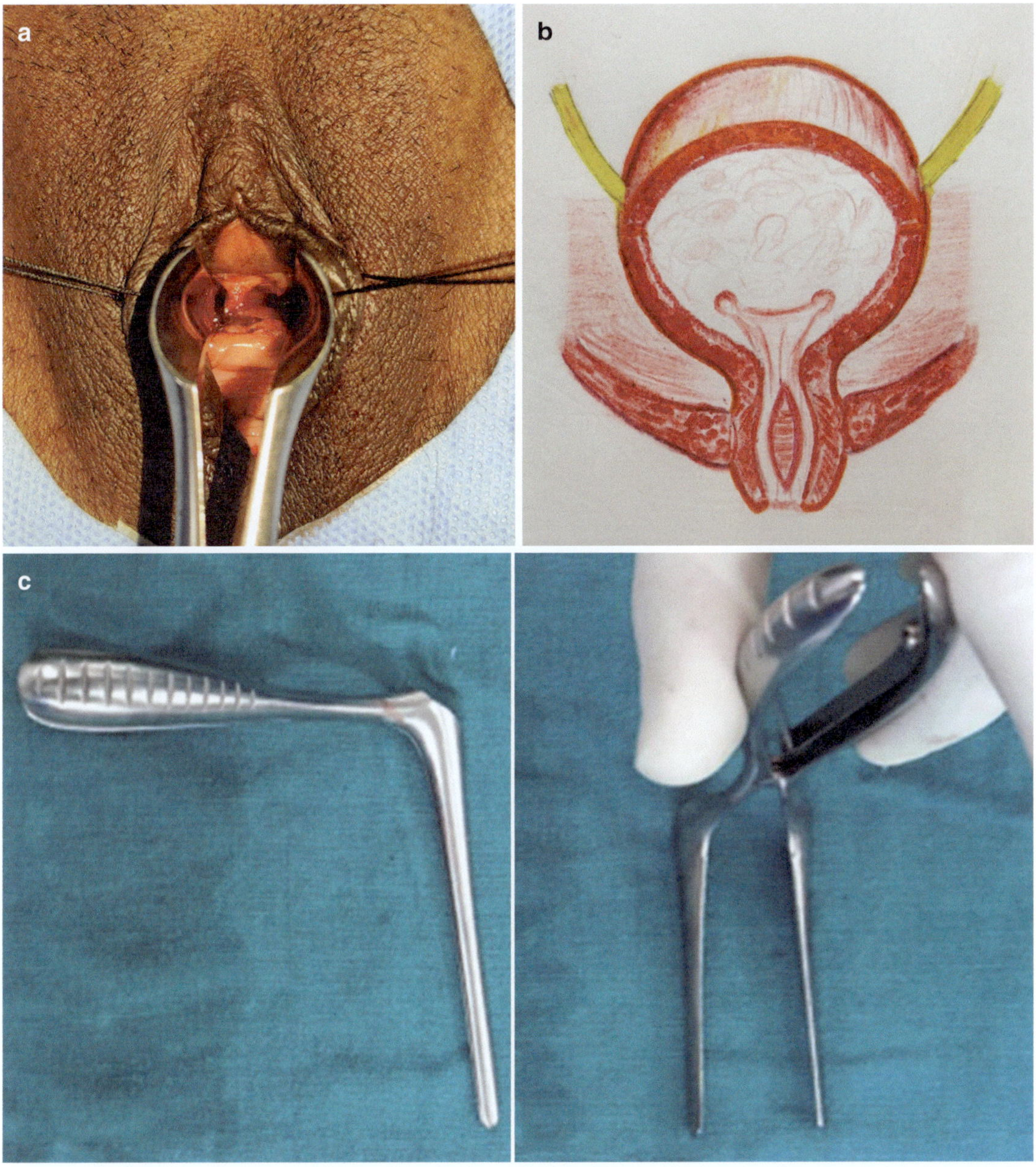

Fig. 17.1 (**a**) Urethra after incision of stricture, (**b**) illustrative diagrams of the urethra after incision of stricture, (**c**) nasal speculum, (**d**) normal needle, (**e**) Curved needle, (**f**) buccal mucosa with proximal two sutures, (**g**) illustrative diagrams of the buccal mucosa with proximal two sutures, (**h**) after fixing the buccal mucosa distally to the bed, (**i**) final appearance of the buccal mucosa attached to the bed

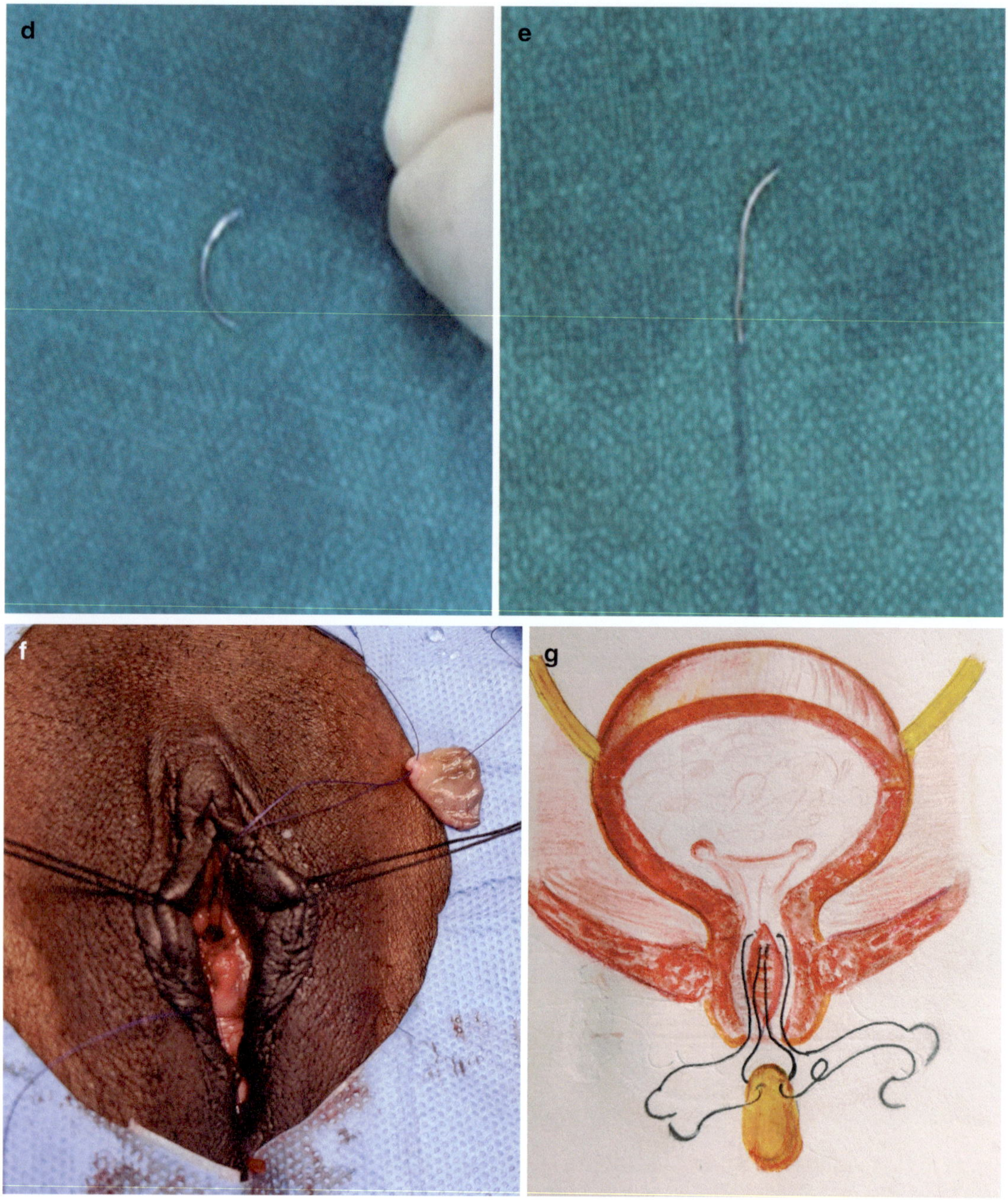

Fig. 17.1 (continued)

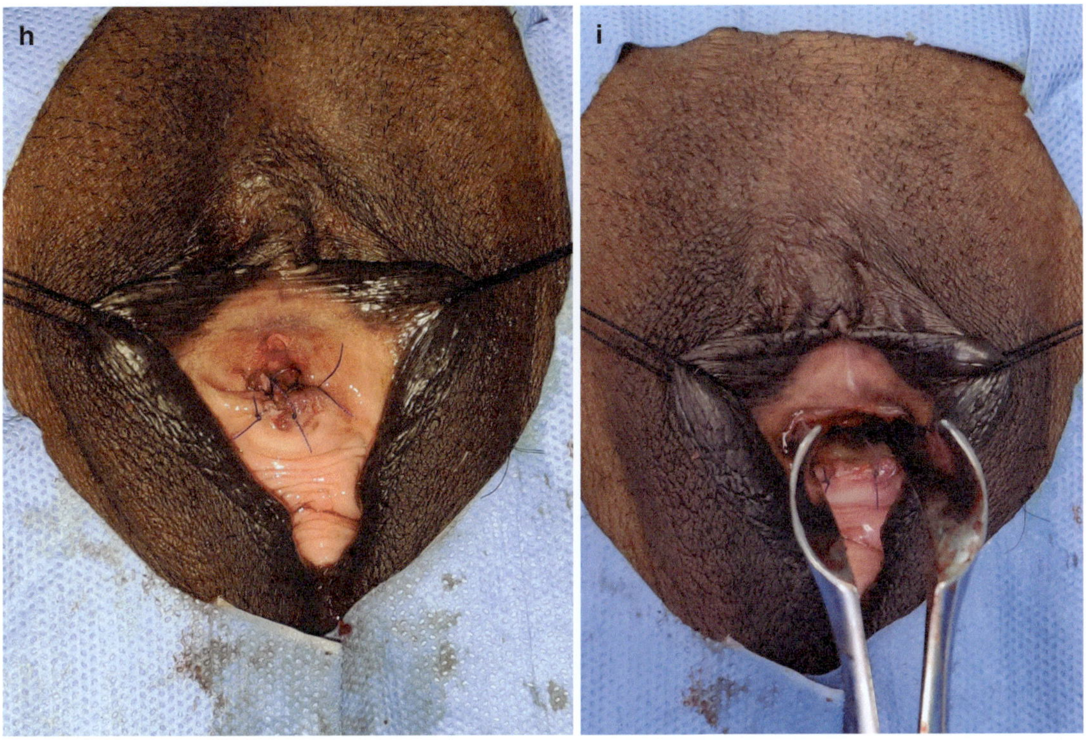

Fig. 17.1 (continued)

Catheter removal is done after 1 month. Uroflowmetry and USG for post-void residue is obtained after a week to ascertain good flow and completeness of voiding.

17.4 Follow-Up

The follow-up protocol includes uroflowmetry and ultrasonography for measurement of post-void residue every 3 months for the first year and annually thereafter for 3 years. Further follow-up visits would be dictated by the presence of symptoms.

17.5 Results

In our case series of 19 cases, the length of the stricture varied from 1 to 4 cm. While nine had distal urethral, six had distal and midurethral stricture, and four had a pan-urethral stricture. Stricture etiology was inflammatory in 11 women and iatrogenic in 8 women. Two women had recurrence of symptoms in our series of 19 cases. One of them had a proximal recurrence due to inadequate proximal reach of the graft and the other had an undiagnosed underactive detrusor. Therefore, failure of the technique to ameliorate the stricture was seen in one woman. She was treated by urethral dilatation followed by institution of a self-dilatation regimen and is doing well in follow-up.

17.6 Limitations of Ventral Inlay Technique

Taking the proximal stiches are at times difficult and possibly needs a little experience with the procedure to gain confidence.

The bevelled Killian's nasal speculum is a useful additional instrument required in the armamentarium for ventral inlay.

Meatus always needs incision in inlay techniques irrespective of stricture site and length.

References

1. Hoag N, Gani J, Chee J. Vaginal-sparing ventral buccal mucosal graft urethroplasty for female urethral stricture: a novel modification of surgical technique. Invest Clin Urol. 2016;57:298–302.
2. Nayak P, Mandal S, Das M. Ventral inlay buccal mucosal graft urethroplasty for female urethral stricture. Indian J Urol. 2019;35(4):273–7.

Labial and Vaginal Flaps for Female Urethroplasty

18

Divakar Dalela and Ravi Lohani

Learning Objectives

- To introduce the reader to various procedures for female urethral reconstruction using local genital and periurethral tissues and their expected outcomes.
- To familiarize with the selection process for using local tissues for female urethral reconstruction to enable individualization for each situation.

18.1 Introduction

Female urethral stricture (FUS) is described as a fixed anatomical narrowing between the bladder neck and urethral orifice [1]. The first-line treatment consists of dilatation but the long-term cure rates are disappointing [1, 2]. The relative rarity of the disease, the lack of experience and the fear of urinary incontinence usually preclude urologists from performing female urethroplasty. This chapter attempts to review the preoperative evaluation plan and to provide an insight into the surgical techniques and outcome of various flaps used for the reconstruction of FUS. Many surgeons prefer using buccal mucosal grafts in similar situations. The selection of graft vs. flap is largely based on operator experience.

D. Dalela (✉) · R. Lohani
Department of Urology, King George Medical University, Lucknow, India

18.2 Clinical Assessment

In women with symptoms of bladder outflow obstruction, a detailed genito-pelvic examination followed by calibration with a 14 Fr urethral catheter should be the first step. In absence of a strict definition of normal calibre of female urethra, the ability to pass a 14 Fr urethral catheter in a well-relaxed adult lady is a reliable way of excluding urethral stricture that might deserve a surgical reconstruction.

Overall, a detailed preoperative evaluation to ascertain site, length, degree of narrowing of stricture; health of vestibular and vaginal tissues (e.g. lichen sclerosus, post-menopausal changes and genital prolapse); co-associated local complications like infection; co-associated urinary complications like back pressure changes must be taken a note of before contemplating surgery using cysto-urethroscopy, retrograde and voiding cystourethrography, uroflowmetry, urodynamic evaluation and measurement of post-void residual urine volume.

Lichen sclerosus could significantly impact decision making as it alters the quality of genital tissues to be used for reconstruction. The prevalence of lichen sclerosus is 1.7% in general gynaecological practice [3]. It may result in resorption of labia minora, entrapment of clitoris and in extreme cases may even cause obliteration of vaginal introitus resulting in problems with micturition and intercourse. An extensive litera-

N. Khattar et al. (eds.), *Female Bladder Outlet Obstruction and Urethral Reconstruction*,
https://doi.org/10.1007/978-981-15-8521-0_18

ture search and our own experience do not consider lichen sclerosus as a cause of female urethral stricture disease. However, caution need to be exercised while undertaking reconstruction in these patients as usage of perigenital tissues may result in failure.

The palpation of urethra through anterior vaginal wall gives an insight into the adequacy of vaginal access, degree of urethral fibrosis, quality of vestibulo-vaginal and juxta-urethral tissues that might be utilized for urethral reconstruction.

18.3 Preoperative Counselling

An idea about the age of the patient, degree of sexual activity, concern for genital cosmesis and freedom of genital violation allowed to surgeon must be obtained from every patient. Use of vaginal flaps could concern unmarried females. Similarly, possibility of temporary dyspareunia should be explained to a sexually active female if a vaginal flap is planned. This may be of concern to a lady with higher degree of sexual activity (Fig. 18.1).

In patients where surgical reconstruction is going to involve caliber, positioning and direction of the external urinary meatus, its influence on her urinary stream and its likely direction must be discussed with the patient.

By the time the patients become candidate for reconstruction, they have already undergone one or two dilatations. The poor outcome as well as repetitiveness of that compels them to accept urethral reconstruction [1]. Some patients even after reconstruction may need self-dilatation for some time after the surgery [1]. Therefore, this must be talked about beforehand.

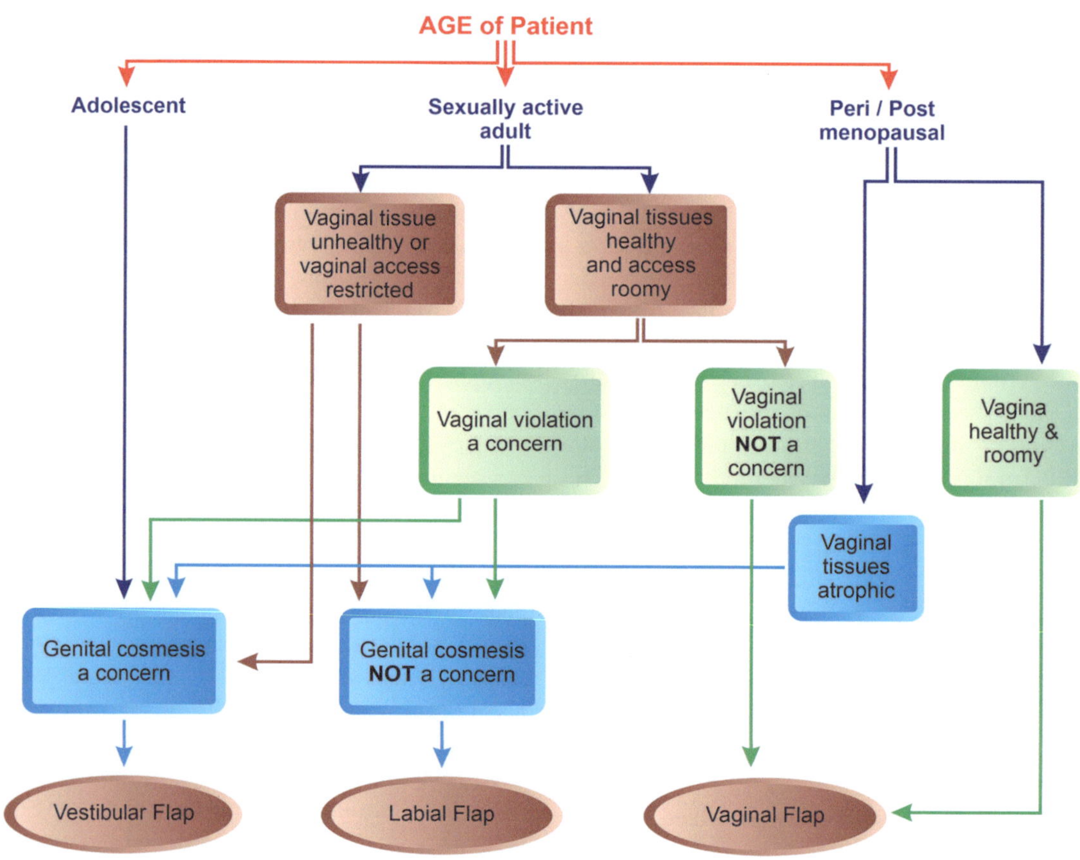

Fig. 18.1 Systematic approach for choice of flap according to age, sexual activity and post-menopausal status

18.4 Preoperative Preparation

Any coexisting vaginal infection must be meticulously treated and the reconstructive surgery should be deferred till it is resolved.

In post-menopausal women, topical oestrogens used preoperatively have a role in promoting vaginal health [4]. Topical oestrogens are generally prescribed for a period of 6 weeks preoperatively, but their role in the post-operative period is unclear.

18.5 Surgical Techniques of Flap Urethroplasty

Flap urethroplasty techniques have demonstrated short-term efficacy and safety and, therefore, are preferred for most female urethral strictures that have failed dilatations. Vaginal and labial flap urethroplasty techniques have a mean success rate of 91% [5]. Certain basic things must be remembered before undertaking them

1. The flap will contract with healing in due course, depending upon patient's own healing characteristics. Thus, to obtain durable results, mobilization of a generous flap is paramount.
2. During surgery, preservation of a substantial vascular supply retains tissue viability and may also affect delayed contraction. The surgical planning must focus on this.
3. The most popular and established flap techniques include vaginal wall flaps. The few appealing plus points of local vaginal wall flaps are that they are naturally wet, elastic, well vascularized, freely mobile and abundantly available. Furthermore, use of the vaginal wall has the lowest morbidity of any flap-based procedure. The vestibular flaps are evolving and long-term results are awaited.

Figure 18.2 shows various sites from where the flaps can be harvested.

18.5.1 Anterior Vaginal Wall Flap (Blandy Flap)

An inverted U-shaped incision is made in the anterior vaginal wall, keeping the tip of flap just below the urethral meatus [1, 2, 6–8] (Fig. 18.3a). The flap is sharply dissected away from the posterior urethral wall for about 3 cm, preserving its sub-mucosal vascular supply (Fig. 18.3b). The ventral side of urethral meatus and the urethra are incised with Pott's scissors until healthy proximal urethral mucosa is recognized. Pass a 20 Fr catheter to see adequacy of urethrotomy. Stay sutures, placed on both edges of the opened urethra, improve the exposure. The tip of U flap is sutured to the proximal part of the opened urethra with three interrupted polygalactin sutures, keeping the mucosal surface inside the urethra (Fig. 18.3c). The edges of the flap are subsequently sutured to the edges of opened urethra using continuous sutures on both sides up to the external meatus (Fig. 18.3d). The remaining base of the flap is utilized for local closure of the vaginal wound.

Anterior vaginal wall flaps can be used in case of meatal strictures or short (<2 cm) distal urethral strictures. The meatus must be involved in stricture process as this procedure involves mandatory meatus splitting. This method is fairly simple and also allows placement of slings if required [6].

Blaivas et al. [9], in a series of 10 patients who underwent anterior vaginal flap urethroplasty, demonstrated a success rate of 80%. The mean duration of follow-up was 53 months. Five women in the cohort also had concomitant pubovaginal sling procedure. The two women who developed recurrence were managed by buccal mucosal graft urethroplasty and were stricture free subsequently.

Gormley et al. [10] published similar results in his series of 12 stricture patients with a success rate of 83% and mean duration of follow-up of

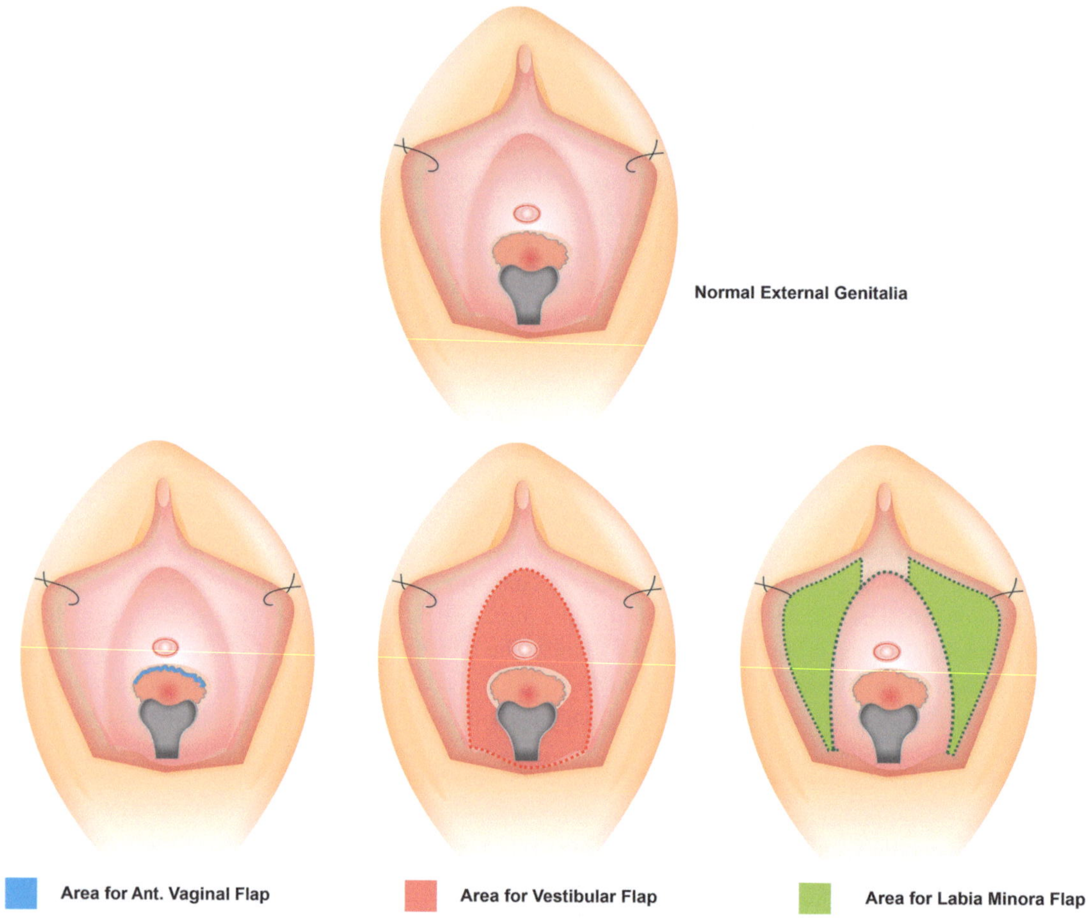

Fig. 18.2 Sites from where various flaps used for reconstruction of female urethral stricture are harvested

30 months. Two women had concomitant pubovaginal sling surgery.

Onol et al. [11] demonstrated 100% success rate with anterior vaginal flap urethroplasty in his cohort of 10 patients with mean follow-up of 36 months.

However, in our experience, the anterior vaginal wall flap mostly results in retrusive meatus, an inwardly directed urinary stream, which, in turn, creates vaginal voiding and irritation (Fig. 18.4).

18.5.2 Vestibular Flap (Montorsi Flap)

An inverted Y incision is made in the vestibular mucosa on the anterior side of the external meatus [12] (Fig. 18.5a). The distal urethra is dissected away from the adjoining anterolateral periurethral tissues but without accessing the posterior urethrovaginal plane (Fig. 18.5b, c). Once the anterior urethral wall is exposed sufficiently, a midline anterior urethral incision is made (Fig. 18.5d). The strictured urethra is opened until healthy proximal urethra is visible. A urethroscopic examination at this stage is useful. Stay sutures are placed on both edges of the opened urethra to improve the exposure. According to the length of stricture, a 1.5–3 cm long and 1-cm wide vestibular flap is mobilized from the right or left side by extending the vestibular incision as shown in Fig. 18.5e. The tip of the flap is sutured to the proximal end of the urethrotomy slit with three separate absorbable sutures (Fig. 18.5g). The edges of the flap are subsequently sutured to the edges of the opened

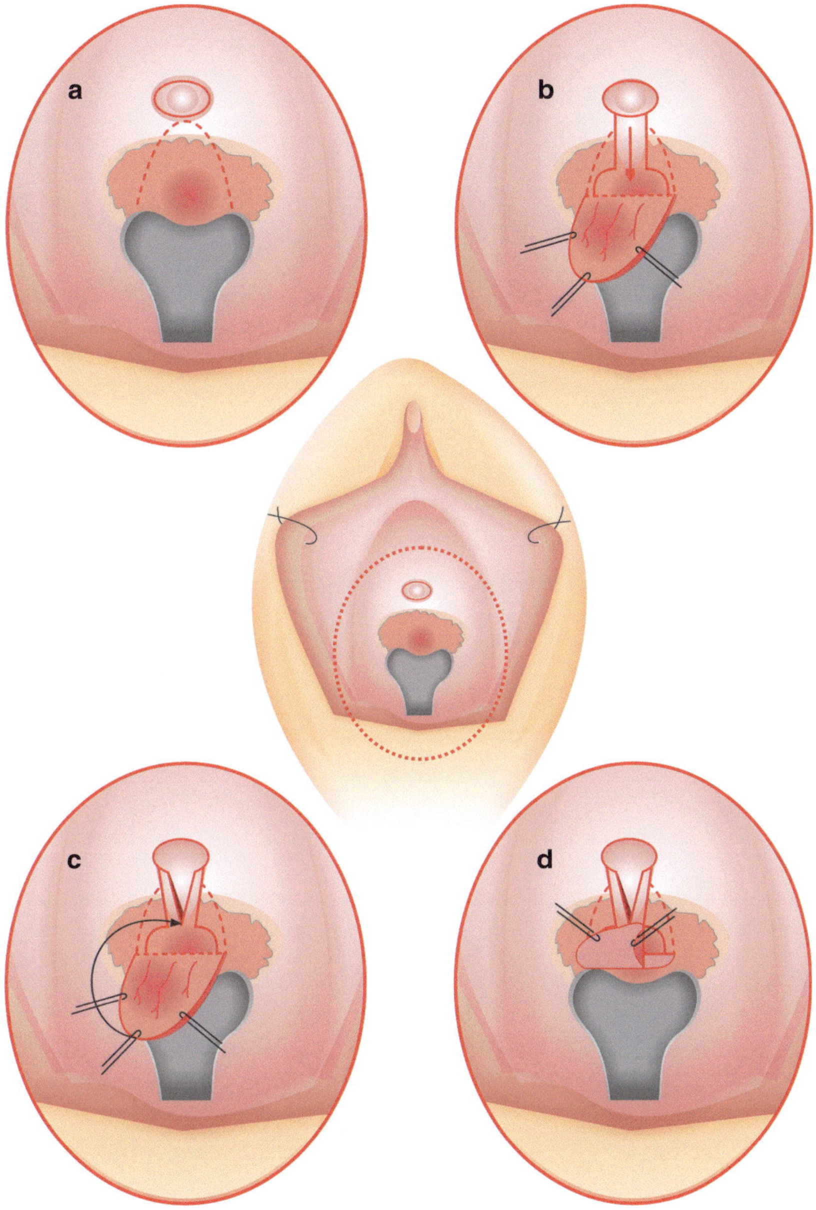

Fig. 18.3 Blandy anterior Vaginal wall flap (**a**) An inverted U-shaped incision made in the anterior vaginal wall; (**b**) vaginal wall flap is dissected off from the posterior urethral wall; (**c**) the posterior wall of urethra is incised at 6 o' clock position till healthy proximal urethral mucosa is visualized; (**d**) the tip of the U-shaped flap is sutured to the proximal cut end of the urethra and the lateral edges to the corresponding edges of the incised urethra

urethra using continuous sutures (Fig. 18.5h). Rest of the flap is rotated appropriately to achieve local closure of the vestibular mucosa with interrupted sutures.

Montorsi et al. [12] performed vestibular flap urethroplasty in a cohort of 17 patients with distal urethral or meatal strictures. At 12-month follow-up, 15 patients demonstrated sustained relief of symptoms while 2 patients developed recurrence.

In our view, the vestibular flap has the disadvantage of spraying and antero-lateral deflection of the urinary stream. Also, it is not suitable for strictures >2 cm or more proximal strictures.

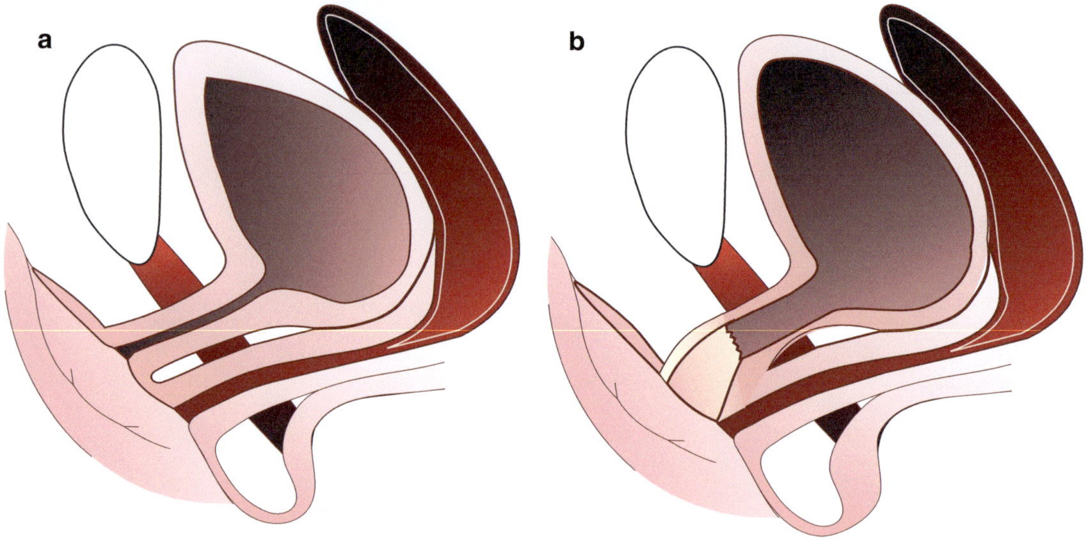

Fig. 18.4 (**a**) Normal central female urethra; (**b**) posteriorly directed urethra in case of vaginal flap

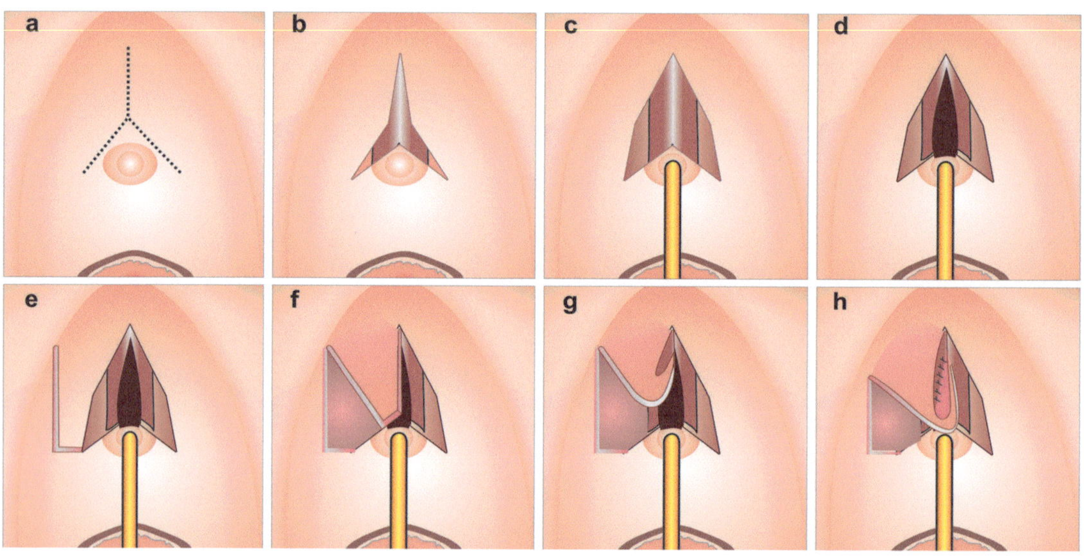

Fig. 18.5 **Montorsi Flap** (**a**) An inverted Y shaped incision made anterior to urethral meatus; (**b**, **c**) distal 3 cm of the urethra dissected free from the surrounding tissues from 3 o' clock to 9 o' clock position; (**d**) the dissected urethra incised longitudinally at 12 o' clock position with scissors; (**e**, **f**) vestibular flap mobilized from right side; (**g**, **h**) the tip of the flap is sutured to the proximal end of the incised urethra and each lateral margin to the cut edges of urethra

18.5.3 Lateral Vaginal Wall Flap (Orandi Flap)

A slightly curved C-shaped incision is made in the anterior vaginal wall [8, 13] (Fig. 18.6a). A guide wire or a thin infant feeding tube kept through the urethra helps in urethral identification. The posterior side of urethra is carefully dissected and the urethra is opened at the level of stricture (Fig. 18.6b). The stricture is slit open, both proximally and distally, along the guide wire until healthy proximal urethra is visible. A 2 cm wide island of vaginal wall with length and breadth adjusted according to the gap noted in

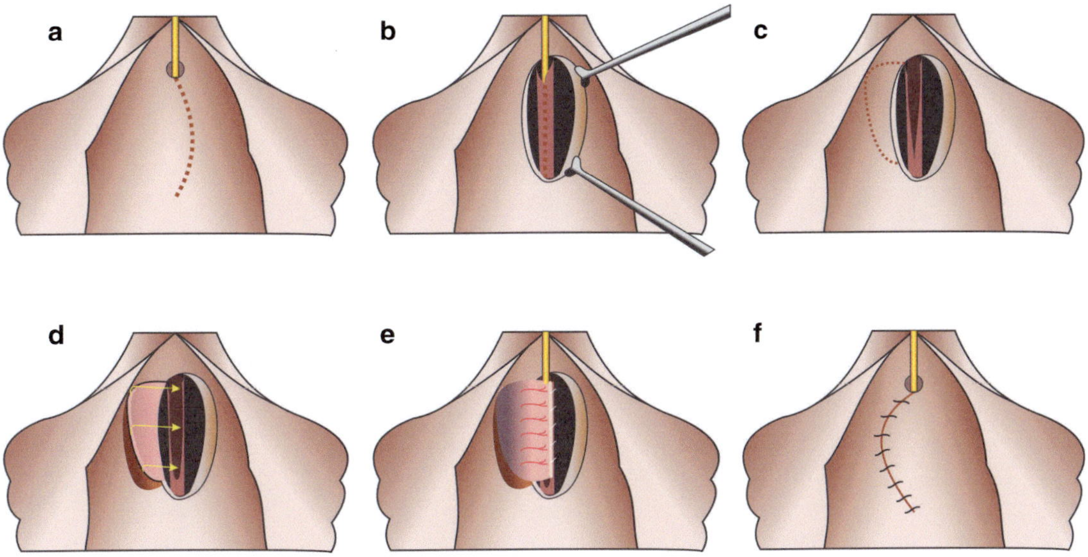

Fig. 18.6 **Orandi Flap** (**a**) A "C"-shaped incision is given on the anterior vaginal wall; (**b**) flap raised laterally; (**c**) urethra incised ventrally; (**d**) medial margin of the flap is sutured to the ipsilateral margins of the incised urethra; (**e**) lateral margins of the flap sutured to the contralateral margins of the incised urethra; (**f**) vaginal defect is closed with interrupted sutures

opened urethra is harvested from the lateral side (Fig. 18.6c). Medial to the flap, the dissection is performed along the peri-urethral plane. Laterally, the dissection is carried along a much superficial submucosal plane to create a lateral vascular pedicle. The mobilization of this pedicle should be sufficient enough to allow the mucosal island to be turned and sutured into the opened urethra (Fig. 18.6d). The medial surface of the flap is sutured with the ipsilateral side of the urethra. The mucosal surface of the flap is turned inwards towards the urethral lumen and the initial lateral side of the mucosal island is sutured to the contralateral side of the urethra (Fig. 18.6e). The lateral vaginal defect is closed with interrupted or continuous sutures (Fig. 18.6f).

The success of this flap depends upon the pliability, thickness and overall health of vaginal wall. Tension on the contralateral urethro-vaginal suture line must be guarded by adequate mobilization.

Simonata et al. [14] used the Orandi flap in a series of 6 patients with a mean follow-up of 58.5 months. All the females had good flow with none complaining of de novo incontinence postoperatively.

This procedure can be used for midurethral strictures where meatus is normal as meatus splitting is not essential in this technique.

18.5.4 Labia Minora Flap

A pedicled island flap from inner labia minora can also be used for reconstruction of distal strictures. First, the urethra is exposed through an incision in the anterior vaginal wall, separating the vagina from the urethra via periurethral dissection [15] (Fig. 18.7a). A vertical rectangular island of inner portion of labia minora skin is created (Fig. 18.7b). The breadth and length of island may be adjusted as per the length and calibre of stricture. An ipsilateral urethrotomy slit is made from the meatus to healthy, nonfibrotic urethra (Fig. 18.7b, c). Two stay sutures are placed on the upper edge of flap, which is meant to go into the proximal end of urethrotomy slit (Fig. 18.7d). The mobilized island of the labia minora is rotated through a tunnel created underneath the vaginal wall to the urethra by dragging the two aforesaid stay sutures (Fig. 18.7e, f). This island derives its vascularity from underly-

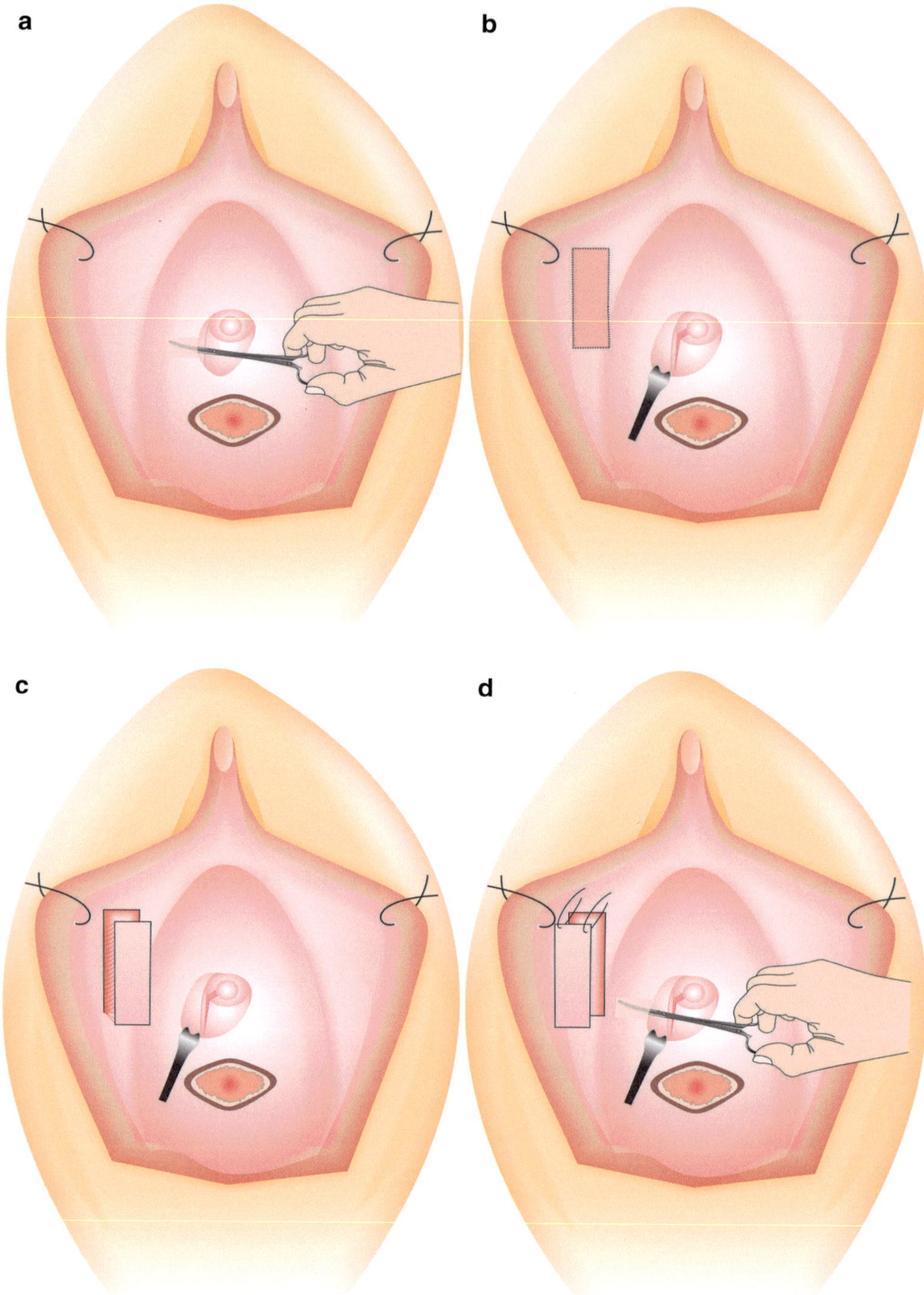

Fig. 18.7 Labia Minora Flap (**a**) Urethra exposed through incision in the anterior vaginal wall; (**b**) lateral urethrotomy done from meatus to healthy non-fibrotic urethra and site of flap marked on the inner side of labia minora; (**c**) the rectangular island flap is dissected off the surrounding tissues; (**d**) two stay sutures applied on the upper edge of the flap and a tunnel is created underneath the vaginal wall to the urethra; (**e, f**) the island flap is dragged through the tunnel by holding these stay sutures; (**g**) the tip of the flap is sutured to the tip of the urethrotomy slit; (**h**) the lateral edges of the flap are sutured to the corresponding edges of the urethrotomy slit

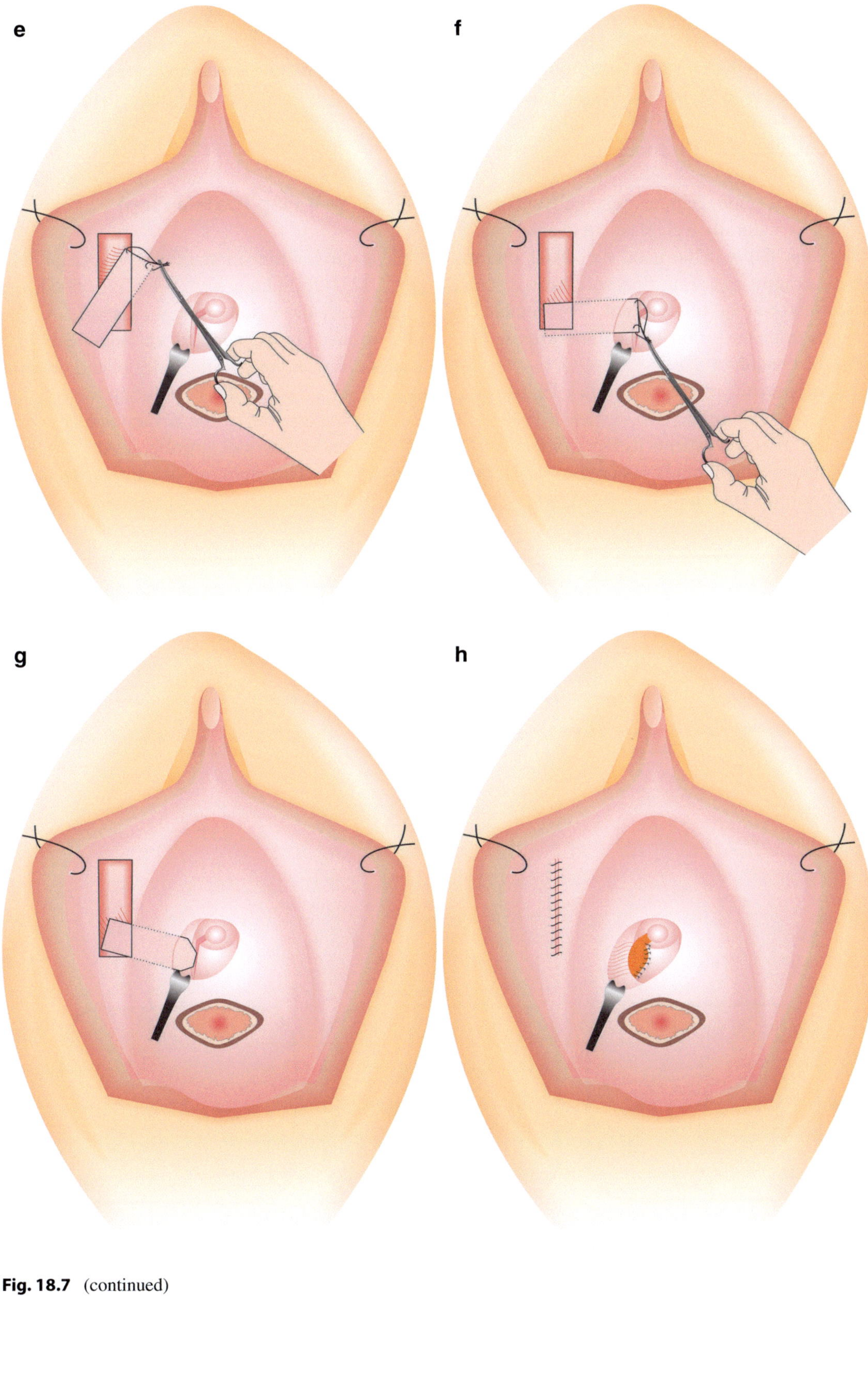

Fig. 18.7 (continued)

ing undefined soft tissue, so care must be exercised in maintaining its supply. The flap is sutured to the edges of the urethrotomy, with the epithelial surface toward the urethral lumen and the vaginal wall closed (Fig. 18.7g, h). The labial defect is closed with continuous subcuticular sutures.

The labia minor flap has many advantages. It is hairless, naturally wet, elastic and easily available. This flap can be used for distal urethral strictures only as a long flap will have vascular compromise at the tip. It is not very suitable for patients who have thin labia minora as it may limit the breadth of flap.

Tannello et al. [15] used the pedicle labia minora flap for urethroplasty in two women with urethral strictures. Both the patients had satisfactory micturition stream with normal cystourethrography findings in subsequent follow-up visits.

Our experience with this flap is not very pleasant as the flap necrosed in the small subset of patients in whom we used it. Since the vascularity of this flap is not very well defined, the delayed contraction of this flap is inevitable.

18.5.5 W-V Flap (Dalela Flap)

This is our modification of the vestibular flap [16]. This technique has been described for totally occlusive distal urethral strictures. A 'W' shaped area is demarcated on the vestibular mucosa in front and on the sides of the urethral meatus, with base of the W pointing towards the clitoris and each half of the W descending nearly 2.5 cm on either side of the urethral orifice (Fig. 18.8b). This marking is incised, deepened and flaps are raised as two separate and indepen-

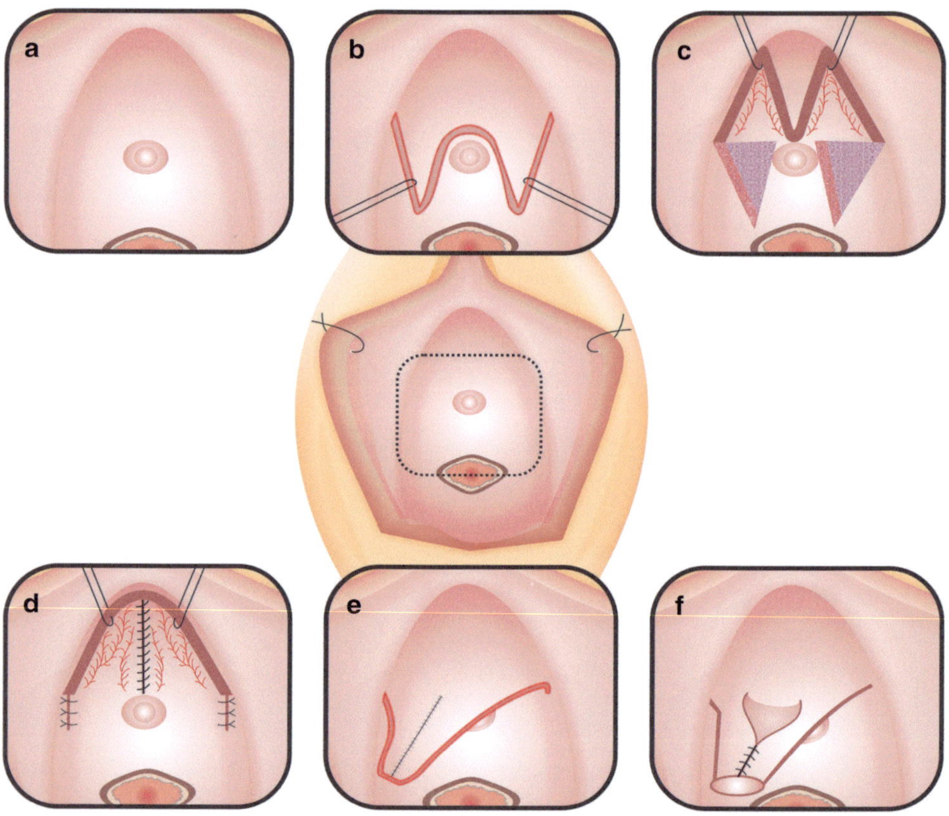

Fig. 18.8 **Dalela W-V Flap** (**a**, **b**) W-shaped incision is marked in front and on sides of the urethral meatus; (**c**) two separate V-shaped flaps raised; (**d**) medial margins of these V-shaped flaps sutured converting W into V-shaped flap; (**e**, **f**) tip of the W-shaped flap anastomosed with the spatulated urethra and the remaining flap tubularised creating a neourethra

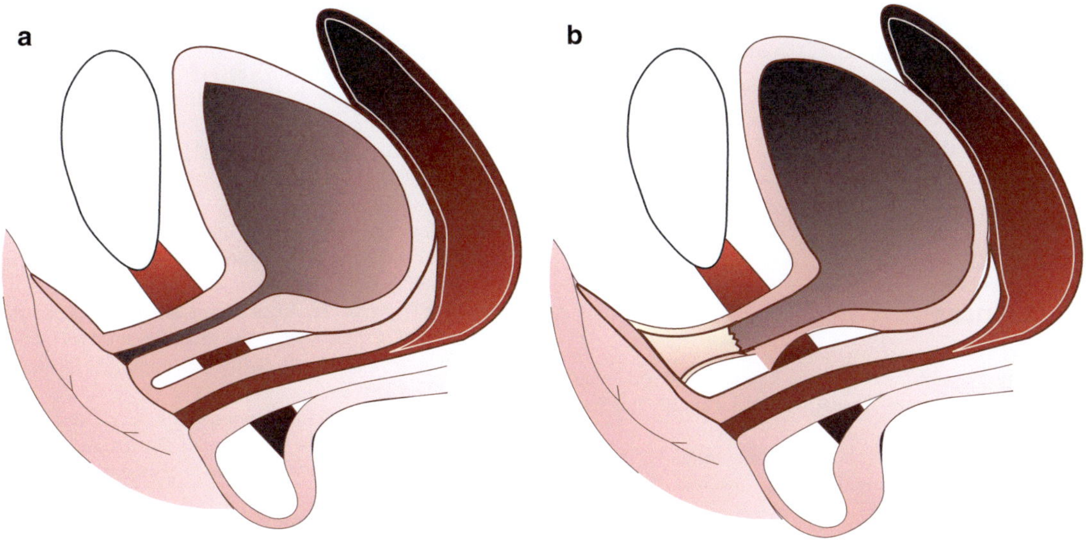

Fig. 18.9 (**a**) Normal central anteriorly directed female urethra; (**b**) anteriorly directed and centrally located urethra in case of Dalela W-V flap

dent V-shaped flaps on either side sequentially (Fig. 18.8c). The lips of the external meatus are grasped and the distal 2 cm of the urethra is circumferentially dissected in the periurethral plane. A curved metallic bougie is passed through the suprapubic tract and guided into the urethra antegradely proximal to the stricture. The urethra is opened posteriorly over the tip of the bougie and two stay sutures are placed on the edges of the healthy urethra at 5 o' clock and 7 o' clock locations. After this, the rest of the urethral circumference is excised. The medial edges of both the flaps are approximated by continuous sutures, thus converting the 'W' to 'V' (Fig. 18.8d). A small dorsal slit is given in the urethra at 12 o' clock location for spatulation. The tip of the V flap is approximated to the edge of the spatulated urethra and the remaining circumference of the distal urethra. The remaining flap is tubularized, keeping the mucosal inwards, to create a neourethra (Fig. 18.8f).

This method is useful only for distal urethral strictures less than 2.0 cm but simple to perform and does not create any donor site morbidity. It may be used either as a dorsal inlay flap or tubularised as neourethra. Since the identical amount of vestibular tissue is taken from both the sides, a centrally located cone-shaped tube is created, which is forwardly directed and therefore the direction of the urinary stream remains as before (Fig. 18.9). Some spraying of stream is, however, inevitable.

18.6 Conclusion

Since FUS remains an uncommon cause of BOO in women, the operating techniques are continuously evolving. A multitude of techniques ranging from dilatations to flaps and grafts are available, a single best technique is yet to be established. Overall, an individualized approach based on patient factors, stricture characteristics and surgeon experience is most appropriate.

Key Learning Points

- The outcomes of use of local genital and periurethral tissues for urethral reconstruction in women are comparable to using grafts. Hence, familiarity with the techniques increases the tools available with the reconstructive surgeon.
- The choice of procedure has to be individualized for each patient depending on local tissues, sexual activity status and whether obvious genital violation is a concern.

- Prevalence of lichen sclerosus involving external genitalia is up to 1.7% and make the use of local tissues unsuitable for use.
- As the outcome of all the techniques is dependent on the vascularity of the flap, need for meticulously following the surgical principles cannot be overemphasized.

References

1. Hoag N, Chee J. Surgical management of female urethral strictures. Transl Androl Urol. 2017;6(Suppl 2):S76–80.
2. Faiena I, Koprowski C, Tunuguntla H. Female urethral reconstruction: a review. J Urol. 2016;195(3):557–67.
3. Fistarol SK, Itin PH. Diagnosis and treatment of lichen sclerosus: an update. Am J Clin Dermatol. 2013;14:27–47.
4. Rahn DD, Good MM, Roshanravan SM, et al. Effects of preoperative local estrogen in postmenopausal women with prolapse: a randomized trial. J Clin Endocrinol Metab. 2014;99:3728–36.
5. Osman NI, Mangera A, Chapple CR. A systematic review of surgical techniques used in the treatment of female urethral stricture. Eur Urol. 2013;64:965–73.
6. Rosenblum N, Nitti VW. Female urethral reconstruction. Urol Clin N Am. 2011;38:55–64.
7. Kowalik C, Stoffel JT, Zinman L, et al. Intermediate outcomes after female urethral reconstruction: graft vs flap. Urology. 2014;83(5):1181–5.
8. West C, Lawrence A. Female urethroplasty: contemporary thinking. World J Urol. 2019;37(4):619–29.
9. Blaivas JG, Santos JA, Tsui JF, et al. Management of urethral stricture in women. J Urol. 2012;188:1778–82.
10. Gormley EA. Vaginal flap urethroplasty for female urethral stricture disease. Neurourol Urodyn. 2010;29(Suppl 1):S42–5.
11. Onol FF, Antar B, Köse O, et al. Techniques and results of urethroplasty for female urethral strictures: our experience with 17 patients. Urology. 2011;77:1318–24.
12. Montorsi F, Salonia A, Centemero A, et al. Vestibular flap urethroplasty for strictures of the female urethra. Impact on symptoms and flow patterns. Urol Int. 2002;69:12–6.
13. Romero-Maroto J, Verdú-Verdú L, Gómez-Pérez L, et al. Lateral-based anterior vaginal wall flap in the treatment of female urethral stricture: efficacy and safety. Eur Urol. 2018;73(1):123–8.
14. Simonato A, Varca V, Esposito M, et al. Vaginal flap urethroplasty for wide female stricture disease. J Urol. 2010;184:1381–5.
15. Tanello M, Frego E, Simeone C, et al. Use of pedicle flap from the Labia minora for the repair of female urethral strictures. Urol Int. 2002;69(2):95–8.
16. Dalela D, Gupta P, Dalela D, et al. W-V flap: a new technique for reconstruction of female distal urethral stricture using vestibular mucosa. BMJ Case Rep. 2016;2016:bcr2016215309.

Female Pelvic Fracture Associated Urethral Injury and Stricture: Principles of Management

19

Rishi Nayyar, Devanshu Bansal, and Bharti Uppal Nayyar

Learning Objectives

- To understand the clinical presentation of female pelvic fracture-associated urethral injuries.
- To learn the evaluation of traumatic urethral injuries and strictures in females.
- To learn the factors governing the management of obliterate urethral strictures in females.
- To review the management options for pelvic fracture associated urethral injury and stricture.
- To understand the principles and indications for various surgical techniques of urethral reconstruction for obliterate urethral strictures in females.

19.1 Introduction

Female urethral injury seen along with pelvic fracture (PFUI) due to trauma is rare and there is no consensus in the literature on its management [1, 2]. Emergency management of PFUI is usually dictated by coexistent life-threatening injuries, while definitive management of these injuries is dependent on various factors, such as etiology, length, site and density of stricture, associated fistulae and genital injury, injury to pelvic floor muscles, bladder capacity, local tissue availability, renal function, patient expectations, and lastly surgeon preference and expertise. It is expected then that management on each such case needs to be individualized.

19.2 Epidemiology and Pathophysiology

Pelvic fractures are the main cause of blunt urethral trauma. **Reported incidence of female PFUI ranges from 1 to 6%** [2]. Compared to males, female traumatic urethral injury is less common and is seen with almost 1/10th the frequency as in males [3]. Multiple reasons have been proposed for this, including shorter length and greater inherent elasticity of female urethra and flexibility provided by the vagina [4]. Also, pelvic fractures are less severe and more frequently stable in females and the location of female urethra behind pubic bone offers protection compared to males [5]. By themselves, less severe injuries (stretch injury or partial lacerations) may be missed or simply get splinted with insertion of a urethral catheter, because catheterization in a short and straight female urethra is relatively straightforward compared to males. A high index of suspicion for urethral injury should

R. Nayyar (✉) · D. Bansal
Department of Urology, All India Institute of Medical Sciences, New Delhi, India

B. U. Nayyar
Department of Obstetrics and Gynecology, All India Institute of Medical Sciences, New Delhi, India

N. Khattar et al. (eds.), *Female Bladder Outlet Obstruction and Urethral Reconstruction*,
https://doi.org/10.1007/978-981-15-8521-0_19

therefore be kept in cases of unstable pelvic fractures as there may be coexistent life-threatening visceral injuries and urethral injury might be missed in up to 40% cases during initial patient assessment [5].

Female PFUI is more commonly seen in children than adults. This observation may be due to the fact that adults are less likely to survive associated injuries. Bladder neck injuries are also more common in children than adults, likely due to the exposed abdominal location of bladder in childhood [6].

Depending on the degree, female PFUI may be classified into two types—longitudinal- or partial-type injuries, presenting as lacerations within the urethra, and transverse- or complete-type injuries, presenting as urethral transection. Longitudinal-type injuries are more commonly missed, whereas complete urethral transection-type injuries are more commonly associated with severe trauma. However, both type of injuries can be associated with vaginal and/or bladder injuries [7]. Female PFUI may also be classified based on the location into proximal urethral with or without bladder neck injuries, midurethral injuries, and distal urethral injuries. **Concomitant vaginal, perineal, or pelvic floor injury is very common in most cases of PFUI**. Vaginal laceration occurs in 75–87% cases [2, 6], and therefore any evaluation or reconstruction attempt must encompass and take care of all pelvic or perineal injuries as well for best overall outcomes.

19.3 Diagnosis

As mentioned earlier, a high index of suspicion is required to diagnose urethral injury in females suffering a pelvic fracture. Female PFUI is most commonly associated with vaginal laceration, pelvic circle disruption, multiple pelvic fractures, and sacral spine injury, and any female with these findings should be carefully evaluated for the presence of PFUI [8]. Other concomitant examination findings include blood at the vaginal introitus, hematuria, urethrorrhagia, labial swelling, urinary retention, or difficulty passing a urethral catheter [4]. Unlike males, retrograde and voiding cysto-urethrography (RGU/VCUG) is inadequate for diagnosis of female PFUI, both during acute injury or delayed phase. In a review, only 29% cases could be diagnosed by radiologic studies [2]. Similarly, physical examination with or without attempted catheter placement could diagnose only one-fifth of cases (21%) [2]. **The diagnosis is best carried out via examination under anesthesia with cysto-urethroscopy and vaginoscopy**. It has been strongly recommended by the European association of urology (EAU) 2019 guidelines [4]. All attempts should be made to gather maximum details about the injury (or stricture in delayed repair setting) as possible. Salient examination features of a female PFUI that may guide the subsequent surgery or management are given in Table 19.1. Simultaneous visualization through suprapubic cystostomy (SPC) and urethroscopy or a properly placed bougie at one end with endoscopy from the other end gives best estimation of urethral stricture length through per-vaginal palpation. Density of stricture, adherence to underlying bone, expanse of fibrotic/bony scar tissue, associated genitourinary fistula, loss or thinning of adjoining genital tissue, bladder capacity, relation to ureteric orifices can all be ascertained during the same examination. MRI or CECT rarely add much to evaluation of female urethra. A CT cystogram may however be recommended for evaluation of suspected bladder injury and intra-abdominal urine leak.

Table 19.1 Important examination findings that have a bearing on management in a case of female PFUI

1.	Length of stricture/injury
2.	Density of stricture or viability of tissues
3.	Obliterate/nonobliterate stricture
4.	Expanse of fibrotic/bony scar tissue or hematoma
5.	Adhesion of urethra or vagina to underlying bone
6.	Relation to bilateral ureteric orifices
7.	Genito-urinary-fecal fistulae
8.	Vaginal cicatrization and health of vaginal/perineal tissues
9.	Pelvic floor muscle injury
10.	Bladder capacity

19.4 Management

Goals of management in every case should be to restore urethral anatomy for normal voiding and continence. Additionally, uro-genital or fecal fistula repair, ureteric reimplantation, pelvic floor repair, or vaginoplasty would be necessary in many cases depending upon the types and extent of injuries with aim to improve overall pelvic health and sexual function. These additional procedures may be done in the same sitting or separately depending upon the approach being used or avoiding fecal contamination during repair.

19.4.1 Emergency Room Management

Female PFUI are usually associated with concomitant severe injuries and management of these life-threatening injuries takes higher priority during emergency management of the patient. Although definitive management of the PFUI is not essential in the emergency room, it is prudent to perform early urinary diversion via per-urethral or suprapubic catheter for various reasons, including urine output monitoring in hemodynamically unstable patients, treatment of symptomatic urinary retention in conscious patients, and to minimize urinary extravasation and its sequelae like infection and fibrosis. In resource-poor countries where trauma care facilities or expertise for emergent or early repair may not be available, a gentle attempt at passing a per-urethral catheter is acceptable [4]. Cases in whom catheterization fails, require a SPC. Insertion of SPC catheter may be done under ultrasound guidance or by laparotomy (if being undertaken for other injuries). Once the patient is hemodynamically stable enough to withstand a reconstructive surgery, an early repair may be undertaken. If left as such, a large proportion of cases with SPC would end up with a completely obliterate stricture and significant urethral loss.

19.4.2 Definitive Management

The definitive management of female PFUI may be classified depending upon the time after trauma at which repair is undertaken as *(a) Early realignment; (b) Early repair (within 7 days), and; (c) Delayed repair (after 7 days).*

19.4.2.1 Early Realignment

Early realignment of PFUI involves passing a urethral catheter under endoscopic or open surgical control. Bladder neck must be identified through antegrade approach from the bladder side, to prevent joining into the bladder through a false tract. It relies on the assumption that placing a catheter will keep the urethra aligned, reduce the length and density of stricture, or prevent fistula formation. However, similar to early realignment in males, the results of early realignment in females are not encouraging. It has been seen that stricture rate and fistula formation rates can be as high as about 60% and 15%, respectively, with early realignment alone [2, 4]. There have not been any reports of immediate or persistent stress urinary incontinence following early realignment. Based upon current evidence, EAU 2019 guidelines do not recommend early realignment for female PFUI [4].

19.4.2.2 Early Repair

Unlike male pelvic trauma patients where early realignment or repairs have shown poor results and more complications, there is a relative consensus favoring early repair for female PFUI. **Early repair has shown least short-term restricture (3%) or other complication rates (5–10%)** [2, 4] **compared to early realignment or delayed repair**. Vaginal stenosis is also rare with early repair. Thus, if expertise is available, early repair of urethral trauma with primary anastomosis is the preferred mode of management [2]. However, it should be ensured that there is no infection, the tissues used for repair have good viability, and other injuries are not compromised.

The approach for repair (vaginal, abdominal, or combined) depends largely on the location of the injury. Retropubic route is usually appropriate for proximal urethral disruptions, whereas mid or distal urethral disruptions may be approached by trans-vaginal route [4]. Location of the urethral defect is usually suggested by the location of the vaginal laceration, which can be extended further if required for exposure. Cystoscopy is performed via SPC to identify the proximal bladder neck accurately and a guidewire is placed across the urethral defect. The bladder neck and proximal urethra are mobilized thereafter and both ends are anastomosed in a tension-free manner by interrupted sutures over a urethral catheter. The vagina is then closed in two layers [2]. However, larger avulsion injuries or tissue loss may necessitate major reconstructive procedures, which must be weighed judiciously against the benefits, taking into account other injuries as well. In case of any uncertainties or nonavailability of expertise, delayed repair is acceptable.

19.4.2.3 Delayed Repair

Despite the expert consensus and recommendations for early anastomotic repair, most cases particularly in resource-poor nations end up with delayed repair due to nonavailability of expertise. A significant proportion of the contemporary female PFUI literature describes various options for delayed repair and the evidence is gradually building up. Nonetheless, it remains a rare disease reported in form of case reports and retrospective case series of few cases. As discussed earlier, **the management largely depends on the site, length and density of the stricture, and the presence of associated genital injuries**. Management of passable urethral stricture follows the same principles as discussed in a previous chapter. However, delayed repair with SPC in situ often leads to complete urethral obliteration with extensive fibrosis. This necessitates complex urethral reconstruction using native tissue "tubed" grafts or flaps and risks complications like urinary incontinence (30%), restricture (3%), fistula (4%), and vaginal stenosis (4%) [2]. Basic principles for a good urethral repair are given in Table 19.2. Although a repair beyond 1 week has been considered as a delayed repair, once beyond this approximate time limit, it is our opinion to repair only when full tissue healing has been achieved, that is, around 3 months. Some patients with severe obstetric injuries and genital fistulae may also end up with obliterate urethral and bladder neck contracture, requiring management similar to PFUI with obliterate stricture. Available native tissues and their vascularity may vary in every index case requiring best judgment on the part of treating surgeon to select the type of tissue repair. Renal function, patient preferences, and surgeon's preferences/expertise may ultimately guide the choice of treatment.

Table 19.2 General principles for reconstruction of post-traumatic urethral stricture in females

Repair after full tissue healing has been achieved
No infective focus (colonization with uro-pathogens may require treatment)
Changing SPC or urethral catheter and bladder wash
Use of tubed vascularized flaps or grafts with vascularized base or support
Minimize direct apposition of suture lines
Use advancement vaginal flap to cover repairs wherever feasible
Dead space should be minimized
Use interposition tissue to reduce fistulization
Continence, vaginal stenosis, and pelvic floor should also be factored in adequately during repair

19.5 Salient Surgical Considerations for Repair of Female PFUI

19.5.1 Blood Supply of Female Urethra

The blood supply of female urethra and lower bladder is illustrated in Fig. 19.1. **The female urethra is supplied primarily by longitudinal branches from inferior vesical artery, bilaterally. There is additional variable supply from bilateral bulbo-urethral, introital and vaginal branches of internal pudendal artery, and twigs from vaginal and obturator arteries** [9]. In the event of a pelvic fracture, pudendal arteries

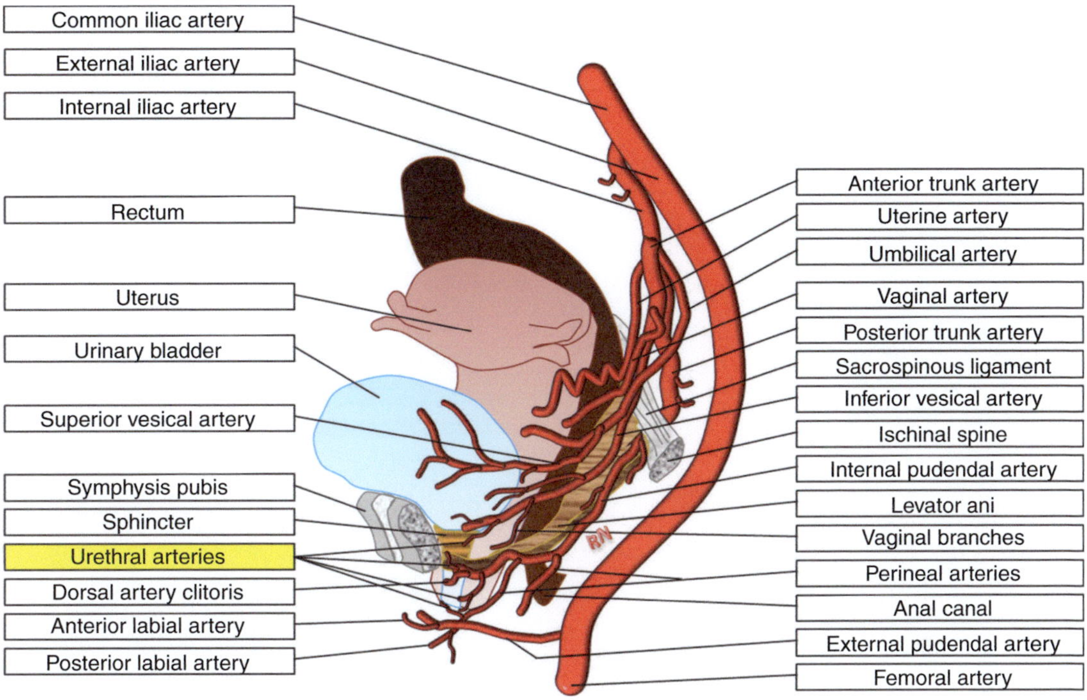

Fig. 19.1 Blood supply of female pelvis and urethra

are at risk in their course through Alcock's canal. Similarly, obturator vessels have close proximity to bony pelvis, possibly making them prone to injury during a fracture. However, given the inputs of arterial supply from multiple origins, complete urethral necrosis as a result of vascular injury is rare, unless the urethra is directly crushed or lacerated during trauma.

The labia are supplied by branches from external pudendal artery anteriorly and internal pudendal artery posteriorly. The Martius flap can therefore be developed based on either anterior or posterior supply of labial fat pad [10, 11].

19.5.2 Sphincter and Pelvic Floor Muscles

Detailed sphincter and pelvic floor anatomy is outside the purview of this chapter. The levator ani, pelvic diaphragm muscles, and anal sphincter may also need repair particularly if torn significantly to reduce subsequent morbidity and repeat surgeries. This is more often the case with early repairs, and it is best to seek gynecologists' help, who are more experienced in post-partum perineal tear repairs. It is our view that restoration of pelvic floor muscle support of uro-genital hiatus also helps in subsequent achievement of continence.

19.5.2.1 Episiotomy/Vaginoplasty/Fistula Repair

A postero-lateral deep episiotomy may occasionally be required for adequate exposure in some cases associated with vaginal cicatrization. It opens the vagina and the pelvic floor allowing easier access and more space to work around (Fig. 19.2). The transverse perineal muscles or the levator muscles must be adequately repaired back in layers. Vaginoplasty may additionally be required in these cases to allow reasonable width of vagina sufficient for copulation. In one such case of severe introital contracture, we required transposition of adjacent thigh flap similar to "Singapore flap" in males [12]. In another case, the deep vaginal cut was left open after incising the contracture band and patient

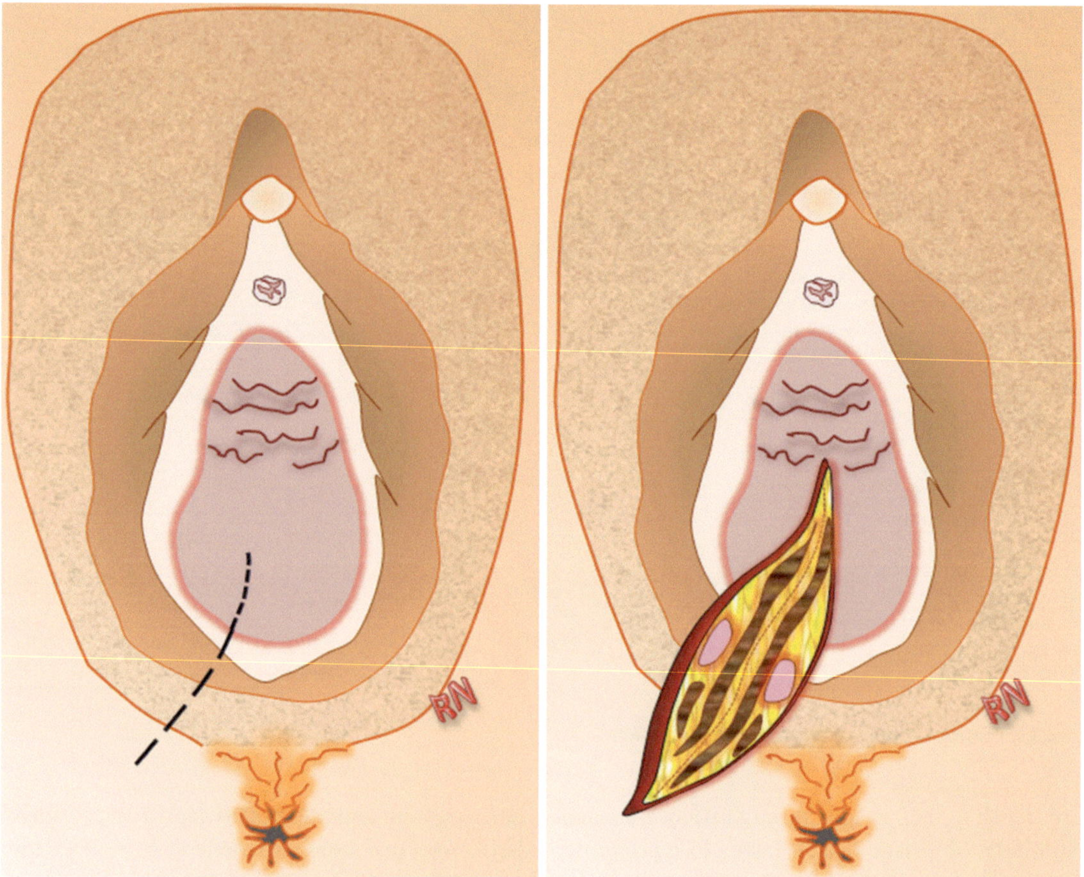

Fig. 19.2 Schematic diagram showing a deep postero-lateral episiotomy incision to improve surgical working space. The incision runs deep across bulbospongiosus, transverse perinei, and if required levator muscles

kept on a vaginal glass mold for 4 weeks followed by frequent self vaginal dilatation. Urogenital fistula is also commonly associated in these cases. Therefore, it is imperative that the urologist himself be well versed in female genital reconstruction or such patients be treated in a multidisciplinary team involving urologists, gynecologists, and plastic surgeons. Urogenital fistula repair, vaginoplasty, tissue transfer, etc. are integral part of any such reconstruction attempts.

19.6 Techniques for Delayed Repair of Female PFUI

Traumatic obliterate strictures in females pose a significant surgical challenge. Various available options have been tabulated in Table 19.3. For patients with intact bladder neck, management options include tubularized flaps or grafts from buccal mucosa, bladder mucosa, vagina or labial tissue. End-to-end anastomosis although may be technically feasible in few cases with short segment stricture, its success is highly dependent upon residual distal urethral blood supply, which may be limited in post-traumatic setting and often not quantifiable. Tubularized vascularized flaps may thus be considered better. Xu et al. have described pedicled tubularized labia minora skin flaps in eight cases with good short-term outcomes [13]. Other options described include tubularized vaginal mucosa covered with a flap of adjacent vaginal wall [14] and tubularized vaginal mucosa covered with a pedicle flap of labia and/or bulbocavernosus muscle [15]. Park et al. first described the use of tubularized buccal mucosal graft for urethral reconstruction in seven patients

Table 19.3 Various available options for traumatic obliterate urethral stricture in females

Procedure	Indication/remarks
Endoscopic procedures • Laser core through. • Cut to light.	For very short obliterate urethral stricture
End-to-end anastomosis	For short obliterate urethral stricture
Tubularized graft procedures with or without vascularized tissue wrap/support • Bladder mucosa. • Buccal mucosa. • Vaginal mucosa. • Skin (Labia minora). Tubularized pedicled flap • Labia minora. • Vaginal wall.	For short obliterate urethral stricture with intact bladder neck. Tubularized flaps may be preferred over tubularized grafts.
Tubularized free graft or flap procedure with pubo-vaginal sling procedure	For obliterate urethral stricture with bladder neck contracture.
Anterior bladder wall flap • Tanagho's tube repair. • Nayyar's tube repair.	For obliterate urethral stricture with bladder neck contracture, particularly long strictures
Salvage procedures • Continent vesicostomy. • Continent pouch. • Augmentation. • Indwelling SPC.	May be indicated in cases with contracted bladder, pelvic floor tear, incontinence issues, previous failed repairs

with cloacal exstrophy and cloacal malformation. The graft was reinforced with peri-urethral tissue. They achieved urinary continence in five patients with the primary procedure and clean intermittent catheterization (CIC) [16]. We have earlier reported use of a tubularized bladder mucosal-free graft for urethral reconstruction with good result in one case [17]. Few authors have also described endoscopic urethrotomy under cystoscopic guidance as a minimally invasive management option for these cases; however, substantial evidence for the same is lacking [6, 18].

Management options for patients with bladder neck obliteration along with urethral loss are very limited and are fraught with concerns for continence. Any tabularized free graft or flap procedure would have to be coupled with some anti-incontinence procedure, usually pubovaginal sling with autologous fascial tissue. Tanagho's tubularized bladder flap procedure provides another good option in these cases [19, 20]. The procedure by itself provides both continence and tissue for reconstruction of the entire urethra. However, longer the length of the tube required, poorer are the chances that continence would be achieved [21]. Tanagho's procedure depends upon utilization of detrusor fibers near the bladder neck for continence. These fibers are circularly arranged unlike haphazard arrangement in rest of bladder and also have neural innervation as per bladder neck. Therefore, when refashioned into a tube, they may be able to aid continence. However, with requirement of a longer tube, the new bladder neck moves further away from site of original bladder neck, being reconstructed using anterior wall detrusor fibers, which are randomly arranged. This may explain the poorer results with the long Tanagho's tube flap. To overcome this limitation, we have described a bladder neck–based anterior bladder flap, which can be tubularized to reconstruct the bladder neck and urethra, without any limitation of the length of the tube and also provide continence at the same time [22]. The entire circumference of detrusor fibers near the bladder neck get incorporated into new bladder neck and urethra unlike Tanagho's repair in which nearly 60–70% of circumference gets excluded from contributing to continence (Fig. 19.3). The new bladder neck also shifts higher up and a posterior redundant recess is formed, which may hinder in adequate voiding and patient may require self-catheterization to void. Since neurological innervation is coming from postero-lateral aspect, making use of posterior 3/4th circumference of fibers and making the base of the flap toward the trigone may be qualitatively better.

For patients with underlying chronic kidney disease, extensive tissue loss, small bladder capacity, or associated neuro-vesical dysfunction salvage procedures like continent stoma or even permanent SPC may occasionally be the most appropriate choice [23]. These

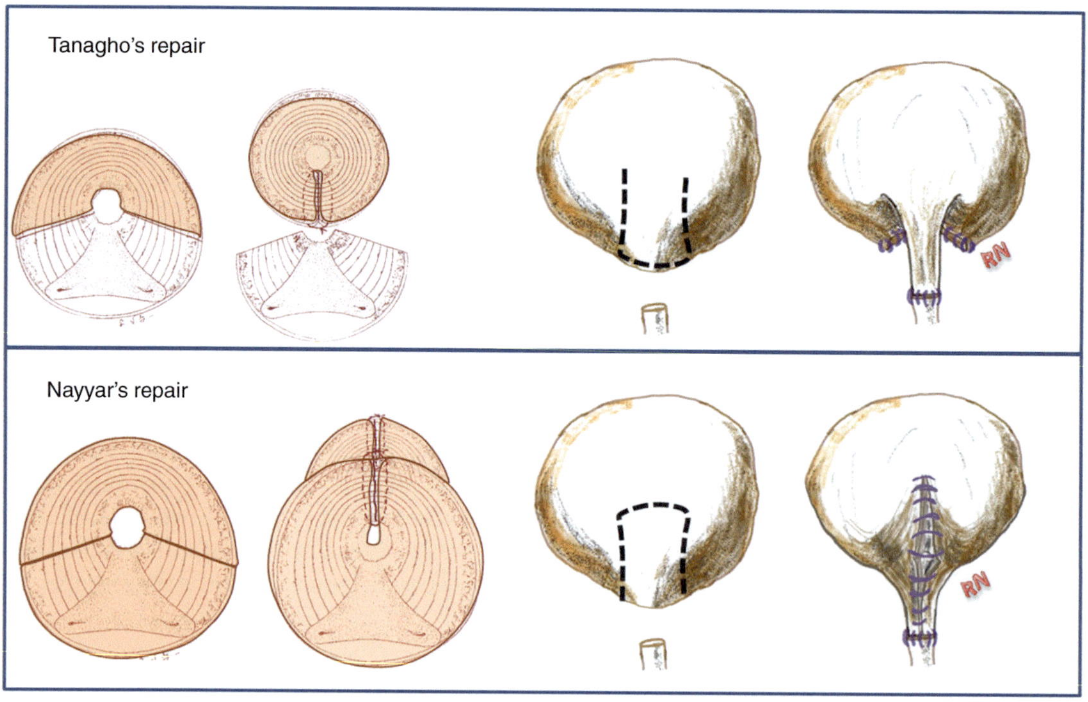

Fig. 19.3 Tubularized anterior bladder flap repairs for urethroplasty of obliterate traumatic urethral strictures involving bladder neck. Shaded region shows the part of detrusor fibers, which finally get included into bladder neck and urethra and help in achieving continence

patients may not be able to tolerate further renal loss in case the reconstructive procedure fails. More extensive reconstruction options need to be discussed with the patient with realistic goal setting for immediate and long-term outcomes.

In conclusion, female PFUI is a rare condition and management options are varied with limited literature support. Immediate patient management should be focused more toward other life-threatening injuries. After patient stabilization, early urethral repair offers the best chance of success with minimal complications. Endoscopic management for obliterate strictures may have poor long-term outcomes compared to tubularized tissue repairs. Pubo-vaginal sling surgery should be added for longer strictures also involving bladder neck. Vaginoplasty, fistula repair, etc. may additionally be required in many cases. Contemporary outcomes of delayed repairs may also improve with our improved understanding of continence and female pelvic anatomy.

Key Learning Points

- Pelvic fracture associated urethral stricture is rare in females.
- Given the common association of urethral injury with genital or bladder neck injury, most experts would agree for an acute repair of injury, provided the general condition of the patient is stable and requisite expertise is available onsite.
- Most cases present with suprapubic cystostomy in situ with an obliterated urethral stricture commonly associated with bladder neck contracture as well.
- Options for reconstruction include endoscopic cut to light, end-to-end anastomosis, tubularized graft, or tubularized flap.

- Continence is an issue for repair of long obliterate strictures, particularly those involving bladder neck as well. Additional concomitant autologous sling procedures are needed for most open surgical repairs.
- Genital reconstruction like urogenital fistula repair or vaginoplasty should be an integral part of any attempts at surgical repair.
- Salvage options include continent Mitrofanoff's vesicostomy or permanent SPC.

References

1. Podestá ML, Jordan GH. Pelvic fracture urethral injuries in girls. J Urol. 2001;165(5):1660–5.
2. Patel DN, Fok CS, Webster GD, Anger JT. Female urethral injuries associated with pelvic fracture: a systematic review of the literature. BJU Int. 2017;120(6):766–73.
3. Bjurlin MA, Fantus RJ, Mellett MM, Goble SM. Genitourinary injuries in pelvic fracture morbidity and mortality using the National Trauma Data Bank. J Trauma Inj Infect Crit Care. 2009;67(5):1033–9.
4. Kitrey ND, Djakovic N, Hallscheidt P, Kuehhas FE, Lumen N, Serafetinidis E, Sharma DM, Abu-Ghanem Y, Sujenthiran A, Waterloose M. EAU guidelines. Urological trauma. Presented at the EAU Annual Barcelona Spain 2019. ISBN 978-94-92671-04-2. https://uroweb.org/guideline/urological-trauma/#4_4.
5. Black PC, Miller EA, Porter JR, Wessells H. Urethral and bladder neck injury associated with pelvic fracture in 25 female patients. J Urol. 2006;175(6):2140–4.
6. Hemal AK, Dorairajan LN, Gupta NP. Posttraumatic complete and partial loss of urethra with pelvic fracture in girls: an appraisal of management. J Urol. 2000;163(1):282–7.
7. Venn SN, Greenwell TJ, Mundy AR. Pelvic fracture injuries of the female urethra. BJU Int. 2001;83(6):626–30.
8. Delaney KM, Reddy SH, Dayama A, Stone ME, Meltzer JA. Risk factors associated with bladder and urethral injuries in female children with pelvic fractures: an analysis of the National Trauma Data Bank. J Trauma Acute Care Surg. 2016;80(3):472–6.
9. Delancey JOL. True pelvis, pelvic floor and perineum (Chapter 73). In: Standring S, editor. Gray's anatomy E-book. 41st ed. Amsterdam: Elsevier; 2016. p. 1221–36.
10. Martius H. Die operative Wiederhellstellung der volkommen fehlenden Harnhohare unde des Sclessmuskels derselben. Zentralbl Gynakol. 1928;52:480–6.
11. Wilson A, Pillay S, Greenwell T. How and why to take a Martius labial interposition flap in female urology. Transl Androl Urol. 2017;6(Suppl 2):S81–7.
12. Clifton MM, Gurunluoglu R, Pizarro-Berdichevsky J, Baker T, Vasavada SP. Treatment of vaginal stenosis with fasciocutaneous Singapore flap. Int Urogynecol J. 2017;28(3):493–5.
13. Xu Y-M, Sa Y-L, Fu Q, Zhang J, Xie H, Jin S-B. Transpubic access using pedicle tubularized labial urethroplasty for the treatment of female urethral strictures associated with urethrovaginal fistulas secondary to pelvic fracture. Eur Urol. 2009;56(1):193–200.
14. Barnes R, Hadley H, Jacobs E. Transvaginal and distal urethroplasty for treatment of urinary incontinence in women. J Urol. 1974;112(5):605–7.
15. Symmonds RE, Hill LM. Loss of the urethra: a report on 50 patients. Am J Obstet Gynecol. 1978;130(2):130–8.
16. Park JM, Hendren WH. Construction of female urethra using buccal mucosa graft. J Urol. 2001;166(2):640–3.
17. Singh R, Kaushal D, Khattar N, Nayyar R, Manasa T, Sood R. Pediatric pelvic fracture urethral distraction defect causing complete urethrovaginal avulsion. Indian J Urol. 2018;34(1):76.
18. Dogra PN, Nabi G. Endourologic reconstruction of post-traumatic obliterated urethral stricture in a young female: a point of technique. Urology. 2001;58(6):1053–5.
19. Tanagho EA, Smith DR. Clinical evaluation of a surgical technique for the correction of complete urinary incontinence. J Urol. 1972;107(3):402–11.
20. Tanagho EA. Bladder neck reconstruction for total urinary incontinence: 10 years experience. J Urol. 1981;125(3):321–6.
21. Blaivas JG. Vaginal flap urethral reconstruction: an alternative to the bladder flap neourethra. J Urol. 1989;141:542–5.
22. Nayyar R, Jain S, Sharma K, Pethe S, Sharma P. A novel anterior bladder tube for traumatic bladder neck contracture in females: initial results. Urology. 2020;139:201–6. pii: S0090-4295(20)30161-8.
23. Nayyar R, Bansal D, Singh P, Jain S, Seth A. Individualized management of obliterative urethral stricture in females—four patients four management strategies. J Clin Urol. 2020;13(4): 261–6.

Female Anastomotic Urethroplasty 20

S. B. Viswaroop and Ganesh Gopalakrishnan

Learning Objectives
- To understand why anastomotic urethroplasty in females is uncommon.
- Indications for performing anastomotic urethroplasty in females.
- Advantages and disadvantages of primary anastomotic urethroplasty.
- How to circumvent problems.
- Preventive steps to improve continence.

20.1 Introduction

Female urethral injuries differ in many ways compared to men, more so in its management. One of the treatment options is anastomotic urethroplasty. Anastomotic urethroplasty was not considered as a feasible operation due to short urethral length and fear about continence [1].This is particularly true for idiopathic strictures. In traumatic strictures, this was not considered, as incidence was very low, most of the injuries were diagnosed late, and many of them had urethral loss with or without urethrovaginal fistula. With better understanding and awareness of the female urethral injury, the paradigm is changing with emphasis on primary treatment [2], albeit need for delayed repair remains for many cases not receiving primary treatment.

20.2 Indications (Fig. 20.1)

1. Primary repair of urethral avulsion or complete injury at mid or proximal urethra (with or without bladder neck involvement).
2. Short segment, obliterative, stricture of any aetiology (idiopathic, post-traumatic, iatrogenic, or obstetric).

Types of Anastomotic urethroplasty in females: (1) Non-transecting, (2) Excision and anastomosis (a) Primary repair, or (b) Delayed repair, and (3) As part of endoscopic primary realignment [3].

20.3 Technique

Non-transecting urethroplasty—It is an option for obliterative or near-obliterative strictures of idiopathic or iatrogenic aetiology (Fig. 20.1a, rarely Fig. 20.1b). Even though non-transecting urethroplasty as a procedure has not been described in literature, in the cases where we

S. B. Viswaroop
Vedanayagam Hospital and Postgraduate Institute, Coimbatore, Tamil Nadu, India

G. Gopalakrishnan (✉)
Vedanayagam Hospital and Postgraduate Institute, Coimbatore, Tamil Nadu, India

Department of Urology, Christian Medical College, Vellore, Tamil Nadu, India

N. Khattar et al. (eds.), *Female Bladder Outlet Obstruction and Urethral Reconstruction*,
https://doi.org/10.1007/978-981-15-8521-0_20

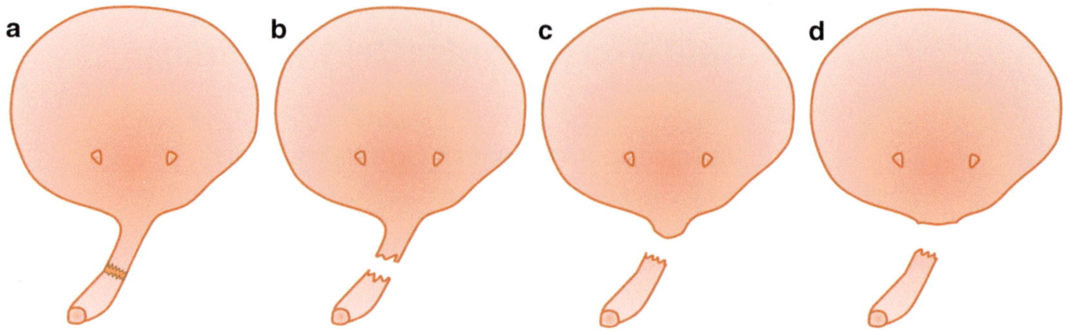

Fig. 20.1 Types of urethral stricture (**a**) Idiopathic stricture, (**b**) mid-urethral avulsion, (**c**) proximal urethral avulsion with dimple of bladder neck, and (**d**) bladder neck injury

have done this procedure indicates that it is possible in females. Unlike in men, the procedure is not standardized but extrapolating from the experience in male urethra, one can say that non-transecting anastomotic urethroplasty in females is possible for obliterative strictures of <1.0 cm and anastomotic urethroplasty for defects of <2.0 cm. We have done non-transecting anastomotic urethroplasty in two cases. Both had obliterative strictures with multiple prior interventions in form of urethral dilation and or visual optical urethrotomy. One of the two was primary voiding dysfunction misdiagnosed as urethral stricture (Fig. 20.2a–c). Both had retention with inability to be catheterized and presented to us with suprapubic catheter. Patients were positioned in lithotomy. After initial cystoscopy from below and from suprapubic cystostomy (SPC) site, we made a lower midline incision. Bladder was partly kept distended for initial identification and dissection. The bladder is decompressed and with blunt and sharp dissection drop the bladder neck and urethra from pubic symphysis. Once sufficient length of urethra is exposed, strictured segment is identified by passing bougie from below. Urethra is opened longitudinally at that site. This is facilitated by keeping cystoscope or a bougie through SPC tract. If suprapubic scopy was difficult and unsure of Bougie not in place, a formal cystotomy is made to facilitate proper identification of obliterated segment from above. Longitudinal incision is made extending to healthy mucosal portion on either side of the strictured segment. Strictured segment is excised circumferentially (peel away). Initially posterior mucosa-to-mucosa approximation is done by interrupted sutures using 5–0 PDS. 16Fr Silastic catheter is placed and longitudinal incision is then closed transversely (Figs. 20.3 and 20.4).

20.4 Excision and Anastomotic Urethroplasty

In an *acute trauma situation*, the patient should be haemodynamically stable, and might have had suprapubic catheter placement. Repair within 7 days of injury is defined as *acute primary repair*.

Under anaesthesia, examine the vagina for type of injury and perform careful cystoscopy. Partial or longitudinal injuries can be sutured over stented urethra [4]. Distal urethral injuries can be left hypospadiac. If there is complete or avulsion injury, anastomotic repair is done and the steps are described in detail under delayed repair. Objective is to ensure tension-free mucosa-to-mucosa approximation. Urethra is short and in order to prevent loss of length debridement should be bare minimum. Moreover, urethral injuries almost always have associated vaginal lacerations and mobilizing the urethra and vagina as a unit is preferred to bridge the gap and also to reduce tension on anastomosis. If mucosa is too fragile and suture ligatures are cutting through, then this would necessitate the bladder being mobilized from the anterior vaginal wall. During this manoeuvre, care must be

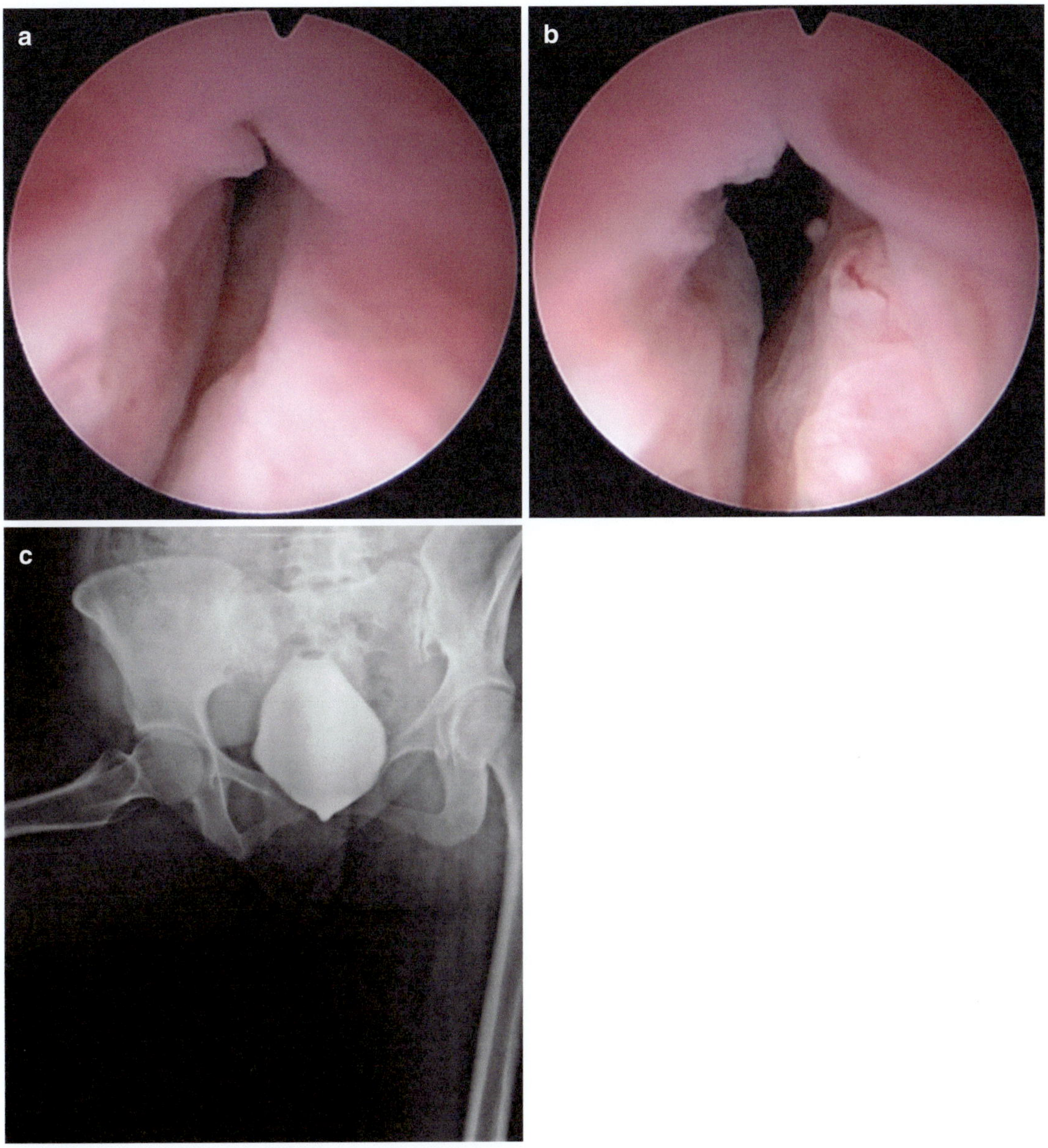

Fig. 20.2 Short obliterated iatrogenic stricture in a female with voiding dysfunction who was subjected to multiple urethral dilatations. (**a**, **b**) Cystoscopy through urethra and through suprapubic tract. (**c**) VCUG of the same patient showing cut-off at proximal portion. Patient was managed with a non-transecting anastomotic urethroplasty

taken to protect the ureters and it would be advisable to place stents or infant feeding tubes to help identification of the ureters and prevent inadvertent injury. In occasional cases during primary repair, one can decide to place 3–4 loose sutures on cut ends with catheter acting as a splint similar to primary realignment. It is advisable to extend the vaginal laceration to check for urethral injury if it is not apparent and to ensure urethral integrity with endoscopy.

If it is a *delayed presentation* with or without diversion, it is good to do imaging studies prefer-

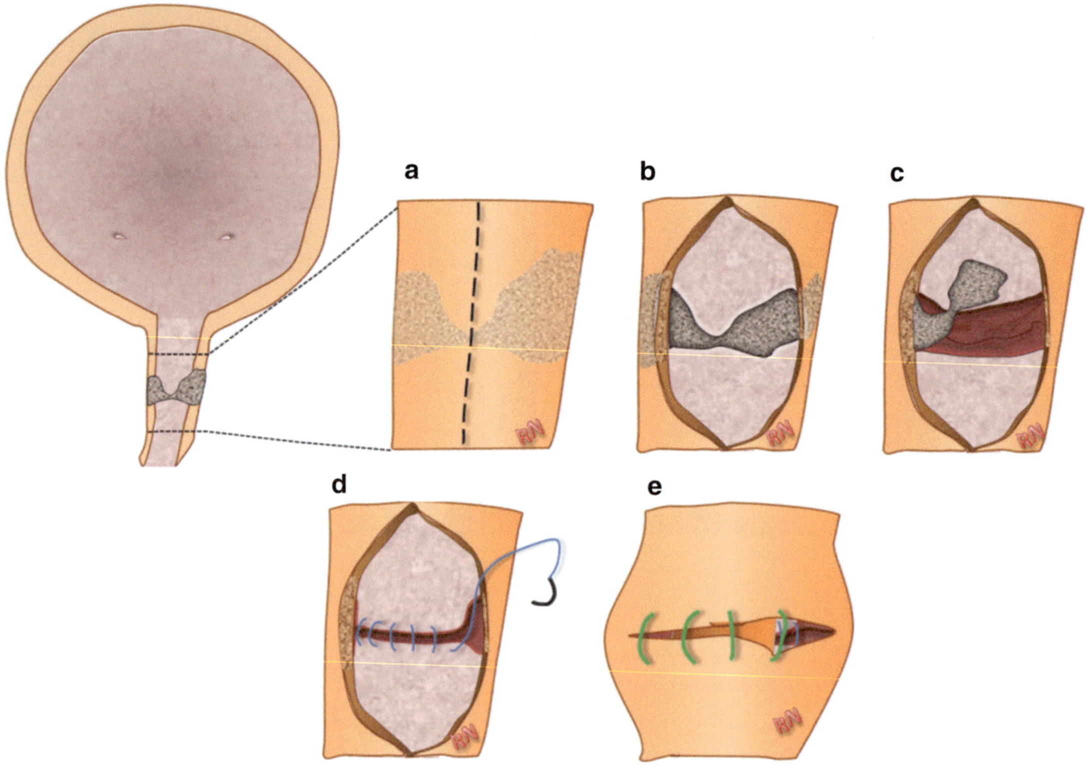

Fig. 20.3 Non-transecting anastomotic urethroplasty: diagram depicting a near-obliterative mid-urethral short annular stricture. (**a**) Exposure and planning of longitudinal incision, (**b**) incised stricturous area, (**c**) removal of fibrosis, (**d**) mucosal approximation, and (**e**) completed anastomosis over a urethral catheter

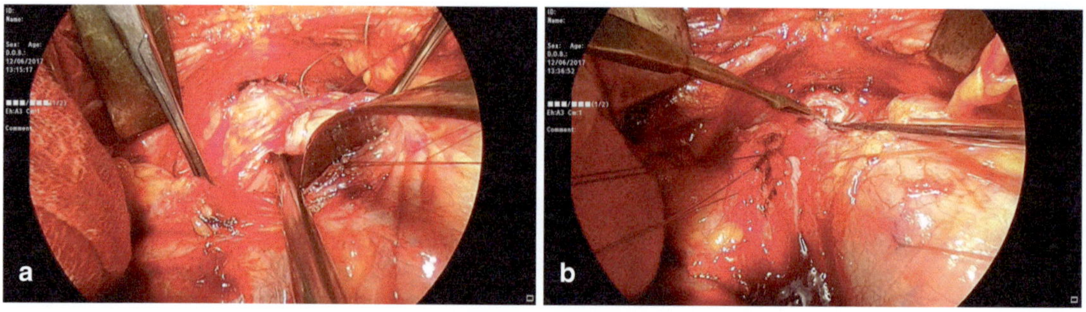

Fig. 20.4 Clinical pictures showing steps of non-transecting anastomotic urethroplasty. (**a**) Identification of obliterative segment on table with help of bougies. (**b**) Incision up to urethral lumen. (**c**) Opening the distal urethra. (**d**) Placement of feeding tube with eversion of mucosal sutures. (**e**) Opening of proximal urethra, calibrating with the dilator. (**f**) Stricture segment displayed between two catheters (feeding tube and Foley's catheter). (**g**) Excision of fibrosed unhealthy mucosa. (**h**) Suturing posterior wall with placement of silastic catheter into bladder. (**i**) Closure of anterior wall

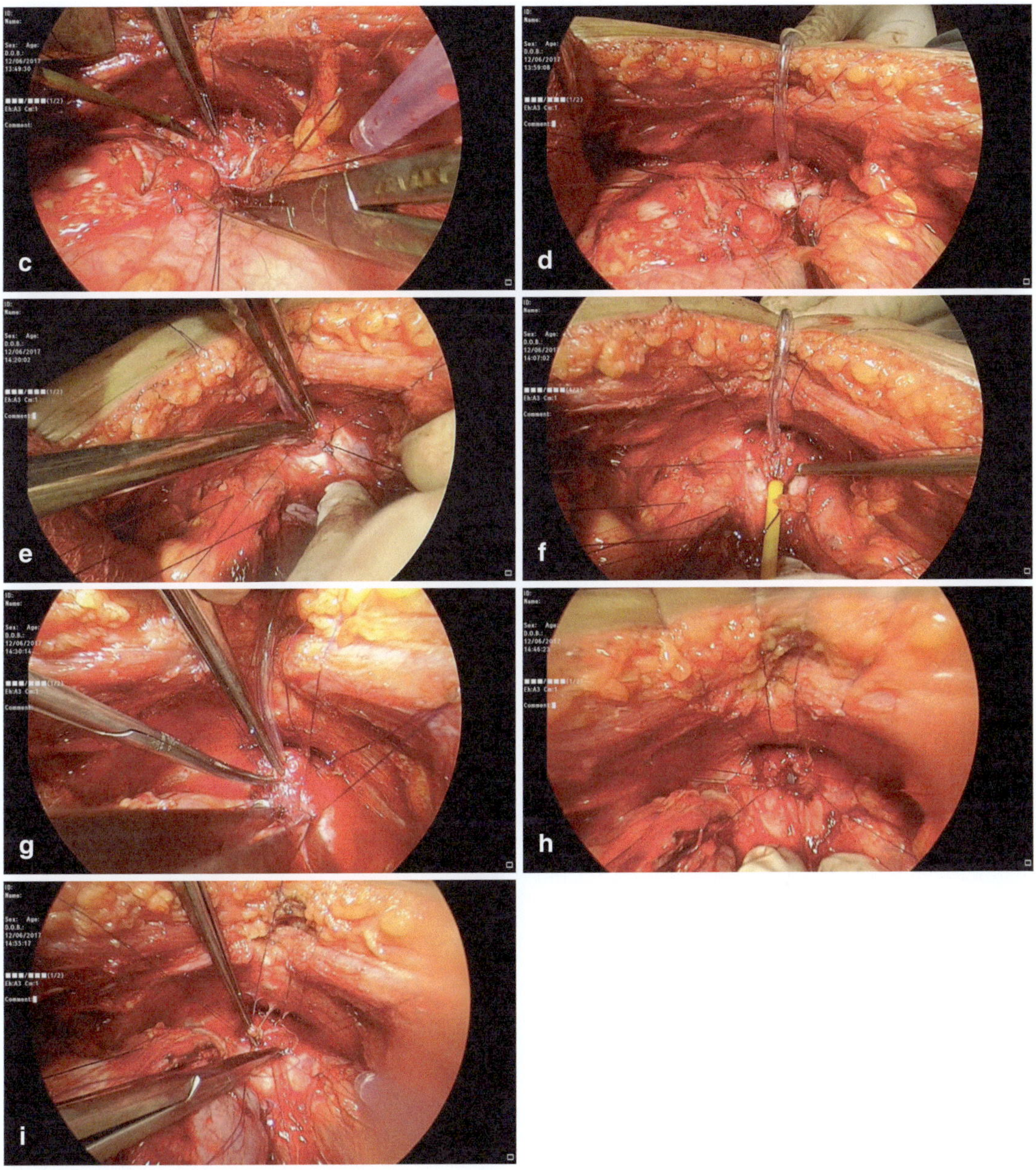

Fig. 20.4 (continued)

ably voiding cystogram or MRI prior to surgery. Cystoscopic examination under anaesthesia should be performed with emphasis on suprapubic cystoscopy to assess bladder neck and proximal urethra. If distal urethra is intact, length of defect may be noted per vaginum by keeping Hegar's dilator or cystoscope or Nelaton catheter in situ.

Once the feasibility of repair is assessed vaginal, abdominal or a combined abdominal and vaginal approach is planned based on adequacy of vagina, level of defect, length of defect, proximity to bladder neck or involvement of bladder neck.

Combined approach is preferred in delayed repair as there is extensive fibrosis and also due to distal vaginal stenosis. Moreover, the combined approach is versatile in handling unforeseen situations.

In delayed primary repair, if vaginal approach is deemed possible, then jackknife-prone position provides easier access for repair. However, lithotomy position has its own advantages.

If an abdominal repair is contemplated, then we would suggest low lithotomy position using Allen stirrups. Midline suprapubic incision encircling the SPC (if it is present) is made and bladder is identified. Bladder neck and posterior bladder wall is dissected off from scar tissue and vagina (Figs. 20.5 and 20.6). This step is necessary to ultimately ensure a tension-free end-to-end anastomosis (EEA). The initial step requires sharp separation to find the exact plane of dissection. Depending on the nature of the accident, the anterior bladder wall could be adherent to posterior surface of pubic bone. If access to the proximal urethra is limited, then a symphysiotomy or superior pubectomy may be necessary. Transpubic approach may be required in a select few. The fibrous tissue and callus, if present, is excised completely. To facilitate urethral identification and mobilization, either a Nelaton catheter or a bougie or a cystoscope can be used as a guide. Due to close adherence of the urethra to the vagina, this kind of injury invariably results in a fistulous communication to the vagina. If the bladder neck (BN) is completely cut off and stenosed there is no incontinence. However, if there is injury to BN, the patient develops vesicovaginal fistula (VVF).

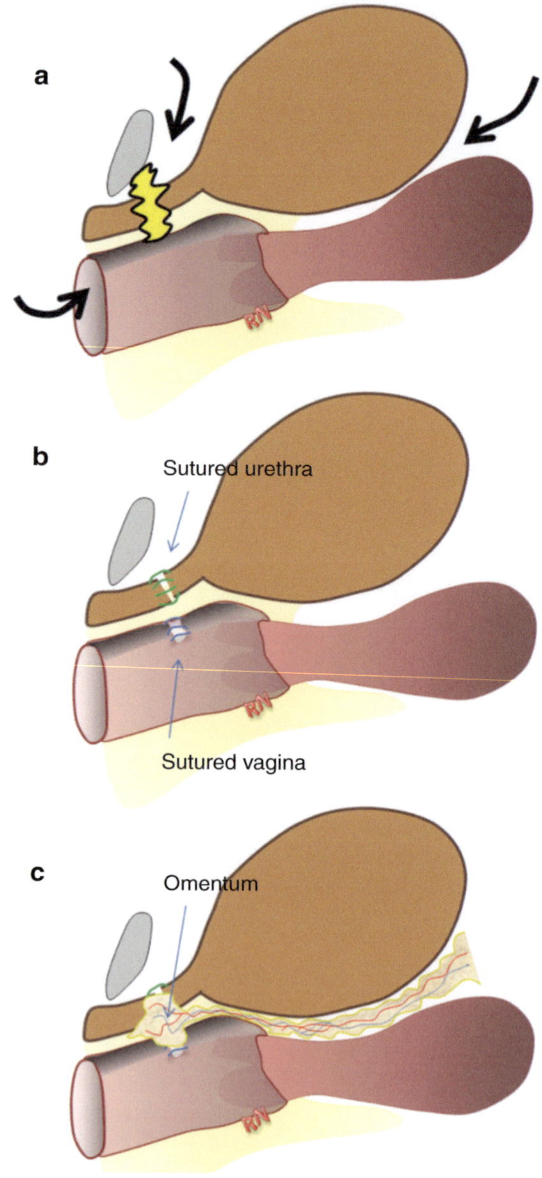

Fig. 20.5 Line diagram of anastomotic urethroplasty. (**a**) Suprapubic or transvaginal or combined approach may be required. Plane of dissection between bladder and vagina is used to mobilize bladder and urethra on posterior aspect and isolate the fistula. (**b**) Fistula is repaired and circumferential urethral anastomosis is done. (**c**) Omentum is passed to the site of repair

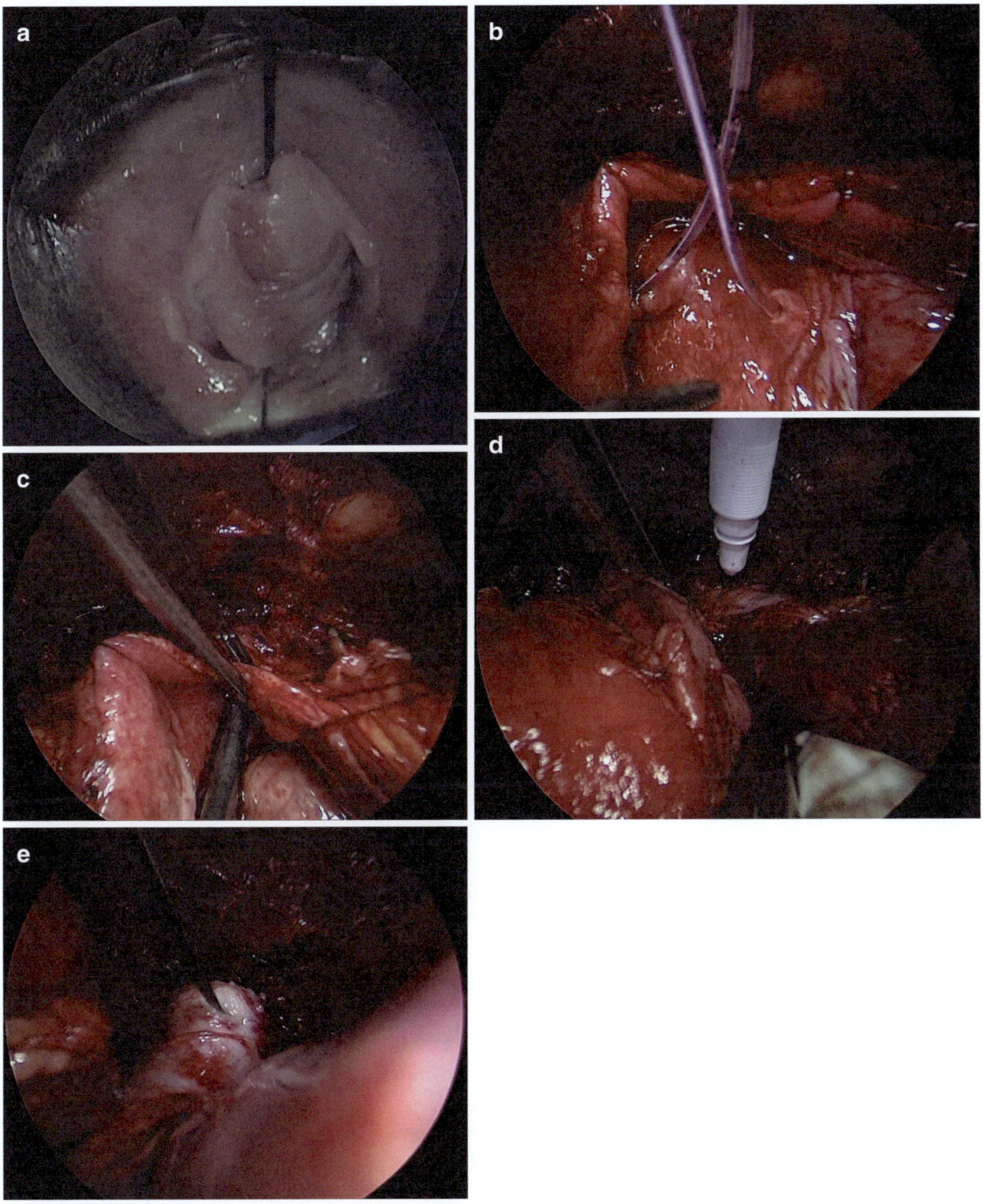

Fig. 20.6 Clinical pictures showing steps of excision and anastomotic urethroplasty. (**a**) Placement of guide wire through distal urethra demonstrating urethrovaginal fistula. (**b**) Splinting of ureters after formal cystotomy. (**c**) Placement of bougie proximally and distally to identify the ends. (**d**) Marking the site of stricture. (**e**) Opening of the obliterated urethra

In the vast majority of patients, the external urethral meatus and distal 1.5–2.0 cm of the urethra are patent. This segment of the urethra is anatomically closely opposed to the vagina. To isolate this portion requires careful sharp dissection. This separation is additionally necessary to obtain an inferior vaginal wall to effect a vaginal closure. If this cannot be done via the retropubic route, then a vaginal approach can be used.

In the event of bladder neck (BN) being stenosed, a formal cystotomy is made to better identify the BN. The site of the BN can be identified as a dimple or can be estimated to be at the apex of an isosceles triangle the base of which is interureteric ridge. This part is opened with a right-angled forceps (Mixter) and widened to accommodate a 16 Fr catheter. The scar tissue around the BN is excised and the mucosal margins are everted in preparation for end-to-end anastomosis to the previously mobilized distal urethral stump. Before the anastomosis, a sheet of omentum is placed over the repaired vagina as an interventing layer (Fig. 20.5).

20.5 Options for Long Segment Gap

In cases where it is not possible to bridge the gap primarily without tension, alternatives are

(a) A Tanagho or Modified Tanagho procedure with or without a sling would be an appropriate choice of procedure. Since continence cannot be assured, we prefer to err on the side of caution and additionally carry out a Burch colposuspension (our preferred adjunctive procedure) for early repairs, and an autologous sling (either the rectus sheath or tensor fascia lata) for delayed repairs.
(b) Appendix along with its blood supply.

One of our patients who had thimble bladder from tuberculosis had additionally urethral loss and vaginal fistula due to iatrogenic injury from an endoscopic intervention. As part of the ileocaecal augmentation, the appendix with its blood supply was found favourable and was used as a urethral substitute akin to a Mitrofanoff (Barosso) [5].

Post procedure, both urethral and suprapubic catheter are kept for 4 weeks following which pericatheter-voiding studies (Fig. 20.7a, b) are carried out to confirm healing of anastomosis.

20.6 Literature Review

In a systematic review of female urethral injuries associated with pelvic fracture, Patel et al. [6] studied 158 patients. Children to adult ratio was 2:1. Of the 53% managed in acute setting, only 20% (17/83) had primary alignment with only 2 of them having partial injuries, rest 15 had complete or avulsion-type injuries. Nine of 15 patients developed stricture after initial realignment and formal delayed repair was done in 5. Anastomotic repair in acute injury setting was done in 80% (66/83). Of the 66 patients, 41% were adults and 59% were children with 68% (45) being complete or avulsion injuries. Vaginal, abdominal or combined approach was followed in 53%, 17% and 30%, respectively. Indications for abdominal approach were complete bladder neck transaction, severe bladder neck injuries and necessity for concomitant abdominal exploration. Follow-up ranged from 8 months to 7 years. Outcome was good with stricture rate of 3%, VVF in 6%, and stress urinary incontinence (SUI) in 9%.

On the contrary, in delayed repair all had abdominal or combined abdominal and vaginal approach. Common reasons mentioned were extensive fibrosis with limited accessibility or damaged bladder neck. Most common delayed repair was a retropubic or transpubic urethroplasty. In comparison to primary anastomotic repair in 80%, only 43% (32/75) had anastomotic repair with rest requiring either anterior bladder wall flap or in a miniscule, management by endoscopic approach or continent diversion. Stricture recurrence was seen in 3% with one

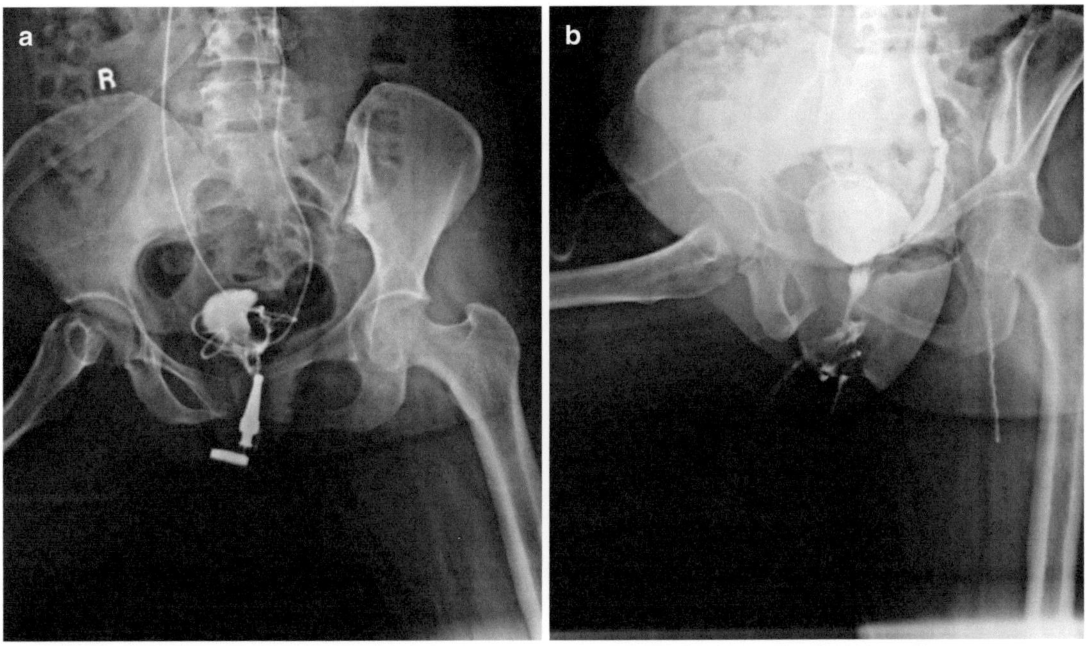

Fig. 20.7 Pericatheter study (**a**) and voiding study (**b**) following catheter removal after anastomotic urethroplasty

requiring repeat transpubic anastomotic urethroplasty. The incidence of urethrovaginal fistula was 4%, distal vaginal stenosis 4% and SUI in 31%.

Hosseini et al. [7] in a series of 7 cases of urethral injury in girls performed delayed retropubic anastomosis with good outcome. The gap ranged from 1.0 to 2.5 cm with median of 2.0 cm. They advocated use of flexible cystoscope to identify the urethral cut margin. This is also emphasized by Patil et al. [8] in an illustrated case report.

We have done non-transecting repair in two, anastomotic repair in six and Tanagho's repair in three. The aetiology and outcomes are given in Table 20.1.

In conclusion, anastomotic urethroplasty is the choice of treatment in primary as well as in delayed repair of traumatic female urethral injuries and in certain cases of short segment obliterative strictures. Primary treatment is preferable, but if patient is haemodynamically unstable or the expertise is not available, suprapubic diversion and delayed repair should be done. Delayed anastomotic repair is possible only in 50% of cases and has good outcome with respect to stricture recurrence and fistula occurrence but has higher rate of stress incontinence as compared to primary anastomotic repair.

Key Learning Points

- Anastomotic repair is indicated during primary repair of urethral avulsion injuries and repair of short obliterative strictures.
- A non-transection anastomosis is also possible in specific situations with very short near-obliterative strictures.
- Acute primary repair (with in first week) should be undertaken after urethral avulsion injuries if the patient is hemodynamically stable.
- Associated genital injuries need simultaneous repair and omental interposition is required between the two walls.
- One must be prepared for progression from vaginal to combined vaginal/suprapubic to transpubic repair.
- A Tanagho procedure or its modifications and alternatively, an appendix can be used to bridge long gaps.

Table 20.1 Various procedures done and their outcomes

Case no	Age (years)	Aetiology	Surgery	Outcome	Follow-up (months)
1	54	Iatrogenic, faulty UD, EIU	Non-transecting	VPU (Fig. 20.8)	18
2	66	Iatrogenic	Non-transecting	VPU, needs 3 monthly cystoscopy ± UD, primary voiding dysfunction	36
3	22	RTA	EEA with autologous PV sling	VPU	6
4	6	RTA	EEA	VPU, small UVF after 2 years	30
5	29	Obstructed labour, forceps + suction, emergency VH urethral injury	EEA with Burch colposuspension	VPU, VVF 2 years later, abdominal repair, minimal stress leak	48
6	35	Fall on stool	EEA	VPU	12
7	5	RTA	EEA	VPU	72
8	24	RTA at 3 years of age, multiple procedures	EEA	VPU with stress leak FBC—120 mL	24
9	20	Obstetric	Tanagho repair with Burch colposuspension	VPU	36
10	2	Iatrogenic	Tanagho repair with sigmoid vaginoplasty	VPU, minimal stress leak	12
11	25	RTA	Tanagho repair	VPU	86

UD urethral dilatation, *EIU* endoscopic internal urethrotomy, *VPU* voiding per urethra, *RTA* road traffic accident, *PV* pubovaginal, *UVF* urethrovaginal fistula, *FBC* full bladder capacity

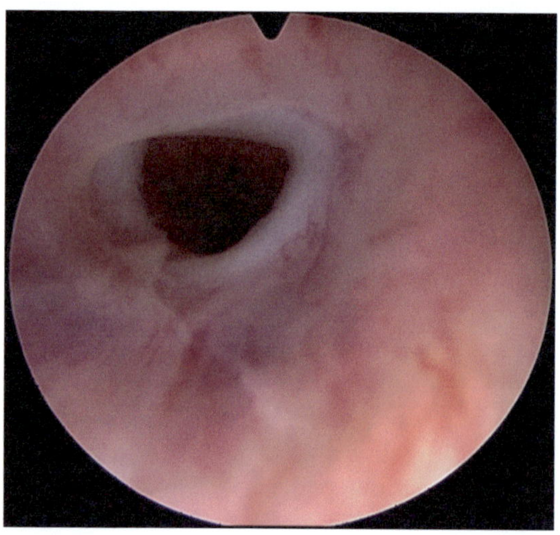

Fig. 20.8 Follow-up scopy at 18 months of a patient who had non-transecting urethroplasty

References

1. Anast J, Brandes SB, Klutke C. Female urethral reconstruction (Chapt 27). In: Brandes SB, editor. Urethral reconstructive surgery. Totawa: Humana Press; 2008. p. 304–5.
2. Black PC, Miller EA, Porter JR, Welles H. Urethral and bladder neck injury associated with pelvic fracture in 25 female patients. J Urol. 2006;175:2140–5.
3. Dorairajan LN, Gupta H, Kumar S. Pelvic fracture-associated urethral injuries in girls: experience with primary repair. BJU Int. 2004;94:134–6.
4. Bredael JJ, Kramer SA, Cleeve LK, Webster GD. Traumatic rupture of the female urethra. J Urol. 1979;122:560.
5. Barroso U Jr, Duel B, Barthold JS, Gonzalez R. Orthotopic urethral substitution in female patients using the Mitrofanoff principle. J Urol. 1999;161(1):251–3.
6. Patel DN, Fok CS, Webster GD, Anger JT. Female urethral injuries associated with pelvic fracture: a systematic review of the literature. BJU Int. 2017;120(6):766–73.
7. Hosseini J, TavakkoliTabassi K, Razi A. Delayed retropubic urethroplasty of completely transected urethra associated with pelvic fracture in girls. Urol J. 2009;6(4):272–5.
8. Patil S, Dalela D, Dalela D, Goel A, Sankhwar P, Sankhwar SN. Anastomotic urethroplasty in female urethral stricture guided by cystoscopy—a point of technique. J Surg Tech Case Rep. 2013;5(2):113–5.

MIX
Papier aus verantwortungsvollen Quellen
Paper from responsible sources
FSC® C105338

If you have any concerns about our products,
you can contact us on
ProductSafety@springernature.com

In case Publisher is established outside the EU,
the EU authorized representative is:
Springer Nature Customer Service Center GmbH
Europaplatz 3, 69115 Heidelberg, Germany

Printed by Libri Plureos GmbH
in Hamburg, Germany